The Sex of Men in Premodern Europe

How were male bodies viewed before the Enlightenment? And what does this reveal about attitudes towards sex and gender in premodern Europe? This richly textured cultural history investigates the characterization of the sex of adult male bodies from ancient Greece to the seventeenth century. Before the modern focus on the phallic, penetrative qualities of male anatomy, Patricia Simons finds that men's bodies were considered in terms of their active physiological characteristics, in relation to semen, testicles and what was considered innately masculine heat. Reorienting attention from an anatomical to a physiological focus, and from fertility to pleasure, Simons argues that women's sexual agency was perceived in terms of active reception of the valuable male seed. This provocative, compelling study draws on visual, material and textual evidence to elucidate a broad range of material, from medical learning, high art and literary metaphors to obscene badges, codpieces and pictorial or oral jokes.

PATRICIA SIMONS is Professor, History of Art, at the University of Michigan, Ann Arbor. She has curated several exhibitions including *Seeing is Healing? The visual arts of medicine* (2000), and her previous publications include *Patronage, art and society in Renaissance Italy* (co-editor, 1987).

Cambridge Social and Cultural Histories

Series editors:
Margot C. Finn, University of Warwick
Colin Jones, University of Warwick

New cultural histories have recently expanded the parameters (and enriched the methodologies) of social history. Cambridge Social and Cultural Histories recognises the plurality of current approaches to social and cultural history as distinctive points of entry into a common explanatory project. Open to innovative and interdisciplinary work, regardless of its chronological or geographical location, the series encompasses a broad range of histories of social relationships and of the cultures that inform them and lend them meaning. Historical anthropology, historical sociology, comparative history, gender history and historicist literary studies – among other subjects – all fall within the remit of Cambridge Social and Cultural Histories.

A list of titles in the series can be found at:
www.cambridge.org/socialculturalhistories

The Sex of Men in Premodern Europe: A Cultural History

Patricia Simons

CAMBRIDGE
UNIVERSITY PRESS

CAMBRIDGE UNIVERSITY PRESS
Cambridge, New York, Melbourne, Madrid, Cape Town,
Singapore, São Paulo, Delhi, Tokyo, Mexico City

Cambridge University Press
The Edinburgh Building, Cambridge CB2 8RU, UK

Published in the United States of America by Cambridge University Press, New York

www.cambridge.org
Information on this title: www.cambridge.org/9781107004917

First published 2011

Printed in the United Kingdom at the University Press, Cambridge

A catalogue record for this publication is available from the British Library

Library of Congress Cataloguing in Publication data
Simons, Patricia.
The sex of men in premodern Europe : a cultural history / Patricia Simons.
p. cm. – (Cambridge social and cultural histories)
ISBN 978-1-107-00491-7 (hardback)
1. Human body – Social aspects. 2. Human body – Symbolic aspects.
3. Men – Physiology. 4. Men – Sexual behavior. 5. Sex role – History.
6. Generative organs, Male – Social aspects. 7. Generative organs, Male –
History. I. Title. II. Series.
GN298.S54 2011
305.31–dc22

2011009936

ISBN 978-1-107-00491-7 Hardback

To the Gang of Four

Contents

Illustrations

Acknowledgements

It is a special pleasure to thank a cadre of stalwart friends who read the first, unwieldy draft of this book in its entirety. Without the astute comments and constant support over the years from the Gang of Four, Louise Marshall, Timothy McCall, Sean Roberts and Monika Schmitter, the project would not have come to fruition. This book is dedicated to them with heartfelt gratitude.

Struggling to balance succinctness against yet more information and ideas, I have tried to take into sufficient account the valuable thoughts of everyone, including Colin Jones and Lyndal Roper. Katharine Park very generously offered useful reflections on an early version of Chapter 4. Margaret Lourie provided valuable editorial guidance, and I also appreciate the work of all the staff at Cambridge University Press.

An incalculable debt is owed to the librarians and institutions that continue to support historical research at a time of funding constraints and short-sighted presentism. In particular, I have benefited from the always awe inspiring collections at the British Library, and the holdings at the University of Michigan Library, including the Taubman Health Sciences Library, as well as interlibrary loans.

Funding to support the publication of the number of photographs necessary in an interdisciplinary, wide-ranging study was gratefully received from the Office of the Vice President of Research, and the Department of History of Art, at the University of Michigan, Ann Arbor. For all the research advantages of the digital age, certain suppliers of images are obstructing the affordable, long-term publication of images in digital form. At the opposite extreme, the semi-automated, free service of the British Museum is a model for all collections wishing to encourage research on their objects.

Kelly has been a constant and beloved companion during the writing of this book, most recently in her makeshift feline hospice on my desk. I provide the room service, she walks over the keyboard on occasion to leave her mark. If any typos remain in this book, say hello to Kelly.

Introduction

When Elena Cumano's maid first purchased wax figurines to aid Elena in wooing back her husband, something vital was missing. In 1588, the Inquisitors at Venice heard that the maid had been sent out one morning to a respected votive maker, whose revision to his usual statuette was satisfactory because it was returned with "a virile member and testicles."[1] Nothing less would do, because the efficacy of love magic was at stake. The wax specialist overcame the deficiency by adding beans, which formed two testicles placed either side of another *fava*.[2] Notably, full manhood had to be signified, and through a complete set of genitals supplied by a hill of beans that amounted to something.

The morphology of the phallus, which can be defined as a culturally weighted sign of masculine power, is based on the male genitals (usually in a significantly exaggerated way), and it has come to be regarded in modern dictionaries and popular culture as the symbol of the penis alone, or the erect penis, or simply to be an alternative word for that organ. However, the premodern phallus encompassed the male genitals *in toto*, and for people like Elena and the votive maker testicular signifiers necessarily accompanied the penis. In the words of Michel Foucault, when summarizing medical theory of the first and second centuries but presenting a view that I will show long ruled, and in a broad range of languages and materials, "the male is preeminent because he is the spermatic animal par excellence."[3] Citing the authority of a renowned physiologist, the provincial French physician Jacques Duval opined in 1612 that "man is entirely semen."[4] I argue that the best model for early modern masculine anatomy and

[1] Guido Ruggiero, *Binding passions: tales of magic, marriage, and power at the end of the Renaissance* (Oxford University Press, 1993), p. 71.

[2] The smooth, round bean (*fava*) was a commonplace in the obscene lexicon: Valter Boggione and Giovanni Casalegno, *Dizionario storico del lessico erotico italiano* (Milan: Longanesi, 1996), pp. 295–96. It also produced wind that was linked with pneumatic ejaculation.

[3] Michel Foucault, *The history of sexuality*, 3 vols., trans. Robert Hurley (New York: Pantheon Books, 1981–86), vol. III, p. 112.

[4] Jacques Duval, *Des hermaphrodits* (Rouen: David Geuffroy, 1612), "Advertissement au lecteur": "*homo totus semen est*."

patriarchal action was projection, from protruding beans to external genitalia and ejaculation, from medical theory into the world of public exploits and commercial aggression.

This book is about the neglected realm of semenotics, a neologism I have coined to suggest that in premodern Europe there was substantial meaning (or semiotic valence) to three non-penile factors: semen, testicles and what was considered the concomitant matter of innately masculine "heat." The word's tongue-in-cheek reference to semiotics tries to evoke the humor of various jokes and images made about the adult male body from ancient Greece to the mid-seventeenth century. With some attention to classical and medieval precedents, I concentrate on the fifteenth and sixteenth centuries in Italy, but with examples drawn from England, France, Germany, the Netherlands and Spain. In large part, the communality is due to broad-reaching ideological institutions like the Church and medical learning, but also to the circulation of oral traditions and the movement of people, books and other objects between linguistic groups through such conduits as warfare, trade, adventure and education. Also key was a distinctive rise in translations and the spread of literature, knowledge and images through print technology.

Although it can be said that "bodies are local," as Mary Fissell has stated, there are other ways in which those bodies are inflected by and impact upon broader material cultures.[5] Regional differences – the German interest in the scatological, for example, or the Italian fascination with anal copulation – are not the focus here because I am elucidating wide-ranging cultural patterns. So too religious differences do not feature because, overall, Catholic, Protestant and Jewish systems shared standard medical models (inherited from the ancient Greeks) and hence certain cultural metaphors. One emphasis here is the degree of continuity, revival or adaptation from antiquity, evident not only at the elite Latinate level during the Renaissance but also in "popular" or vernacular forms such as ribald word play and creatures on secular badges (figs. 10–13). Of course, not all vernaculars generated exactly the same jokes and images, but the overlap is striking, whether in the phallic form inherited from antiquity or numerous verbal and pictorial references in different regions to semen as coin, for example, or soup and sauce, from ancient Greece to seventeenth-century Holland. Artifacts like illustrated anatomical books, bollock knives and phalliform drinking vessels (figs. 23, 30–32, 44) were used in more than one linguistic region, and codpieces (figs. 16–18) were an international fashion.

[5] Mary Fissell, *Vernacular bodies: the politics of reproduction in early modern England* (Oxford University Press, 2004), p. 248. One example that requires more than "local" knowledge: the ballad of 1633 discussed on p. 217 is actually a variant on the theme of Shooting at Father's Corpse, which circulated through Europe in story and image from the twelfth century. The variations evident in the lyrics and image are "local" while larger issues like fidelity and inheritance amongst men are premodern.

Differing ideas co-existed, mingled and held on. Scholars often characterize their object of study as new, yet such claims sometimes betray a lack of understanding regarding historical precedents. The long premodern focus on semen waned and the age of sperm began over the course of the second half of the seventeenth century with the rise of new anatomical research and the aid of the microscope. At the end of the sixteenth century, resistance was mounted against the notion that male and female reproductive systems were anatomical inversions of each other (what has been called since 1990 the one-sex model). Notably, these two intellectual changes occurred many decades apart, and there seems little point in selecting either as the key signal of the modern era to come. Instead, I suggest, it is more fruitful to concentrate on the premodern endurance of a semen-centered and humoral way of conceiving of sexed bodies, and the ways in which those ideas produced non-modern notions of masculinity and of sexual action and pleasure.

Even so, the ongoing existence of particular traditions and images does not indicate an unchanging, ahistorical understanding of human bodies. Whereas Foucault focused on medico-legal theories and practices, my study of the history of masculinity includes not only that field but also turns to vernacular, material and cultural history, to lived metaphor and what I will call "social iconography." This is about the mutual feedback loop and reinforcement between imagery and its context, in which the imaginative construction of metaphors and signs to convey meaning is informed by social and ideological assumptions, everyday activities, familiar objects and corporeal experiences more than by elite knowledge and textual sources alone.[6] Sexual metaphors were often grounded in an understanding of the adult male body's fluids, heat and projective more than penetrative capacity. It was best to marry, argued Martin Luther in 1522, because "if it does not pour into flesh, it will pour into your shirt," choosing a verb that applied only to fluids.[7]

In 1990 Thomas Laqueur claimed that "it is probably not possible to write a history of man's body and its pleasures because the historical record was created in a cultural tradition where no such history was necessary."[8] Indeed, it is the case that, always with great expenditure, patriarchal systems strive to maintain the perfect male body as the stable term against which female bodies are

[6] According to Guido Ruggiero, "Introduction," the essays in Sara Matthews-Grieco (ed.), *Erotic cultures of Renaissance Italy* (Aldershot: Ashgate, 2010) also show the omnipresence of erotic culture and the intertwining of licit and illicit. This book reached me too late for anything more than cursory use.

[7] Gerard Strauss, *Luther's house of learning* (Baltimore: Johns Hopkins University Press, 1978), p. 103: "fleusset es nicht ynn das fleisch, sso fleusset es ynns hembt" (but my translation). The verb is *fliessen*, to flow, pour, gush.

[8] Thomas Laqueur, *Making sex: body and gender from the Greeks to Freud* (Cambridge, MA: Harvard University Press, 1990), p. 22.

measured. However, much of the anxiety discerned in current interpretations of the history of masculinity only comes to the fore due to the ongoing assumption that phallic stability is the ideal state and that anything less proves male vulnerability. The phallus is posited as universal, fixed and always-already hegemonic, whereas I point to ways in which it can be historicized and redefined. If it were to be thought of as less central to everyone's desire and more historically contingent, the phallus could not undergird patriarchal domination or the logocentric privileging of a certain construction of masculinity.

A plethora of sophisticated studies have emerged recently on the history and character of masculinity, but I believe it is time to return to men's physical bodies and consider them as performers of power more than vessels of anxiety, situated in a particular rather than universal set of discourses that engaged anatomy, physiology, metaphors, festivities, jokes and images in a very material way. Since Laqueur's claim was made, histories of the penis, of circumcision, castration and impotence have been written, and authors have chiefly considered male bodies when studying masturbation.[9] Over the last several decades, scholars have studied the premodern system of humoral medicine and bodily fluids like blood and milk, but semen remains little investigated.[10] The few studies that have begun to acknowledge the importance of semen and testicles have not grasped the broader historical context and full ramifications.[11] I argue that the central tenets of the semen-centric system illuminate the sex of premodern men in two senses, morphological and performative, one could say, for the principles were central to both the understanding of male genitals and sexed

[9] For example, David Gollaher, *Circumcision* (New York: Basic Books, 2000); Gary Taylor, *Castration: an abbreviated history of western manhood* (New York: Routledge, 2000); David Friedman, *A mind of its own: a cultural history of the penis* (New York: The Free Press, 2001); Thomas Laqueur, *Solitary sex: a cultural history of masturbation* (New York: Zone, 2003); Leonard Glick, *Marked in your flesh: circumcision from ancient Judea to modern America* (Oxford University Press, 2005). For impotence, see Ch. 2 below.

[10] Studies of the modern representation of sperm include Emily Martin, "The egg and the sperm: how science constructed a romance based on stereotypical male–female roles," *Signs* 16 (1991), 485–501; Lisa Jean Moore, *Sperm counts* (New York University Press, 2007). On blood and milk see Peggy McCracken, *The curse of Eve, the wound of the hero: blood, gender and medieval literature* (Philadelphia: University of Pennsylvania Press, 2003); Rebecca Zorach, *Blood, milk, ink, gold: abundance and excess in the French Renaissance* (University of Chicago Press, 2005); Bettina Bildhauer, *Medieval blood* (Cardiff: University of Wales Press, 2006); Caroline Walker Bynum, *Wonderful blood: theology and practice in late medieval northern Germany and beyond* (Philadelphia: University of Pennsylvania Press, 2006).

[11] See Gianna Pomata, "Vollkommen oder verdorben? Der männliche Samen im frühneuzeitlichen Europa," *L'Homme* 6 (1995), 59–85; Taylor, *Castration*; Rebecca Ann Bach, "Tennis balls: *Henry V* and testicular masculinity, or, according to the OED, Shakespeare doesn't have any balls," *Renaissance Drama* 30 (2001), 3–23; Sarah Toulalan, *Imagining sex: pornography and bodies in seventeenth-century England* (Oxford University Press, 2007), pp. 72–77; Cathy McClive, "Masculinity on trial: penises, hermaphrodites and the uncertain male body in early modern France," *History Workshop Journal* 68 (2009), 45–68.

identity, and to acts of sex. Rather than focus on objects of desire, my study considers the imagining and enacting of physical desire more broadly.

I sketch out a synoptic framework, integrating metaphor and medicine, erotic imagery and practice, representation and experience in order to show that male and female bodies were ontologically distinct and unequal in both medical theory and political reality. Yet they were also interconnected categories according to premodern schemes of medical thought and cultural representation. Often overlooked material like carnival songs, drinking vessels, diaries and obscene badges is placed alongside mainstream anatomical illustration and high-end paintings such as Botticelli's *Birth of Venus* (fig. 33), where the goddess is wafted to shore by foamy waves which, I will show, signal the myth's focus on parthenogenesis by semen.

The importance of semenotics

The inseminating fluid that Aristotle defined for European medicine as "vital spirit," comprised of fluid and "air" (*pneuma*), was fundamental to premodern notions of masculinity. Considered essential for virility and sexual pleasure (male and female) as well as reproduction, in some ways semen played the role now granted to the hormone testosterone, regarded as the marker of libido, vigor and strength. But the testicles where semen was thought to be either produced or stored were also essential. Medical authors well into the seventeenth and even eighteenth centuries echoed the belief that the testicles "witness strength and man-hood."[12] Virility was located in the semen-producing testicles rather than the penis. The latter was a delivery system (figs. 29–31), "principally ordained that it might cast seed into the bottom of the Womb" as Johann Vesling's popular textbook of anatomy summarized standard opinion in 1641. The state of naturally more "heated" male bodies was a third crucial element, for it led to the exterior situation of male genitals, the extrusion of male hair like beards and the proper concoction then expulsion of semen.

Hence, the Catholic Church scrutinized three criteria when considering charges of male impotence: erection (caused by semen and its spirit), penetration (important for the uterine placement of seed) and ejaculation (caused by the build up of heated semen).[13] Significantly, the capacity to father children was not a factor, and the same principles informed the opinion of most civil

[12] Johann Vesling, *Syntagma anatomicum*, 2nd edn. (Padua: Pauli Frambotti, 1651), p. 62; Johann Vesling, *The anatomy of the body of man: wherein is exactly described every part thereof, in the same manner as it is commonly shewed in publick anatomies*, trans. Nicholas Culpeper (London: Peter Cole, 1653), p. 23, hereafter quoted from p. 25 (p. 64 in the Latin edn.).

[13] Joseph Bajada, *Sexual impotence: the contribution of Paolo Zacchia (1584–1659)* (Rome: Editrice Pontificia Università Gregoriana, 1988), pp. 15, 20. The exact weighting of these three factors was much debated.

lawyers.[14] Beyond marriage, Christianity through Christ's body established a male ideal that was only potentially generative. Divinity incarnate and necessarily male, his sex was commonly visualized by way of a babe's naked genitals, as Leo Steinberg pointed out in his classic study on the "sexuality of Christ."[15] He wisely avoided the term "phallus" on the whole and referred accurately to the penis as a specific organ or more often used terms like genitals, genitalia, privy parts or groin, which encompassed what was considered the full manly apparatus. Rather than sexuality, Steinberg really considered Christ's sex, as a sign of God's advent in human, mortal flesh, and thus the chaste savior's anatomy was not exceptional.

Humoral medicine was central to the understanding of all male bodies. This medical system of explanation and treatment operated for millennia, explored by the ancient Greek Hippocratics during the fifth and fourth centuries BCE, then elaborated and synthesized by the renowned second-century CE physician Galen. Bodies were conceived of in terms of humors, that is, certain fluids and their fluxes, the balance of which determined health and temperament. It was believed that humors governed emotions but also that passions could be somewhat controlled, chiefly by managing the "non-naturals" like diet, rest and sexual activity (especially in men whose ideal masculinity centered on rationality and constancy). What modern culture has, until recently, divided into the separate spheres of psychology and physiology were instead interactive elements in a complex *soma*. While semen was not one of the four humors, it was a crucial fluid mainly concocted from the most vital humor, blood; a build up of semen gave rise to sexual desire, and its management was a crucial aspect of men's health.

The humoral system underpinned a Neoplatonic analogy for divine love offered by the Jewish physician Leone Ebreo written around 1501–02.[16] In his *Dialoghi d'amore* the "paternal love of Heaven" was likened to the motions and humoral processes of human reproduction. The feminine body of Earth was vivified and impregnated through the intromission and reception of moisture and heat in the form of dew, rain and sunshine. The paternal, heavenly agency was produced in a process akin to how "semen is produced by the whole body of man." The catalogue of seven organs that together bring semen into being began

[14] Aidan McGrath, *A controversy concerning male impotence* (Rome: Editrice Pontificia Università Gregoriana, 1988), pp. 22, 36–38, 42–47, 55–56 and passim, addressing canon law since the twelfth century as well as an influential papal brief of 1587. For civil law in Italy, see pp. 58–67. According to most authorities, sterile men and women were allowed to marry.

[15] Leo Steinberg, *The sexuality of Christ in Renaissance art and in modern oblivion*, 2nd edn. (University of Chicago Press, 1996).

[16] Leone Ebreo, *Dialoghi d'amore*, ed. Santino Caramella (Bari: Laterza, 1929), pp. 80–85, *The philosophy of love*, trans. F. Friedeberg-Seeley and Jean Barnes (London: Socino Press, 1937), pp. 89–95. It was first printed in Rome in 1535.

with the heart and ended with the genitals. It depended "sixthly on the testes, in which the constitution of the semen is perfected and it receives its spermatic genital nature (*natura seminale generativa*); seventh and last on the penis (*virga*) which conveys the semen to the female." As in anatomical conceptions of the human body, the celestial penis is less important than the testicles. The male body covered and surrounded (*copre e circonda*) the receptive woman, and the delivery system of the penis infused or afforded (*influisce* and *porge*) rather than penetrated. While Leone's analogy virtually literalized Lacanian phallogocentricism when it likened the penis to the tongue or speech (*lingua*), the model of sexual concourse did not. His allegory was Hippo-Galenic: "the testes of Heaven are Venus, which plays a great part in providing a good and perfect humor to ensure fertility . . . The male member of heaven is Mercury, sometimes advancing, sometimes retreating, now actually causing the rains, now impeding them." The mercurial penis was a figure of repetitive action, moving back and forth (*diretto* and *retrogrado*), and its chief purpose was to bring or cease the rains (*le pioggie*, which are the flow of both male and female seed).[17]

The most outrageously entertaining championing of the testicles came from the pen of the monk turned physician and satirist François Rabelais, who published the four parts of his popular *Gargantua and Pantagruel* between 1532 and the mid-1540s. This doctor's attention to the male body and to the richness of the French vernacular led him to concentrate more on the balls than the penis when following Pantagruel's contemplation of marriage while obsessing on the likelihood that he would thence be cuckolded.[18] In all, the text "names the penis . . . 45 times, but the testicles . . . 336 times," as though profligate use of the word mimics a man's outpouring of seed.[19] So one character "shall preach a new Crusade. God keep my pill-grims safe in my ball-bag!" The book then offers standard medical opinion and cites authorities like Galen when pointing out that "in the testicles, as in a sacred repository, lies the germ which preserves the whole human stock." As he piles up testicular metaphors and lists of

[17] For rain, see Eric Partridge, *Shakespeare's bawdy*, 3rd edn. (London: Routledge, 1990), p. 171; Boggione and Casalegno, *Dizionario*, pp. 357, 502; Ch. 7 below. Jean Toscan, *Le carnaval du langage: le lexique érotique des poètes de l'équivoque de Burchiello à Marino* (Lille: Presses Universitaires de Lille, 1981), p. 1733 and passim (*pioggia*, *piova*), reads it as menses, which was often conflated with female seed and hence could refer to sexual pleasure rather than only menstruation (see Ch. 6 below). A homoerotic text of *c*. 1630 likened the distasteful "concorso de' semi" of heterosexual intercourse to a stormy, troublesome downpour ("d'intempestiva importuna pioggia"): Antonio Rocco, *L'Alcibiade fanciullo a scola* (Rome: Salerno, 1988), p. 66.

[18] The following is drawn from François Rabelais, *Œuvres complètes*, ed. Mireille Huchon and François Moreau (Paris: Gallimard, 1994), pp. 217–22, 371–76, 432–43, 448–55; François Rabelais, *The histories of Gargantua and Pantagruel*, trans. J. M. Cohen (Harmondsworth: Penguin, 1955), pp. 172–74, 305–10, 360–68, 373–79.

[19] Taylor, *Castration*, p. 50.

adjectives (from "stumpy" to "tumbling," "musty" to "unloaded"), Rabelais occasionally alludes specifically to the liquid output of testicles, which are likened to "the pot of milk" or called "milky" ball-bags.[20] The text delights in logocentric virility centered on praising fecund male seed and balls, without waxing about fatherhood or domesticity. In this case, and many others, virility consisted of much more than the capacity to become a parent; prolific erection, copulation and ejaculation was the chief aim, numerous children an incidental sign of vigor and manliness.

So vital were testicles that it was believed that a ceremony of inspection was devised for a newly elected pope. To prove his masculinity, it was claimed, a specially designed seat facilitated the ritual performed by a young deacon, "the touching of the testicles" as it was called.[21] In the words of the Florentine merchant Giovanni Rucellai, probably echoing those heard from a guide when he visited Rome in the Jubilee year of 1450, a hole in the seat enabled someone "to determine if [the Pope] was male or female."[22] Even when reporting that Pope Julius II's coronation in 1503 did not involve such a tactile investigation, the Venetian ambassador Antonio Giustiniani still imparted knowledge of a "ceremony, vulgarly said to be that of putting a hand underneath" to find "evidence of the virility of popes."[23] Whether it was true or not, the idea of the ritual was eagerly relayed. In gossip and pasquinade, chronicle and guide-book, the notion that papal genitals were subjected to ritual inspection, and that testicles were the essential element, circulated from at least the thirteenth to the seventeenth centuries.

Sex and projective virility

Modern assumptions about sex and genitals primarily insist on a model of male penetrative action by an erect penis. Yet, evidence from premodern culture demonstrates more variety in sexual practice and theory. The shape, parts, history and function of the phallus are complex and variable, so much so that the concept may not always prove a useful tool of historical analysis, or not without fundamentally reconceiving its components. The commonplace notion

[20] Rabelais, *Gargantua*, pp. 309, 360, 363. See also Gordon Williams, *A dictionary of sexual language and imagery in Shakespearean and Stuart literature* (London: Athlone, 1994), pp. 885–86; Boggione and Casalegno, *Dizionario*, p. 354; Gordon Williams, *A glossary of Shakespeare's sexual language* (London: Athlone, 1997), p. 207.

[21] Peter Stanford, *The legend of Pope Joan* (New York: Berkley Books, 2000), p. 33, Bernardino Coreo's *Patria historia* of 1503, regarding the coronation of Alexander VI in 1492.

[22] *Giovanni Rucellai ed il suo zibaldone*, vol. I, ed. Alessandro Perosa (London: Warburg Institute, 1960), p. 71.

[23] Sergio Bertelli, *The king's body: sacred rituals of power in medieval and early modern Europe* (1999), trans. R. Burr Litchfield (University Park: Pennsylvania State University Press, 2001), p. 184.

that an arrow is phallic often misses the mark, in that another factor in the weapon's operation, the bow, was also crucial, metaphorically considered a potent delivery system for the ejaculatory, semen-laden arrow. *Eiaculatus*, Latin for "shot out," arose from *iaculum*, a little spear or javelin.[24] The taut strings of a bow or musical instrument were likened to the sinews and "nervi" that generated an erection and were vital components of manhood.

The most famous assertion of the penetrative, penile model occurs in psychoanalysis, encapsulated in Sigmund Freud's emphasis on what was later dubbed "vaginal orgasm," as distinct from another over-drawn category "clitoral orgasm."[25] Despite the success of feminist argumentation and scientific research in establishing the importance of the clitoris for most women's sexual pleasure, modern Euro-American popular culture is dominated by the notion of "penetration intercourse and the centrality of the thrusting penis," a focus which still informs much scholarship too.[26] But a third framework for female pleasure is delineated in premodern discourse, for it was utero-centric. The "vagina" was not a term used of female bodies, and the clitoris was only announced as an anatomical discovery in the mid-sixteenth century.[27] The womb was thought to be avid to receive male semen, and female fluids were read as similar to yet lesser than male ejaculate, in both substance and reproductive function. I will show that, rather than typecasting femininity as "passive" in the classic Aristotelian sense, the Hippo-Galenic understanding of uterine agency led to the more nuanced model of receptivity, in which female bodies remained dependent on superior male capacities. A return to such ideas would hardly be progressive since they bolstered patriarchal privilege, but their existence suggests that there are ways to break away from the false vaginal/clitoral binary, which is itself an historically contingent and changeable notion.

The very idea of the phallus and its actions needs to be rethought, here attempted with the aid of historical materials which demystify and denaturalize the word, object and effect that was the phallus. As long as "the phallus"

24 Toscan, *Carnaval*, p. 741; John Scarborough, *Medical terminologies: classical origins* (Norman: University of Oklahoma Press, 1992), p. 212.

25 For Freud's theory that female maturity necessitated a shift from the clitoris, "with its virile character," to the more properly internal and feminine vagina, see "Three essays on the theory of sexuality" (1905), in *The standard edition of the complete psychological works of Sigmund Freud*, ed. James Strachey in collaboration with Anna Freud, assisted by Alix Strachey and Alan Tyson, 24 vols. (London: Hogarth Press, 1953–74), vol. VII, pp. 220–21, "Female sexuality" (1931), vol. XXI (1961), pp. 225, 228, "Femininity" (1933), vol. XXII (1964), pp. 118, 126–30 passim. Mary Roach, *Bonk: the curious coupling of science and sex* (New York: W. W. Norton & Co., 2008), provides an accessible summary regarding current understanding of the complexity of physical factors that play a role in female orgasms.

26 Peter Lehman, *Running scared: masculinity and the representation of the male body*, new edn. (Detroit: Wayne State University Press, 2007), p. xi.

27 On the clitoris see Chs. 4 and 6 below. Vagina in the modern sense is first noted for Italian usage in 1775 in Boggione and Casalegno, *Dizionario*, p. 401.

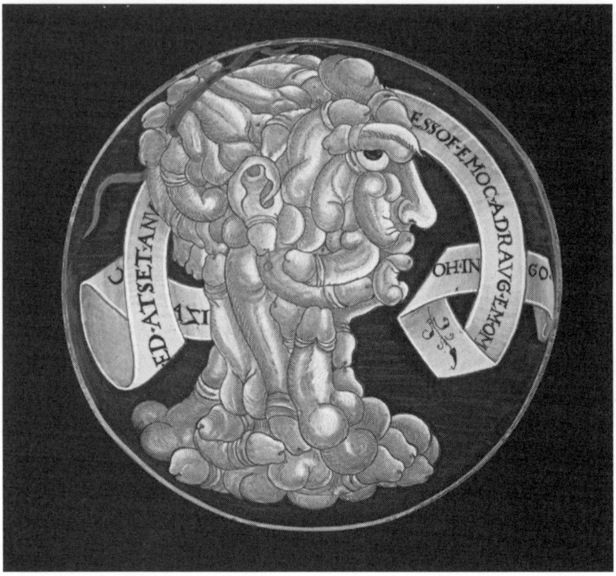

Figure 1 Francesco “Urbini” (attributed), maiolica dish with a composite “head of dicks,” dated on reverse 1536, diameter 23.2 cm, Oxford, Ashmolean Museum

remains monolithic and undifferentiated, subsuming the entire male genitals under a single penile sign, numerous aspects of pleasure, concepts of manliness and sexual dynamics are not given cognizance. Different areas like the glans and foreskin, or various actions like “juggling with little balls” as the renowned, sometimes obscene writer Pietro Aretino put it in 1534, tend to be neglected, especially in theoretical discourse.[28] A penetrative presumption ignores or devalues too many practices, past and present, between people with either the same or different genital configurations.

From ancient Greece to well past the Renaissance, the standard visual signifier of male sex was the ensemble of testicles, penile shaft, foreskin and glans, as seen for example in the labeled *testa de cazzi* painted in Gubbio on a shallow maiolica bowl in 1536 (figs. 1, 8).[29] The classical profile reminiscent of a laureated athlete or bather (hair tied up by a green ribbon), is transformed into a satirical composite of genitals that ingeniously shape a face, attracting the very

[28] Pietro Aretino, *Ragionamento: dialogo*, ed. Paolo Procaccioli (Milan: Garzanti, 1984), p. 24; Pietro Aretino, *Aretino's "Dialogues,"* trans. Raymond Rosenthal (New York: Stein and Day, 1971), p. 25; and another reference to ball play is on pp. 229/175.

[29] Timothy Wilson, “Un ‘intricamento’ tra Leonardo ed Arcimboldo,” *CeramicAntica* 15 no. 2 (2005), 10–44.

attention announced in the banderole: "every man looks at me as if I were a head of dicks." Cleverly, a vital element in the *testa* or *capo* is the multiplicity of punning bared "heads of dicks," that is, glans with foreskins retracted.[30] Two drawings by Leonardo da Vinci and a print of the type do not survive, but its popularity remains evident in a drawing and several medals, one on the reverse of Aretino's portrait. All these represent male heads, as seems to be the case on the dish, judging by the bushy eyebrows and jutting chin.

On the other hand, an earring dangles from a glandular lobe, which brings to mind the outsider status of Jewess, although it is more likely that it recalls Greek infibulation but, primarily, the small bell that hangs from the neck of phallus birds (figs. 12, 14).[31] A mock academic discourse about pricks written in the previous decade observed that they were adorned with a rattle or bell, and that graffiti on university walls and benches showed them with details like wings, feet, beaks and little hands.[32] A seed causes the rattle of small round bells, which hence refer to testicles, and in a secondary sense to semen, as is implied by the golden droplet pictured on the dish. Assertively visible, proudly self-sufficient or, in the case of the maiolica image forming a homoerotic fraternity, the early modern sign of genital masculinity was prolific but focused on more than fertility, staking a claim to power that was grounded in a broader, often humorous sense of virility and one-upmanship.

My study is about the sex of bodies, rather than gender or what is taken to mean sexuality in the modern sense. The theory and practice of male sex provided the underpinnings for gender and for the medico-legal comprehension of male sodomy. When sexuality was about acts as much as sexual identities or categories of perversion, and when those deeds entailed pleasure as well as (though only at certain times) reproduction, then language and imagery celebrated more than single-minded penile penetration of the orifices of vagina or anus. Characters with a penis are visually represented or textually recorded in past European cultures doing mundane things like "pissing" or ejaculating alone, placing that organ in the armpits or mouths of partners of either sex, between breasts or thighs, or ejaculating without any aid except visual stimulation and / or fantasy. In many of these cases, friction, male sexual fluid and projection were important parts of the act and its pleasure for the man; female sexual pleasure was constructed within the same orbit.

Ruth Mazo Karras has remarked of people in medieval Europe that "for the most part, [they] understood sex acts as something that someone did to someone

[30] For *capo* and *testa* see Boggione and Casalegno, *Dizionario*, pp. 26, 308, 312; Ch. 8 below for Michelangelo and "hood."

[31] On Jews see Diane Owen Hughes, "Distinguishing signs: ear-rings, Jews and Franciscan rhetoric in the Italian Renaissance city," *Past and Present* 112 (1986), 3–59.

[32] Antonio Vignali, *La cazzaria*, ed. Pasquale Stoppelli (Rome: Edizioni dell'elefante, 1984), pp. 125–26.

else," and that the very differently constructed roles of active and passive partner (a hierarchy evident in both same-sex and cross-sex behavior but always privileging what was considered properly masculine initiative) meant that words for sex acts were transitive verbs.[33] "Mutuality was not important," and the same is somewhat true for much of the early modern period, although the receptive model of female bodies granted more internal agency to the yearning womb. The Aristotelian notion that women did not produce seed was largely overtaken by the counter-idea that a woman's "seed" was vital to reproduction (what I call the "unequal two-seed theory"). The sense that female seed played some role in generation was present in much medieval discourse too, though it rose to predominance after the printing and translation of Hippo-Galenic texts around 1525–35. But it did not necessarily always lead to a fundamental rethinking or new comprehension of a woman's orgasmic pleasure. Normative sex remained a matter of the delivery device of the penis conveying semen from the testicles to the uterus.

Vaginal intromission was nevertheless avoided for a variety of reasons, to prevent pregnancy and avert disease, for instance, to maintain virginal status, or to preserve one's sense of honor and chastity. A major model for sexual interaction focused on friction and on repetitive, rhythmic motion, without the end goal of penetration or ejaculation into the vagina. Recalling his profligate youth, the English writer Ben Jonson described in 1619 one woman who "lay diverse tymes" with him and "shew him all that he wished except the last act, which she would never agree unto."[34] Court records from early seventeenth-century Somerset suggest that "heavy petting became an end in itself" amongst the "largely illiterate lower orders," and the restricting of premarital sexual acts "to mutual masturbation or to the manipulation of the female genitals … may have been so effective that it became an ingrained male response or desire."[35] Sexual courtship before marriage was similarly overt but not predominantly penetrative amongst the lower classes in preTridentine Venice and elsewhere.[36] Engaging in numerous acts besides penetration was not necessarily regarded as a deprivation; in the 1520s one of the fantasies drawn in an account book by a Ferrarese clerk pictured coitus, but another imagined a man and a woman seated side by side on a bench, with the woman masturbating

33 Ruth Mazo Karras, *Sexuality in medieval Europe: doing unto others* (New York: Routledge, 2005), pp. 3–4.

34 C. H. Herford and Percy Simpson (eds.), *Ben Jonson*, vol. I (Oxford: Clarendon Press, 1925), p. 140.

35 G. R. Quaife, *Wanton wenches and wayward wives: peasants and illicit sex in early seventeenth century England* (London: Croom Helm, 1979), pp. 5, 169.

36 Cecilia Cristellon, "Public display of affection: the making of marriage in the Venetian courts before the Council of Trent (1420–1524)," in Matthews-Grieco (ed.), *Erotic cultures*, pp. 173–97. For a case in Augsburg in 1533 see Lyndal Roper, *Oedipus and the devil: witchcraft, sexuality and religion in early modern Europe* (London: Routledge, 1994), pp. 69–72.

both of them.[37] Many amateur sketches of naked men or of the phallic animal show them as solitary but ejaculating.[38]

Whereas the female body was characterized as receptive and recessive, colder in nature and marked by internal genitals, the male body was active and radiating, heated and distinguished by extruded genitals and hairiness. Hence, sunshine was a vital force in Ebreo's analogy and the personifications of the ancient gods Sol or Apollo were erotically charged. The humoral heat of male bodies fired an engine that was always focused outwards. In keeping with erection and ejaculation, projection, as much as or more than penetration, was the fundamental principle of masculinity. Both modes are typified by an expansion and protrusion from a central self or State or institution, but the word "penetration" indicates physical piercing and claims to special insight, whereas "projection" suggests a broader impact beyond the singular focus, leading to widespread overlay (Ebreo's *coprire*) and imposition as well as a range of representational, sometimes self-deluding strategies.

Modern reductions

Modern theories have tended to reduce the phallus to a circumcised pole. Castration, commonly misunderstood today to mean the removal of the penis, is in fact the excision of testicles and does not invariably result in feminization.[39] Yet, a singularly penile and penetrative assumption tends to hold today (except, perhaps, in some safe-sex classes and, of course, in the variety of personal practices which do not feature in public, commercial and political stereotypes). The fluidity of oil was hardly the point when former Maryland Lt. Governor Michael Steele set up a chant at the Republican National Convention on 3 September 2008: "drill, baby, drill, and drill now." At a time of rising oil prices and Republican support for offshore drilling during a Presidential campaign, the oil was a politicized excuse for sexist aggression, predicated upon everyone thinking of phallic, potent action in terms of insistent, violent penetration by a long pole (into compliant, dependent Mother Earth).

Words have power, and modern terms have often eradicated the testicles. Jean Toscan's magisterial compilation of erotic words in Italian poetry of the fifteenth through seventeenth centuries is marred by a focus on finding penile and penetrative (called phallic) connotations in nearly everything, even when the sense points more to testicular or semen-laden interests

37 Guido Guerzoni, "The erotic fantasies of a model clerk: amateur pornography at the beginning of the Cinquecento," in Matthews-Grieco (ed.), *Erotic cultures*, p. 63, fig. 2.3.

38 Ibid., p. 87 n. 65, figs. 2.1b, 2.5, 2.8.

39 J. N. Adams, *The Latin sexual vocabulary* (Baltimore: Johns Hopkins University Press, 1982), pp. 69–70; Taylor, *Castration*. If conducted after puberty the patient is infertile but usually capable of erections and ejaculation.

instead.[40] In an excellent translation of the *Priapea*, a collection from ancient Rome of bawdy poems about phallic garden god Priapus and his instrument, the obscene Latin word for balls is instead translated as "cocks."[41] Giordano Bruno's "ser coglione" (Master Balls) of 1582 becomes "Master Dick" in a fine translation, as though it is assumed that jokes about balls no longer make sense to modern readers.[42] While it is true that "the penis is thus centre stage" in seventeenth-century pornographic texts, as it was in sixteenth-century examples by authors such as Aretino and Antonio Vignali, its erection was medically explained in terms of semen, the testicles were necessarily ubiquitous in genital imagery and the very definition of virility, and ejaculation was the goal.[43] Even when the penis seemed to feature on its own, in other words, it was within the context of semen-driven and testicular manhood.

Non-penile aspects of the phallus can be so ignored that in one recent book on the penis, according to the title, the body part was "defined here not merely as the penile shaft and glans, but encompassing the testes, sperm, and all the other parts and products of the male genitalia."[44] The belief in the imperial might and mystery of the organ elided differences and nuances. For example, the claim that the Virgin Mary's sanctity was defined by "her lack of contact with a penis" is only documented by a quotation from the fourth-century Pope Siricius who actually said that she was uniquely not "stained by the presence of male seed."[45] Not only was there no rupture of Mary's virginal seal but Siricius' focus was Christ's parentage. Because the human matter of male seed had not come near Mary's pure body, the conception of Christ was uncontaminated by effluvia, the seed that Augustine proposed was at the core of human mortality. So fundamental was semen to the transmission of the vital spirit in propagation that to Augustine it was the means by which human beings were born already stained by sin and thence doomed to die due to Eve's successful temptation of Adam.[46] Christ, fully human yet divinely fathered, was conceived in Mary's virginal womb, untainted by semen or sin.

40 Toscan, *Carnaval.*

41 *The Priapus poems: erotic epigrams from ancient Rome*, trans. Richard Hooper (Urbana: University of Illinois Press, 1999), p. 56 (*coleis*), which rightly has "balls" for *coleos* on p. 66.

42 Giordano Bruno, "Candelaio," in his *Opere italiane*, ed. Giovanni Aquilecchia (Turin: UTET, 2002), p. 357; Giordano Bruno, *Candlebearer*, trans. Gino Moliterno (Ottawa: Dovehouse, 2000), p. 133.

43 The quotation is from Toulalan, *Imagining sex*, p. 69.

44 Friedman, *Mind of its own*, p. 4. 45 Ibid., pp. 5, 35.

46 Augustine, *Concerning the city of God against the pagans*, trans. Henry Bettenson (Harmondsworth: Penguin, 1984), p. 523; Elaine Pagels, *Adam, Eve, and the serpent* (New York: Vintage, 1988), pp. 109, 112, 131; Elizabeth Clark, "Generation, degeneration, regeneration: Original Sin and the conception of Jesus in the polemic between Augustine and Julian of Eclanum," in Valeria Finucci and Kevin Brownlee (eds.), *Generation and degeneration* (Durham: Duke University Press, 2001), pp. 17–40.

Similar blind spots about the male genital apparatus occur at the academic level. The catchy title of an illuminating study on witches has them stealing penises, even though many of the cited documents speak of plural "genitals" or "members."[47] Before the witchcraze set in, numerous images of popular magic illustrated Hans Vintler's manual on the virtues and vices, printed in 1486, and one of the woodcuts depicts a sorceress stealing a man's genitals in order to add them to the collection in her nearby "basket."[48] Notably, she has removed both penis and testicles, represented as one unit in the visual manner conventional since antiquity. From folk tales and popular images of phallus birds (figs. 12, 14), as well as metaphors for women's genitals as a "nest," "cage" (figs. 2, 23) or container, the foundational witch-hunter's manual the *Malleus maleficarum* (first published in 1486) mistook them as fact and reported that, with the aid of demonic illusionism, witches removed male genitals and stored them in birds' nests or boxes.[49] Furthermore, theorists of witchcraft adopted St. Thomas Aquinas' idea that devilish, feminine succubi stole semen from men, then transported it and disguised themselves as human men in order to impregnate women.[50] Semen was the manual's primary concern in that it was protecting the sacrament of marriage and particularly insistent about the necessity of sanctioned reproduction.[51]

The separation between penis and phallus is often bemoaned, as though a virtual castration, but the replacement of the two with "the soft and hard penis," proposed by English literature scholar Raymond Stephanson, does not, shall we say, stand up. It does not take account of symbolic and social power (which the "phallus" does), particularly when a "brain–testicles homology" discerned in the Enlightenment is at other times described as "mind–yard connections" as though there is no difference between the "yard" (penis) and the testicles.[52] Excising the testicles from the "yard" is actual castration. While I too am critical of feminist

47 Walter Stephens, "Illusion and reality, Part Two: witches who steal penises," ch. 11 in his *Demon lovers: witchcraft, sex and the crisis of belief* (University of Chicago Press, 2001). For the occasional use of the plural "members" in the influential witch-hunters' manual of 1486, see Heinrich Kramer and James Sprenger, *The hammer of witches: a complete translation of the "Malleus maleficarum,"* trans. Christopher Mackay (Cambridge University Press, 2009), pp. 171, 194 n. 384 and passim.

48 Charles Zika, *The appearance of witchcraft: print and visual culture in sixteenth-century Europe* (London: Routledge, 2007), pp. 39–45, 242 n. 22, fig. 2.3.

49 Kramer and Sprenger, *Hammer of witches*, p. 328.

50 For example, Kramer and Sprenger, *Hammer of witches*, pp. 121–39; Francesco Maria Guazzo, *Compendium maleficarum*, trans. E. A. Ashwin, rpt. (New York: Dover, 1988), pp. 30–33; Stephens, *Demon lovers*, pp. 19, 23, 64, 69–70, 80–82, 114 and passim.

51 On the sacrament, see Stephens, *Demon lovers*, pp. 312–21. For sorcery and marital impediment in canon law, see James Brundage, *Law, sex, and Christian society in medieval Europe* (University of Chicago Press, 1987), pp. 131, 145, 290, 291, 512. For a Spanish case in which sorcery was inter-related with the sacrament of marriage, see Ch. 1 below.

52 Raymond Stephanson, *The yard of wit: male creativity and sexuality, 1650–1750* (Philadelphia: University of Pennsylvania Press, 2004), pp. 29, 38, 47, 56, hereafter quoted from p. 45.

and Lacanian projects that arrive at "privileging an ahistorical, symbolic phallus over the material penis," Stephanson forgets to suggest why it would be any more useful to privilege that penis.

Ramifications

Far from a linguistic quibble, the reorientation from anatomy to physiology, from penile focus to semen-centric and testicular complexity has profound ramifications. Rather than applying the modern model in which "penetration symbolizes power," other somatic, biological bases for the institution and maintenance of patriarchal power must also be taken into account.[53] Even when women were regarded as possessors of testicles (actually ovaries) and producers of a kind of seed, female "lack" lay in their lesser quality, along with a "colder" humoral nature, rather than in the absence of a penis.

This book challenges many current assumptions about the European history of bodies. The idea that the female sex was regarded simply as an inversion of the male sex (Laqueur's famous "one-sex" model), for example, is finding its critics. My study goes further; it looks beyond anatomical morphology, past conventional remarks in medieval and Renaissance anatomical texts, to examine the way in which masculinity was defined and distinguished from femininity. I find that an "unequal two-seed" theory more accurately characterizes much about premodern understandings of male and female bodies.

Although this study concentrates on masculinity, women play a central role in several chapters, due to the way in which male bodies were differentiated according to criteria that also defined, by opposition, the female sex. Laqueur's work usefully identified the importance placed on female pleasure in early modern culture, yet it is time we examined more closely the exact understanding of a woman's erotic delight. For instance, in both serious medical literature and playful or obscene texts male sexual action and semen was regarded as a refreshing, arousing cure for a host of female ailments. The inferiority and dependence of women's bodies contributed significantly to the reinforcement of gender norms and patriarchal assurance, while also creating opportunities for more acknowledgement and expression of female desire.

Responding in part to the late twentieth-century focus on a new kind of nurturing fatherhood, some scholars of early modern Europe currently tend to focus on the way in which fatherhood was central to manliness. By contrast, I maintain that a celebration of fertility was more about virility than parenthood, about masculine projection and social power more than parenting. Rebecca Zorach's study of visual culture in Renaissance France reveals the multivalence

53 The quotation is from Karras, *Sexuality*, p. 25.

of abundant, excessive flows of four liquids, blood, milk, ink and gold, which had allegorical, political, national and erotic meanings.[54] The academic and theoretical field of what used to be called without differentiation "the body" now needs to be posited and analyzed in these expansive, plural terms.[55] While my study concentrates on adult male bodies in their active prime, it relies on multifarious evidence about several core genital components and actions of masculinity which are not always presented as ideal or somber.

Much literary analysis of masculinity relies on the psychoanalytic model of anxiety and thus reinscribes, on materials from earlier periods, the conventional, modern concept of the phallus. Supposedly, masculinity is always self-consciously insecure, reliant on the ever-stable phallus to symbolize ideal patriarchal power. Instead, my book argues that "anxiety" is telling ascribed to the masculine gender alone without sufficiently explaining why it is not a driving force for women too. "Anxiety" is a symptom of patriarchal power, manifested by a group privileged both in its historical moment and in historians' interpretations. More importantly, far from offering an explanatory framework particular to any historical period the interpretative device of "anxiety" reinforces the underlying ideological assumption that patriarchal masculinity is always in crisis yet forever triumphantly faces and overcomes every obstacle. "Anxiety" may seem to point to the constructed and precariously maintained nature of patriarchal power, but it occurs in unison with a series of apparati and processes that conquer one "crisis" after another so that authority is rarely damaged or challenged irreparably.

In Judith Butler's terms, "language and materiality are not opposed, for language both is and refers to that which is material, and what is material never fully escapes from the process by which it is signified."[56] The chicken and egg question of whether bodies or language, flesh or subjectivity, experience or discourse, sex or gender came first is unanswerable, and beside the point when working with historical bodies that are always materially and linguistically conditioned and constrained. Moreover, bodies from the past are most available to us in language, images, objects, and other cultural traces.

In some literary and historical studies the materiality of flesh tends to disappear under euphemistic layers or into a cloud of abstraction that assumes a universal psychic or biological framework. Histories of masculinity have become plentiful, though they are primarily about gender not sex, often focus on early modern England, and are mainly written by literature specialists, with some reference to social customs, whereas this book, as the product of an art

[54] Zorach, *Blood, milk, ink, gold.*

[55] Patricia Simons, "Bodies and contexts," *Art History* 10 (1987), 541–49.

[56] Judith Butler, *Bodies that matter: on the discursive limits of "sex"* (New York: Routledge, 1993), p. 68.

historian, is grounded in the materiality of culture and flesh.[57] My goal is to engage with the ways in which verbal language, visual rhetoric, material culture and living bodies constructed each other in multiple feedback loops of interchange and cross-fertilization. For instance, men and women watching and acting in jousts or enjoying the pictorial and literary spectacle of tournaments learned and deployed the sexual symbolism of the broken lance. While a modern emphasis on the penile nature of the weaponry focuses on its solidity and thrust, Renaissance interest lay as much in its orgasmic rupture.

This study contributes to the recent corporeal turn in historical studies, to what I call "embodied history," moving beyond the seeming divide between experience and discourse, tracing ways in which historical agents lived with and understood their bodies.[58] Moments of lived practice are brought into dialogue with cultural artifacts or codes, social scripts and literary tales, and each element inflects the others. From the pissing infant to the cocky youth and bearded elder, men learned how to name and understand their somatic experiences, absorbing and in turn inculcating that formative knowledge through humor and sobriety, images and books, public rituals and intimate encounters.

Metaphors had real influence on people's understanding of their bodies, intertwined as they were with familiar technologies, rebellious attitudes, clever wit, public performances, visceral habits and medical knowledge. The representational informed and reinforced the experiential and practical. People untrained in the literary arts nonetheless structured addresses, such as their accusations in court or pleas for leniency, along the lines of contemporary stories or plays.[59] Historical agents represented themselves with the aid of

[57] For example, Mark Breitenberg, *Anxious masculinity in early modern England* (Cambridge University Press, 1996); Elizabeth Foyster, *Manhood in early modern England: honour, sex and marriage* (London: Longman, 1999); Tim Hitchcock and Michèle Cohen (eds.), *English masculinities 1660–1800* (London: Longman, 1999); Kathleen Long (ed.), *High anxiety: masculinity in crisis in early modern France* (Kirksville, MS: Truman State University Press, 2002); Valeria Finucci, *The manly masquerade: masculinity, paternity, and castration in the Italian Renaissance* (Durham: Duke University Press, 2003); Alexandra Shepard, *Meanings of manhood in early modern England* (Oxford University Press, 2003); Thomas King, *The gendering of men, 1600–1750*, vol. I: *The English phallus* (Madison: University of Wisconsin Press, 2004); Stephanson, *Yard of wit*; Scott Hendrix and Susan Karant-Nunn (eds.), *Masculinity in the Reformation era* (Kirksville: Truman State University Press, 2008). For English material culture see Will Fisher, *Materializing gender in early modern English literature and culture* (Cambridge University Press, 2006).

[58] For example, Roper, *Oedipus and the devil*; Laura Gowing, *Common bodies: women, touch and power in seventeenth-century England* (New Haven: Yale University Press, 2003); Kathleen Canning, *Gender history in practice: historical perspectives on bodies, class, and citizenship* (Ithaca: Cornell University Press, 2006); Lyndal Roper, *Witch craze: terror and fantasy in Baroque Germany* (New Haven: Yale University Press, 2006); Lyndal Roper, "Martin Luther's body: the 'Stout Doctor' and his biographers," *American Historical Review* 115 (2010), 350–84.

[59] On the role of fiction see Natalie Zemon Davis, *Fiction in the archives: pardon tales and their tellers in sixteenth-century France* (Stanford University Press, 1987); Laura Gowing, *Domestic dangers: women, words, and sex in early modern London* (Oxford: Clarendon Press, 1996),

pre-existing narratives that were circulating more widely, and so too did they structure their selfhood in relation to everyday metaphors. Much of my study is interested in finding the overlap or interweaving between seeming fact and fiction, practice and art, noting the porous nature of shared assumptions about sexed bodies.

Identifying the suggestive meaning of words and the double entendre of visual elements is essential to such a project. Recent calls for a catalogue or dictionary of erotic art would certainly fill a gap, although visual vocabularies are necessarily allusive at times and various components can combine in inventive, even contradictory ways.[60] Lexica of erotic or obscene words already exist, yet still many visual jokes and sexual references are not comprehended.[61] More useful is an understanding of the reasoning that informs the signs, and later chapters here map out that logic. Morphology is one key factor, most easily recognizable, but another is action. Hence, for instance, the plumb line suspended over a woman's genitals by an aroused satyr in a print by Agostino Carracci (fig. 2) has only recently been deciphered, for its sexual suggestion by shape is not obvious whereas its motion makes connotative sense.[62] It is a pendulous instrument that sways rhythmically but finds the true vertical, and a carnival song likened it to a cleansing plunger that removes "grease." Even if at first delighted by the riddle, viewers (predominantly male) would have quickly grasped the humor by thinking about penile action. The obvious bulge in the satyr mason's apron is both a satirical comment on censorship and an example of how arousal was frequently displaced visually onto the bestial in order to validate actual, continuing viewing of an art object. Corporeal experience and gestural practice were often part of the sensorium appealed to by erotic imagery. As with the plumb line, stereotypical notions of a solid, rigid penile pole obstruct our decoding of many metaphors, especially when semen-centric references predominate.

pp. 68–69, 249–50; Joanne Ferraro, *Marriage wars in late Renaissance Venice* (Oxford University Press, 2001), p. 7 and passim; Guido Ruggiero, *Machiavelli in love: sex, self, and society in the Italian Renaissance* (Baltimore: Johns Hopkins University Press, 2007).

60 For the calls, see Ruggiero, "Introduction," pp. 5, 6.

61 Such dictionaries and guides include Toscan, *Carnaval*; Adams, *Latin sexual vocabulary*; Frankie Rubinstein, *A dictionary of Shakespeare's sexual puns and their significance*, 2nd edn. (London: Macmillan, 1989); Jeffrey Henderson, *The maculate muse: obscene language in Attic comedy*, 2nd edn. (Oxford University Press, 1991); Boggione and Casalegno, *Dizionario*; the two works by Williams listed in n. 20 above; Claudio Fraccari, "Le parole per dirlo. Glossario," in Costantino Cipolla and Giancarlo Malacarne (eds.), *El più soave et dolce et dilectevole et gratioso bochone: amore e sesso al tempo dei Gonzaga* (Milan: FrancoAngeli, 2006), pp. 340–54.

62 Patricia Simons, "Agostino Carracci's wit in two lascivious prints," *Studies in Iconography* 30 (2009), 201–06; cf. Sara Matthews-Grieco, "Satyrs and sausages: erotic strategies and the print market in Cinquecento Italy," in Matthews-Grieco (ed.), *Erotic cultures*, pp. 31–33, where it is read as a morality print in which "the meaning of the pendulum is unclear."

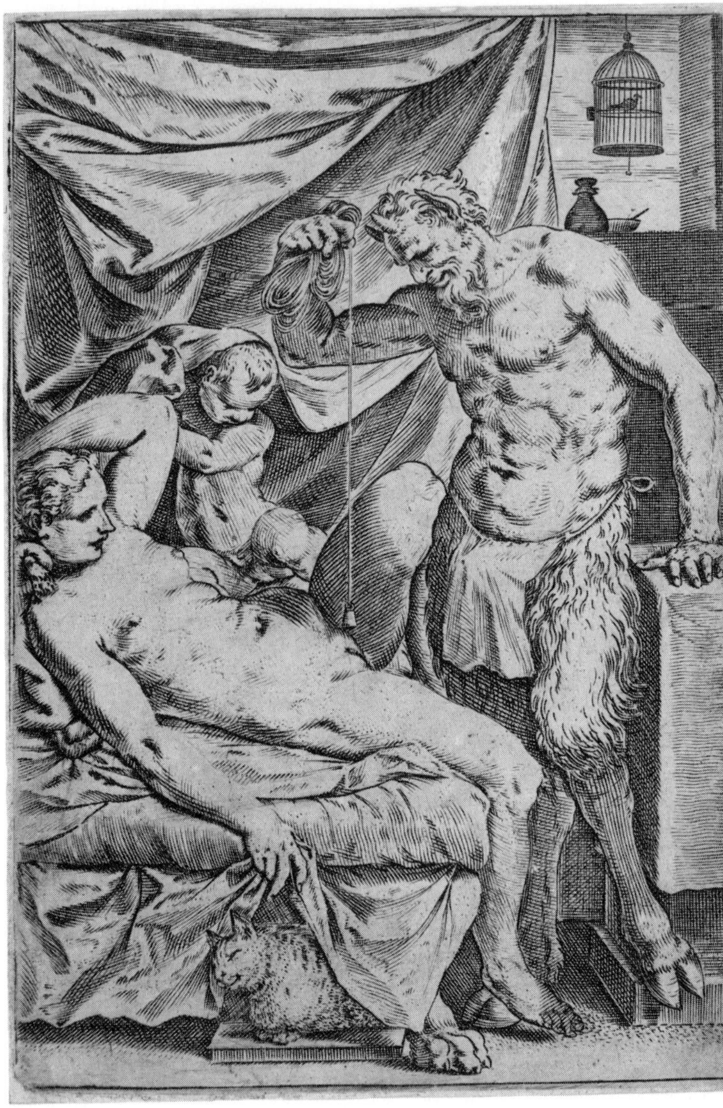

Figure 2 Agostino Carracci, *The satyr mason*, 1585–1600, engraving, 203 × 134 mm, London, British Museum

It is too reductive to summarize the shift from centuries of pre-Freudian notions of sexuality to the brief modern and psychoanalytic period as moving "from scrotum to penis, reproduction to pleasure."[63] Projection and penetration complemented rather than replaced each other and what I describe as the semenotic system was, in fact, deeply engaged in certain kinds of pleasure, for women and men. Reproduction was certainly the most sanctioned, expected result of sex but human fertility was allied with fecundity and pleasurable proliferation in much broader terms, especially advantaging patriarchal power, patrilineal authority and libertine masculinity. Gendered bodies and their actions have histories, and the short moment of the last century or so has its own particular history, from which we cannot generalize about all bodies and every psyche.

Eight chapters follow, divided into two parts. Part I considers the historical and visible nature of masculine bodies, highlighting the centrality of semen and testicles. The first chapter examines what it meant to act "like a man" and be judged to have a male or female body by medical and Church authorities, focusing on the 1580s case of the hermaphrodite Elena/o in Spain, with comparative material drawn from France and Germany. Only after establishing the "embodied" conditions of masculinity does the book turn to the symbolic phallus, in Chapter 2 scrutinizing the history of the phallus as a word, artifact and effect, from ancient Greek rituals and vase paintings to Lacan via Freud, who first used the word in his study of Leonardo da Vinci in 1910. Having stressed the humorous aspects of the phallus, the chapter concludes with a critique of the historical use of the psychoanalytic paradigm of "anxiety." Chapter 3 focuses on material culture in late medieval and early modern Europe, in such forms as phallic beasts on badges and coats of arms with testicular emblems. Not only were so-called "phallic symbols" like lances more varied and complicated than has been assumed but also much imagery concerned itself with overt scrotal signs, from the famous equestrian monument of Bartolomeo Colleoni (General Balls) in Venice to blatantly showy codpieces that are named for the scrota (cods) and are not entirely penile in form or function.

Part II elucidates medical models and metaphors for the male sex, that is, the ideal adult male body that was fundamentally active and projecting. The intellectual history of medical theory about male genitals and masculine "heat" begins in Chapter 4 with the ancient origins in Hippocratic treatises, Aristotelian biology and Galen's humoral physiology. Core ideas are then followed through medieval scholarship and into the Renaissance revival of ancient texts, rendered especially powerful through publication and translation

[63] The quotation from Taylor, *Castration*, p. 97 encapsulates his core argument regarding "the rise of the penis" and the "fall of the scrotum." His dating of the shift is vague and variable.

in printed form and then vernacular dissemination. Here, the unequal two-seed theory is contrasted with the one-sex model. The next chapter demonstrates that semen was regarded as a valuable bodily resource, to be conserved or expended carefully. Certain metaphors about the testicles and semen took this sense of value into the language of economics, presenting them in the context of coins, moneybags and commercial dealings. Chapter 6 reassesses premodern concepts of female sexual pleasure, finding that women's release of fluids was believed to be ejaculatory (within the uterus) and may not always have met modern criteria for orgasmic pleasure. Further, women's delight was theorized in terms of their eager reception of male semen. Medical and semen-centric notions were widely disseminated through textual and visual metaphors, connecting a variety of cultural registers. Curative semen is the subject of Chapter 7, along with various agricultural metaphors set in fields and gardens. From ancient Greek medical analogies to Renaissance fountains of love, the tools, movements and "fruits" of sexual activity are more about plenitude and virility than they are focused on paternity or parenting, let alone anxiety or threat. The last chapter deals with metaphors that represent familiar objects, tools and labor in activities that relate to the social, cultural and medical understanding of sexual and semen-driven corporality. Such actions as blowing, ladling, grinding, mixing, stirring, grating, cooking and baking are double entendres in both texts and images. Some of the visual witticisms have gone unrecognized, due in part to a modern preoccupation with penile penetration. The Conclusion offers final thoughts on the interconnectedness of metaphors and bodies, and of ways in which various strata of evidence enable us to approach the texture of bodily experience in the past.

Part I

Witnessing men's bodies: paradigms old and new

1 How to be a man in early modern Europe

While testicles were key signs of the male body and the penis was essential for emission, those markers had to work in conjunction with performative cues, such as standing erect while urinating, growing beards and discharging a certain kind of semen. Some of the most important behavioral signs of the gender of masculinity were thus tied to the biologically sexed male body, and the latter is the focus here. Mutually constitutive, gender and sex were brought into being by anatomy and physiology, and also by actions, as well as being construed through images and words. The Welsh schoolmaster John Owen (d. 1622) neatly encapsulated logocentric virility in his epigram: "God himself is the Word; he made all things with a word. / We men make words; we too are words."[1] Masculinity was an inter-related and variable mix of three main factors: genital signs, somatic deeds (like the mode of pissing), and behavioral indicators (such as choice of dress, and degree of aggressiveness). Case studies examined in this chapter demonstrate the range but not the instability of early modern parameters within which maleness was designated and enacted.

Assigning maleness: the case of Elena/o

At different times, medical professionals, Church officials and acquaintances came to different conclusions about whether the Spanish mulatto born female as Elena de Céspedes but later called by the male name Eleno was male, female or an hermaphrodite.[2] As did contemporary documents, personal pronouns vary here according to the situation of the time, though they mainly follow the

[1] Fred Nichols, *An anthology of Neo-Latin poetry* (New Haven: Yale University Press, 1979), pp. 578–79.

[2] Extracts have been published from over 150 double-sided folios documenting the case before the Toledo tribunal of the Inquisition, partially translated in Richard Kagan and Abigail Dyer (ed. and trans.), *Inquisitorial inquiries: brief lives of secret Jews and other heretics* (Baltimore: Johns Hopkins University Press, 2004), pp. 36–59. Other than the items cited in footnotes here, see also Emilio Maganto Pavón, "La intervención del Dr. Francisco Díaz en el proceso inquisitorial contra Elena/o de Céspedes, una cirujana transsexual condenada por la Inquisición de Toledo en 1587," *Archivos españoles de urología* 60 (Oct. 2007), 873–86. I have not read the novel Agustín Sánchez Vidal, *Esclava de nadie* (Madrid: Espasa-Calpe, 2010).

protagonist's point of view. To this day, grammar rules and terminologies are inadequate for intersexed people. A corpus of impressive historical research and literary analysis now exists on early modern hermaphrodites and other issues of changeable or problematic masculinity. Rather than concentrate on medical theory and natural philosophy in the abstract, I focus here on taking seriously the pragmatics and physical aspects of one case, spotlighting not only the perception of somatic signs by the authorities but also by the subject of their scrutiny. Considered a liar by recent translators of extracts into English, a lesbian by some scholars, a male transsexual by a Spanish urologist, and now the subject of a novel about a defiant person born to a slave mother, Elena/o as seen through the sole lens of trial documents does not easily fit modern categories. On the other hand, there was broad agreement about the cluster of factors that were thought vital to the identification of a male body in the sixteenth century. Elena/o agreed with these, arguing on the basis of surgical knowledge and a personal library of twenty-seven volumes that s/he was instead an hermaphrodite.

Knowledge of the possibility of bodies changing sex from female to male was disseminated widely through rumor, medical theory and printed books. Professional rivalry was sometimes central, as it was in a French case of 1601 discussed below, or when medical men blamed midwives for misidentifying the sex of newborns.[3] Tales circulated of men falling pregnant, and some thought that Jewish men menstruated.[4] The androgyne was an alluring ideal in alchemy, allegory and Neoplatonic philosophy. Fictive literature, including the popular poetry of Ovid and Ariosto, also instilled the impression that female bodies could magically convert to male ones, and that hermaphrodites existed.

However, most men were not thereby anxious on a daily basis about the untrustworthy, unstable nature of their own body and its potential to shift sex. It was the female state that was marked by irrationality and instability and that could oscillate, theoretically always to the more perfect male condition. As Elena/o's case demonstrates, in the early modern period institutional means to manage disruptions of individual sexed bodies were available in law courts and

[3] For example, André du Laurens, *Historica anatomica humani corporis* (Paris: A. Mettayer et Ourry, 1600), p. 360, cites a case mentioned by an earlier physician as occurring in Paris in 1577, repeated in Helkiah Crooke's translation, *Mikrokosmographia: a description of the body of man. Together with the controversies there to belonging. Collected and translated out of all the best authors of anatomy, especially out of Gasper Bauhinus and Andreas Laurentius* (London: William Jaggard, 1615), p. 250.

[4] Roberto Zapperi, *The pregnant man* (Amsterdam: Harwood, 1991); Sherry Marie Velasco, *Male delivery: reproduction, effeminacy, and pregnant men in early modern Spain* (Nashville: Vanderbilt University Press, 2006); William Johnson, "The myth of Jewish male menses," *Journal of Medical History* 24 (1998), 273–95; John Buestein, "Jewish male menstruation in seventeenth-century Spain," *Bulletin of the History of Medicine* 73 (1999), 447–56.

Church tribunals, increasingly supported by the testimony of medical professionals.[5] The current habit of discerning instability, uncertainty and ambiguity everywhere in the early modern world, and of finding the male body perilous and masculinity tenuous, needs to be balanced by an awareness of limitations both institutional and cultural that provided sufficient assurance and normative grounding. Medical theories varied, but the predominant view about hermaphrodites, those polyvalent bodies that continue to trouble medical and legal orthodoxy today, was increasingly Hippo-Galenic and thence they were placed on a spectrum of Nature's diverse marvels. Social and sexual performance, however, required definition. Courts, medical practitioners and hermaphrodites all had confidence in their ability to categorize individual cases. But those different areas of expertise did not all agree. Whereas self-identification accompanied by consistent gender performance was on the whole acceptable in medieval times, during the sixteenth and seventeenth centuries the individual hermaphrodite was overwhelmed by the authoritative pronouncements of men who were engaged in competing claims to professional status. Hierarchies were asserted, physician over surgeon, Spanish self-educated female surgeon over male surgeons serving royalty, Parisian professor over regional practitioner, judge over a person deemed fraudulent and sinful. Institutions of control asserted their right to interpret what was natural, thereby delimiting capricious Natura.

In 1562, at the approximate age of sixteen, Elena, the daughter of an African slave, bore a legitimate son, but due to the strain of childbirth what she thought of as a penis emerged from her body. Thereafter Eleno at first partially dressed as a man and then did so entirely and, taken by many to be an hermaphrodite or still a woman, he was not noticed by punitive authorities.[6] He lived for years as an itinerant male weaver, hosemaker, soldier and tailor who had sexual affairs with women. By 1584, he was practicing as a successful surgeon and in December applied for a marriage license, at which point the vicar of Madrid queried the beardless face and thought Eleno might be a eunuch (*capon*).[7] Yet, both an immediate inspection by several men, and a physician's examination at Toledo determined that Eleno was male, as did a third inspection by "surgeons

[5] Lorraine Daston and Katharine Park, "The hermaphrodite and the orders of Nature: sexual ambiguity in early modern France," in Louise Fradenburg and Carla Freccero (eds.), *Premodern sexualities* (New York: Routledge, 1996), pp. 117–36.

[6] Rumors that Eleno was an hermaphrodite or a woman were common, and the lifestyle was largely acceptable when s/he cross-dressed. For example, he passed the guild exam for tailors and was allowed to practice, though only under the sign "seamstress": Kagan and Dyer (ed. and trans.), *Inquisitorial inquiries*, p. 41.

[7] Marie-Catherine Barbazza, "Un caso de subversión social: el proceso de Elena de Céspedes (1587–1589)," *Criticón* 26 (1984), 21–23; Israel Burshatin, "Written on the body: slave or hermaphrodite in sixteenth-century Spain," in Josiah Blackmore and Gregory Hutcheson (eds.), *Queer Iberia* (Durham: Duke University Press, 1999), pp. 430–31.

and doctors and other people of good repute . . . ten men in all," and a fourth conducted in February 1586 by a surgeon (Francisco Díaz) and a physician employed at the royal court of Madrid.[8] Witnesses adamantly noted the presence of manly penis and testicles.[9]

Assessed as male, Eleno married María, but after a year or so the couple moved to a different town, and there a fellow veteran reported to the governor in June 1587 that Eleno had been known in the army as either a woman or an hermaphrodite. What had not caused consternation in the military was now a different matter, for marriage had taken place. That very month, and in response to a letter from the Nuncio in Spain sent in May 1586 that expressed concern about the common practice of castrated men being allowed to marry, Pope Sixtus V sent a brief to his legate in Spain condemning marriage with eunuchs, who usurped the title of "husband" and thereby ridiculed the sacrament of marriage.[10] Sixtus' decree of 27 June 1587 declared that only men with testicles and who had "the power of emitting true seed (*verum semen*)" within the female vessel were capable of marriage.

Eleno consistently avowed that he was a man and therefore had not engaged in unnatural or fraudulent practices with a woman. However, in a further round of examinations three midwives declared her a virgin, and physicians discerned a vagina (*vasso natural*) but not "any sign of being a man (*señal nynguna de hombre*)."[11] Considered female, he was found guilty of having "fooled (*engañó*) another woman and married her."[12] Devilish enchantment, disrespect for the sacrament of marriage, bigamy and sodomy are all implied. The documents frequently use nouns like *embustes* (lies, frauds), *enbelecos y ynvençiones* (machinations and inventions), *engaños* (deceits, ploys), *ficçion* (fiction) or the verbs *engañar* (to deceive) and *fingir* (to feign, to pretend) to

[8] Burshatin, "Written on the body," pp. 432–33; Kagan and Dyer (ed. and trans.), *Inquisitorial inquiries*, pp. 43–45. In the very first examination, "three or four men looked at me from the front, though I didn't let them look at me from the back, so they wouldn't be able to see my woman's parts" (p. 43). The editors take this as a sign of "Elena's disappearing penis" and hence its "fiction" (n. 21), but male genitals were discerned, and because she did not bend over the men did not see the vaginal opening. Even if later medical professionals were "befriended or bribed, or both," as Kagan and Dyer suggest, this first test was made on the spot, before any chance to influence witnesses.

[9] Burshatin, "Written on the body," pp. 428, 433.

[10] McGrath, *Controversy*; misread in Finucci, *Manly masquerade*, pp. 263–64, for procreation was *not* the issue. Rather, manliness was, and the issue of satisfying female desire (see Ch. 6 below).

[11] Israel Burshatin, "Elena alias Eleno: genders, sexualities, and 'race' in the mirror of natural history in sixteenth-century Spain," in Sabrina Petra Ramet (ed.), *Gender reversals and gender cultures* (London: Routledge, 1996), pp. 106–08.

[12] Israel Burshatin, "Interrogating hermaphroditism in sixteenth-century Spain," in Sylvia Molloy and Robert McKee Irwin (eds.), *Hispanisms and homosexualities* (Durham: Duke University Press, 1998), pp. 14–15.

characterize the effect Elena/o had had on the wife and on a range of people from female lovers to renowned surgeons.[13]

Skepticism about a woman of a lower social and racial status was due, in part, to what Eleno admitted were changes to his body. The penile member that emerged after childbirth had disappeared in the course of 1587, so the surgeons, including Díaz again, blamed the prisoner for her inherently feminine wiles and sorcery, because she must have used "an art so subtle that it sufficed to fool him by sight and by touch" on the previous occasion.[14] Devilish illusion was not only a convenient excuse for the professional men's inconsistency but also deployed a theory familiar to Inquisitors, because canon law as well as witchcraft manuals had long addressed sorcery as a cause for marital impediment and the theft of male genitals. Elena/o instead presented a physical explanation: due to a riding accident the member became weak and spongy, and self-administered surgery had gradually cut it off.[15] Nevertheless, s/he said wounds at that site remained, and the court did not instantly discount the story, perhaps because it was understood that male genitals were often injured by war, disease and other causes.

There were further ways in which masculinity could be verified. The court immediately asked about testicles, which Elena/o had "in a particular form," but hand gestures did not clarify the matter and Céspedes said that a doctor would understand. Ovaries, which were considered internal "stones" or testicles, might have been meant, or Eleno may have been trying to articulate manually an unusual configuration like the labia/testicles of what modern medicine classifies as female pseudo-hermaphroditism. The lack of facial hair and "his ears pierced like a woman" continually troubled investigators, as did occasional menstruation.[16]

It was the beardless face that most disturbed the vicar in Madrid and catalyzed the round of examinations and investigations. Visible facial hair was important in the determination of an adult man's virility. Accused of impotence by his wife in 1599, Baron d'Argenton was inspected on the order of an ecclesiastical judge and it was found that he "had no exterior cullions [testicles], but was like a purse

[13] Burshatin, "Written on the body," pp. 423, 425, 426, 427, 433, 450–51; Lisa Vollendorf, *The lives of women: a new history of Inquisitional Spain* (Nashville: Vanderbilt University Press, 2005), pp. 26–27. Similarly, Elena/o is accused of "fiction," manipulation and inconsistency, as well as "personal creativity and ingenuity" by the modern editors in Kagan and Dyer (ed. and trans.), *Inquisitorial inquiries*, pp. 43 n. 21, 48 n. 30, 57, 59.

[14] Burshatin, "Written on the body," p. 433; Vollendorf, *Lives of women*, pp. 22, 207 n. 47. For the removal and return of male genitals by witches see Kramer and Sprenger, *Hammer of witches*, pp. 194–201, 323–30.

[15] Kagan and Dyer (ed. and trans.), *Inquisitorial inquiries*, p. 49. Testimony from the warden, prisoners and other locals confirmed Eleno's worry and pain at the time: Vollendorf, *Lives of women*, pp. 22–23.

[16] Vollendorf, *Lives of women*, p. 20.

without ammunition."[17] Until his autopsy in 1604, the man's apparently recessive testicles were the talk of France. The Baron proclaimed that he was not a eunuch because he had a bearded chin and his voice was not thin or shrill but resembled that of other men, being strong and manly. The beard was a sure sign because, he said, everyone knows that it springs from the abundance of that humor which flows from the face due to the force of the testicles. As the Italian anatomist Alessandro Benedetti put it in the late fifteenth century, the beard "is contained in the testicles."[18] Facial hair, rather than belonging to what are now considered "secondary" sex characteristics or being a sign of non-genital gender, as Will Fisher has argued, was regarded in the sixteenth century as a genital sign, of healthy, male adulthood and virility. Furthermore, asserted Argenton, just as sexual urges increased during coitus (as semen accumulated), so did the beard grow. The Baron's appeal rested on common knowledge. The onset of a beard signaled the end of one type of homoerotic activity (that between an older man and a beardless youth) and, as Eleno heard from the vicar, the beard was an important indicator that a new husband was capable of producing proper male semen. Various tales of women hairy over many parts of their bodies were miracles, marvels, myths or mistakes, exceptions that proved the rule that normative male bodies were hairy due to extrusion caused by their innately greater heat.[19]

The evidence of bodily fluids was also vital. Urination had been performed through Eleno's member, "as other men do."[20] And, according to Céspedes, sex with women resulted in "abundant pollution," that is, the issue of semen.[21] However, at least one of the female sex partners testified that there had been "no effusion of seed," to which the defense was that other men also failed in this manner, probably referring to temporary impotence.[22] To admit to the permanent lack of seed would have seriously detracted from Eleno's masculine state.

[17] Pierre Darmon, *Le tribunal de l'impuissance* (Paris: Éditions du Seuil, 1979), p. 34 ("une bourse sans boulettes").

[18] Alessandro Benedetti, *Historia corporis humani sive Anatomice*, ed. Giovanna Ferrari (Florence: Giunti, 1998), p. 240; trans. in L. R. Lind, *Studies in pre-Vesalian anatomy* (Philadelphia: American Philosophical Society, 1975), p. 114. The book was first published in Venice in 1502, but written in the 1490s. My reading of beards differs substantially from Will Fisher, "The Renaissance beard: masculinity in early modern England," *Renaissance Quarterly* 54 (2001), 155–87, which misreads his key text because it is not recognized as a translation from a Latin book written by the learned Italian cleric Pierio Valeriano after the Sack of Rome.

[19] For a convenient overview of stories about inappropriate female hair, see Merry Wiesner-Hanks, *The marvelous hairy girls: the Gonzales sisters and their worlds* (New Haven: Yale University Press, 2009), pp. 37–46, 56–58, 131–38.

[20] Kagan and Dyer (ed. and trans.), *Inquisitorial inquiries*, p. 49. On the importance of urination, see Patricia Simons, "Manliness and the visual semiotics of bodily fluids in early modern culture," *Journal of Medieval and Early Modern Studies* 39 (2009), 331–73.

[21] Kagan and Dyer (ed. and trans.), *Inquisitorial inquiries*, p. 50; and in separate testimony, Vollendorf, *Lives of women*, pp. 22, 206 n. 35.

[22] Burshatin, "Elena alias Eleno," pp. 112–13.

One of the disturbing factors about the case must have been that Céspedes' body did not obey the conventional teleology whereby sex changes ascended to male "perfection" and then remained stable in that final state.[23] The mother Elena had been the husband Eleno and then reverted to female virginity. The ambiguous body of a brown-skinned, branded person who had raised their status from manumitted slave to respectable surgeon also subverted standard notions of racial, professional and class categories. In 1599, the Inquisition's physician summed up the case as "deceit by a female slave who pretended to be a man."[24] For unknown reasons, the general populace believed Céspedes to be a miracle worker rather than a malevolent bewitcher, flocking to the hospital in Toledo where s/he was serving out a ten-year sentence by attending to indigent patients.[25]

Informed by her knowledge as a surgeon, Elena/o had submitted a letter to the tribunal rebutting charges and citing Cicero, Augustine and Pliny on the existence of androgynous people who "are called hermaphrodites, who have both sexes."[26] Attention was drawn to the fact that four female lovers said "that I was a man and had the effect (*efectos*) of such," doubtless said by the women in part to defend themselves against possible charges of sodomy, but Elena/o used their testimony to assert intersexual identity. Or, rather, since hermaphroditism was a medical phenomenon but not a legal category, Céspedes consistently acted as a man with "male parts." When trying to grasp how the wife innocently thought she was having sex with a man, the Inquisition not only queried her about sexual position and pregnancy but also whether Eleno had ever "praised his male member," an indication that proper masculinity was expected to evince itself in boasting about the genitals.[27]

Other behavioral effects were also decisive, specified as a telling factor in the statements of two of the three medical men who had recently determined that the prisoner was female.[28] Besides anatomical evidence, one man cited all the "signs (*señales*) of woman, like breast, face, speech, and all the rest," such as height, that provided physical evidence of sex. The other observed that there

[23] See, for example, Albertus Magnus in Joan Cadden, *Meanings of sex difference in the middle ages: medicine, science, and culture* (Cambridge: Cambridge University Press, 1993), p. 160; Baldasarre Castiglione, *The book of the courtier: the Singleton translation*, ed. Daniel Javitch (New York: W. W. Norton, 2002), Book 3, chs. 3 and 15; Ambroise Paré, *Des monstres et prodiges*, ed. Jean Céard (Geneva: Droz, 1971), p. 30; Crooke, *Mikrokosmographia*, pp. 249–50. One of the few medical texts to suggest that men sometimes grew cold enough to turn inward and become women had recently been released (1575): Juan Huarte de San Juan, *Examen de ingenios para las sciencias*, ed. Guillermo Serés (Madrid: Catedra, 1989), pp. 607–09. But this was a rare opinion, and the book was prohibited by 1581 (p. 110).

[24] Burshatin, "Elena alias Eleno," p. 119. [25] Barbazza, "Caso de subversión," 39.

[26] Burshatin, "Elena alias Eleno," pp. 112, 212 n. 13. See Cicero, *De divinatione*, 1.20, 36, 98; Pliny, *Natural history*, 7.15, 34, 36; Augustine, *City of God*, 16.8.

[27] Vollendorf, *Lives of Women*, p. 23.

[28] Burshatin, "Elena alias Eleno," p. 108; Vollendorf, *Lives of women*, p. 26.

was no "sign (*señal*) of being a man, . . . and in the composure (*conpastura*) of body, breast, face, and speech she has the appearance of a woman, as she is, and not a man." Most of the corporeal signs had been listed in the previous decade by the French royal surgeon Ambroise Paré, including not only genitals but face, "virile or shrill" voice, breasts, gendered actions and capacity of the "male rod" to become erect and emit seed.[29]

Current scholarship about the early modern body has been said to show "a world of flexible sex and no secure corporeal basis for gender roles," but it is important that we not assume or imply a contrast with modern certitude and superior knowledge.[30] The body is increasingly becoming again a matter of complexity, flux and change, as knowledge grows about the insecurity of sex tests at the Olympics, for instance, or about pre-adolescents wanting to change the sex they were assigned at birth.[31] Given the humoral intricacy of premodern bodies and the array of possible algorithms that structured prophylaxis and treatment, it is no wonder that a medical system that claimed to be able to explain sex could articulate parameters but not definitive clarity. Elena/o and the examiners were trying to make sense of an exceptional body; as still happens too often today, medico-legal authorities forced that body to fit within polarized standards. Cases such as Elena/o's do not prove that male bodies were thought mutable or provisional. Unlike individual acquaintances and small town populations, medico-legal authorities at regional and Church-wide levels tried to adhere Céspedes' body to one sex and one gender. Not all of these regulatory systems coalesced into a single model, for neither power nor knowledge was totally centralized. But gender was thought to be inflected by sex. Moreover, we must be careful about using such evidence in support of a claim for widespread contestation regarding the parameters of male corporeality. As trial documents, they necessarily speak to different opinions, and what is more striking is that overall they demonstrate a shared understanding, including by Elena/o, of what constituted the comprehensible limits and variations of an adult husband's body.

The best diagnosis was Elena/o's own, that this was an hermaphrodite: "I have quite naturally been a man and a woman, and even though this may seem like a prodigious and rare thing that is seldom seen, hermaphrodites, as I have been one

[29] Paré, *Monstres et prodiges*, pp. 25–26 (first published 1573); Ambroise Paré, *On monsters and marvels*, trans. Janis L. Pallister (Chicago: University of Chicago Press, 1982), pp. 27–29.

[30] The summation is from Gowing, *Common bodies*, p. 3. For modern medical issues, see Suzanne Kessler, *Lessons from the intersexed* (New Brunswick: Rutgers University Press, 1998); Peter Lee, et al., "Consensus statement on the management of intersex disorders," *Pediatrics* 118 (Aug. 2006), 488–500.

[31] See, for example, Patricia Leigh Brown, "Supporting boys or girls when the line isn't clear," *New York Times* (2 Dec. 2006); Jennifer Finney Boylan, "The XY Games," *New York Times* (3 Aug. 2008).

myself, are not against nature."[32] Elena/o made an articulate, learned and reasoned case, and it is probable that s/he genuinely believed the diagnosis of the very first surgeon to examine her/his body, subsequently bolstered by reading natural history books. Hence, no sin was committed in the prisoner's opinion and the wish to marry in the Church, "in God's service," was evidence of sincere piety.[33]

Psychosomatic factors: being "like a man"

Female lovers discerned in Eleno a masculine "effect" (*efectos*), especially when recounting their affairs to the tribunal, yet his wife also found enticing the rumors that Eleno "had the natures of a man and a woman."[34] What motivated desire amongst the various players was surely variable and probably altered over time. Before the marriage, "parents, relatives and neighbors" regarded "him to be neuter and a man, that he was neither the one nor the other."[35] At an earlier time, when still dressed as a woman, she was with a "young and pretty" married woman and "felt like kissing her, and without saying anything, she kissed her." The two then tried to have sex, but "even though she was excited and the head [of Elena/o's member] had come out . . . and [Elena/o] lay down on top of her, she couldn't do any more to her than that demonstration."[36]

Elena/o's unsatisfying encounter with a desirable woman led to the visit to the surgeon Tapia, who diagnosed hermaphroditism and made a cut that released the sensitive organ, "and that was how he began to act as a man (*comenzó usar de onbre*), and he was married."[37] Thence Elena/o was "left with the aptitude (*abtitud*) to have relations with women."[38] For an important part of its adult life the body possessed a male extrusion which had impeded sex with men while enabling sex with women, so the choice for sexual activity with women alone was understandable even on a pragmatic level.[39] To the tribunal, Eleno always

32 Barbazza, "Caso de subversión," 32–33. The condition of his/her body should be taken seriously. Psychologist Suzanne Kessler has suggested female pseudo-hermaphroditism, such as CAH (congenital adrenal hyperplasia): Vollendorf, *Lives of women*, pp. 15–16.

33 Barbazza, "Caso de subversión," 30; Vollendorf, *Lives of women*, pp. 22, 207 n. 43.

34 Burshatin, "Elena alias Eleno," p. 112; Kagan and Dyer (ed. and trans.), *Inquisitorial inquiries*, p. 48.

35 Burshatin, "Interrogating hermaphroditism," p. 8; referred to as *neutro* on p. 10.

36 Ibid., p. 13. Elena/o explained to the tribunal that "when she felt desire and natural excitement it [the "head of a male member"] would come out" (pp. 4, 13); Burshatin, "Written on the body," p. 435.

37 Burshatin, "Interrogating hermaphroditism," p. 10; Kagan and Dyer (ed. and trans.), *Inquisitorial inquiries*, p. 47.

38 Burshatin, "Elena alias Eleno," p. 111.

39 Obstructive *ragadiae*, protuberances usually due to uterine prolapse or an enlarged clitoris, were commonly mentioned, chiefly in surgical literature. See, for example, Avicenna, *Liber canonis* (Venice, 1507), rpt. (Hildesheim: Georg Olms, 1964), 377v (Bk. III, fen. 21, tr. 4, chs. 22–23); Crooke, *Mikrokosmographia*, p. 236.

presented himself as a man who married in order to legitimize sexual acts that he considered natural.

If no "male member" had appeared, or if no surgical incision had occurred, perhaps Elena/o would not have developed the "aptitude" of desiring women. Perhaps the pleasure felt at that part of the body, interpreted as male, directed the body and libido to seek female partners because that was what the Church and Nature decreed. The body part and its pleasures affirmed his masculinity but also fundamentally helped to construct it, giving intelligibility to sexed subjectivity. Rather than having an innate sexual orientation or gender identity, the potential of Eleno's body and his lived experience developed in tandem. Gender effects were a matter of clothing, occupation, economic independence, social rank, sexual action and erotic pleasure, and they were acquired in co-ordination with socialized parameters like Church law, guild regulations and military conscription. The very vocabulary as well as practice of the first surgeon was determinative. It provided both a category and the physical body part through which Eleno then experienced his/her body. Along with the crucial cut of a knife that brought more rather than less into being, naming Eleno an hermaphrodite was a classic instance of a performative speech act that brought her manhood rather than ambiguity fully into existence.

In 1601, in a similar fashion, it was an articulate, detailed description but also the professionalized instrument, in this case an examining finger of the French medical practitioner Jacques Duval, that defined twenty-year-old Marie le Marcis as Marin and saved him from execution as a woman who had had sex with another woman.[40] From Marie/Marin's perspective, the development of a male body justified sexual acts with and desire for a woman. Similar to Elena/o, the prisoner in Rouen was charged with sodomy and sacrilege in relation to marriage plans, and cross-dressing was considered disturbing by the authorities; the female sex partner, in this case a widow with children, found that Marin performed adequately in bed; like Elena/o before surgery, Marin said he had an internal penis that only emerged when aroused. Various issues were weighed, such as how the prisoner urinated, whether testicles were present and whether menstruation occurred.[41]

In the end, Duval's digital penetration brought forth "a virile member, rather large and hard," and friction caused ejaculation of semen that was described as "white genital semen, thick and of mediocre fluidity," that is, unlike thinner

[40] Duval, *Hermaphrodits*, "Advertissement au Lecteur," and pp. 383–447 passim; Katharine Park, "The rediscovery of the clitoris: French medicine and the tribade, 1570–1620," in David Hillman and Carla Mazzio (eds.), *The body in parts: fantasies of corporeality in early modern Europe* (New York: Routledge, 1997), pp. 179–84; McClive, "Masculinity on trial," 53–56.

[41] Duval, *Hermaphrodits*, pp. 388, 394, 401, 422.

female "seed."[42] It was male seed that caused great pleasure and was "so copious and abundant in man, that the learned Fernel had no hesitation in saying that 'man is entirely semen.'"[43] According to Duval's conventional, humoral reasoning, it was Marin's hermaphroditic (that is, feminine) humidity and overly cold complexion during adolescence that caused the male genitals to remain recessed.[44] But an opponent, the Parisian professor of anatomy Jean Riolan, argued on the basis of anatomy rather than physiology that Marie's body was marked by an enlarged clitoris and hence had engaged in sinful female–female sex. Writing eleven years later about the case, Duval was able to report that Marin was occupied as a tailor and had developed a beard. With the publication of books by Duval and Riolan, the case of Marin entered a world of medical knowledge, legal recognition, public print, professional debate and titillating controversy. Words and deeds each had powerful materiality and effect.

Acting like a man

According to the influential work of the royal surgeon Paré, sex was assigned to hermaphrodites due to both physical and behavioral or gendered reasons, including "whether the whole disposition of the body is robust or effeminate; whether they are bold or fearful, and other actions like those of males or of females."[45] His biological reasoning was widespread. The behavioral symptoms he listed, what the postmodern philosopher Judith Butler might recognize as "a stylized repetition of acts," were naturalized.[46] To Paré, boldness, daring or audacity (*hardis*) were explained by manly humoral "heat," and physically involved aggression, projection and initiative.

Literally being on top was a key masculine affect, as noted in Elena/o's trial.[47] In 1405, the legal petition of a French female prisoner represented her former sex partner, the fellow fieldworker Jehanne, as an aggressive hermaphrodite. Masculinity was indicated by action and initiative: "she climbed on her as a man does on a woman, and the said Jehanne began to move her hips and do as a man does to a woman."[48] Notably, the sexual motion regarded as masculine was repetitive friction, not penetration, as it was for numerous episodes of

[42] Ibid., pp. 403, 404. Female seed was different (p. 417).

[43] Ibid., "Advertissement au Lecteur": "que le docte Fervel [sic] n'a fait doute de dire *que homo totus semen est.*" The reference is presumably to Jean Fernel, *The Physiologia of Jean Fernel (1567)*, trans. John M. Forrester (Philadelphia: American Philosophical Society, 2003), pp. 525ff; see also Avicenna, *Liber canonis*, 351v.

[44] Duval, *Hermaphrodits*, pp. 421, 436–37, 441.

[45] Paré, *Monsters and marvels*, p. 28.

[46] Judith Butler, *Gender trouble. Feminism and the subversion of identity* (New York: Routledge, 1990), p. 140.

[47] Vollendorf, *Lives of women*, pp. 16, 23, 24 (*actos como hombre*).

[48] Cadden, *Sex difference*, p. 224.

intercrural sex between men described to a French Inquisitional trial in 1323. In that case, a man placed his penis between another man's buttocks or thighs and, "moving himself as with a woman, his semen flowed."[49]

Initiative and assertion were compelling traits in a fifteenth-century German case too. Those investigating a cross-dressed woman in Speyer, who had had sex with several women, heard that the actions of Katherina Hetzeldorfer successfully mimicked those of a man.[50] During carnival season, the accused "whored like a man," said one female witness in 1477, "and she grabbed her just like a man [. . . and] with hugging and kissing she behaved exactly like a man with women." Another of the sex partners, the married woman Else Muter, similarly had sex with Hetzeldorfer "just like a man" and she observed that "men should be granted such roguery." Only men were that roguish, assertive, insistent and heated in character. Else explained to the court that she was deceived by masculine qualities, including assertive persistence and "manly will" exercised through sex on top, but she also saw manly urination and felt the emission of semen, copious "beyond measure." Else may well have been convinced her sex partner was male. Sex was often conducted in ways that avoided conception, involving external friction rather than penetration, or interruption before ejaculation. And, for a variety of reasons ranging from moral to practical, sex was frequently conducted between people who remained more or less fully clothed.[51] In such circumstances, criteria of manliness did not focus on the penis or penetration alone.

While the sin of male sodomy was defined as the placement of semen in an inappropriate (that is, non-reproductive) vessel, much secular, non-legal material did not overly concern itself with reception. Many male actions and pleasures were conceptualized in much the same way whether due to interaction with a male or female body or done alone, and hence distinctions between homoerotic and heteroerotic acts were passed over in most medical literature. The waste of a precious resource was of concern, and semen was often figured as coin (Chapter 5 below), spent fruitfully or in a manner that might exhaust the body and impoverish the realm. Another metaphor was that it transmitted knowledge from teacher or "master" to eroticized male pupil (typed as "active" in the former case, and "patient" or passive in the latter), a process of infusion and exemplarity that could not involve women for they were usually thought to have little use for learning and were rarely granted an opportunity for public

49 Michael Goodich (ed.), *Other middle ages: witnesses at the margins of medieval society* (Philadelphia: University of Pennsylvania Press, 1998), pp. 122, 134.

50 Helmut Puff, "Female sodomy: the trial of Katherina Hetzeldorfer (1477)," *Journal of Medieval and Early Modern Studies* 30 (2000), 41–61 (subsequent quotations are from the court document, 60–61); Simons, "Bodily fluids," 338–39.

51 John McNeill and Helena Gamer (eds.), *Medieval handbooks of penance* (New York: Columbia University Press, 1938), pp. 211, 336; Simons, "Bodily fluids," 362 n. 28.

action.[52] On the whole, semenotic theory and imagery did not draw distinctions between recipients, all of whom were considered feminine or effeminate. The paramount interest was virility, productivity and pleasure, and the standpoint that of the "active," superior, projecting male agent.

The potential to father a child (preferably a son) was important but the fertility of semen was not essential to masculinity. Today, virility is often understood to signify a capacity to procreate, but in premodern culture that was not necessarily so fundamental. According to the Italian–English dictionary first published in London by John Florio in 1598, *virile* was defined as "manlike, valiant, stout, male, grave, of mankinde, pithie, substantiall"; *virilità* meant "manliness, manhood, courage" and also "the privie parts of a man, mans genitors"; *viripotente* was defined as "ripe for mariage [sic], able to live and lye with a man," corrected in the 1611 edition as "able to discharge the part of a man with a woman."[53] Discharge was a telling term, implying the placement of manly seed in the receptive female vessel of a wife, but none of Florio's entries regarding virility insisted that a proper man had to produce children. The same is true in Randle Cotgrave's contemporaneous French–English dictionary, in which sexual relations with women were not mentioned at all.[54]

As Valeria Finucci has shown for the literature of Renaissance Italy and Mary Fissell for Restoration England, paternity might be a complex, uncontrolled matter, interfered with, for example, by a mother's imagination that reshaped the fetus in an image other than that of the father.[55] But fatherhood need not be in the forefront of all studies of masculinity, for the production and ejaculation of semen symbolized overall virility. Many men, after all, were reluctant to take on the economic and moral burden of recognizing a child born out of wedlock, but were eager to engage in sex beyond the marital bedroom.[56] Paternity was only one factor in the assertion of masculinity through sex acts, along with sexual pleasure and the health of the male body as well as that of the body politic.

52 For "learned seed," see, for example, Bruno, "Candelaio," p. 290 ("mio dottrinal seme"); Rocco, *Alcibiade*, p. 42. Ficino claimed to be rendered fertile by the influence of one pneumatic breath ("uno afflatus") from masculine writings by Bartolomeo Scala: Marsilio Ficino, *Epistolarum*, in *Opera omnia*, 2 vols., facsimile (Turin: Bottega d'Erasmo, 1959), vol. I, bk. 2, p. 865 (Book 8, to the physician Giorgio of Cyprus).

53 John Florio, *A worlde of wordes (1598)*, facsimile (Hildesheim: Georg Olms Verlag, 1972), p. 450; John Florio, *Queen Anna's new world of words* (1611), facsimile (Menston: Scolar Press, 1968), p. 603.

54 Randle Cotgrave, *A dictionarie of the French and English tongues* (1611), facsimile (Menston: Scolar Press, 1968), s.v.: *virile* meant "virile, manlie . . . ; bold, stout, couragious, valiant; strong, substantiall, pithie; grave"; *virilité* indicated "manlinesse, . . . strength, vigor; stoutnesse, courage; also, a mans genitalls."

55 Finucci, *Manly masquerade*; Fissell, *Vernacular bodies*, ch. 7.

56 See, for example, Gowing, *Common bodies*, pp. 177–203.

Male bodies were distinguished by their external genitals, an ability to eject urine and semen and assertive behavior, all of which can be called projective capacities. Adhering to the convention that male and female genitals were somewhat homologous yet situated, respectively, on the outside and interior of the body, the surgeon Paré said that female genitals were "bound to the interior."[57] Sex changes resulted from extraversion, from systemic heat becoming "more robust, vehement, and active" so that the female body was able "to push out what was hidden within" and hence became male. Beards too were extruded by male heat. The French and German women of the fifteenth century used the same criteria as the French and Spanish surgeons did a century later: outward, vehement, roguish action was normative for male bodies, in accordance with humoral theories of masculine "complexion" or physiologically determined temperament.

Acting male: breaking lances

Physical acts in a public, symbolic register also demonstrated Paré's understanding of boldness, and staged spectacles of virility often entailed fluids and projection as well as straightforwardly penile aggression. For example, the long lance aimed at a target with great ferocity was more than a Freudian "long, stiff" pole. It broke. The supposedly phallic characteristics of eternal tumescence and rigidity did not mark the jousting signifier and, rather than thinking of the broken lance as the mere afterlife of the now-absent phallus, the rupture was much of the point. Perhaps in tandem with the growing nature of jousting as a spectacle rather than for the exhibition of military prowess, the aim of jousting was often not so much to unhorse or penetrate an opponent's armor as to break one's own lance and thereby prove that a forceful, skilled hit had been scored.[58] *Rumpo* (to rupture) was an ancient Latin term for aching male sexual desire and ejaculation, but the rise of the technology of the tourney engendered a new metaphor, the bursting, busting, breaking of a lance (*rompere* in Italian, *rompre* in French).[59]

The action was regularly performed at tournaments and it peppered vernacular literature, including comedies performed on the English and Italian stage.[60]

[57] Paré, *Monsters and marvels*, pp. 32–33.

[58] Sydney Anglo, *The martial arts of Renaissance Europe* (New Haven: Yale University Press, 2000), pp. 227, 233, 239, 241, 243, 250, 251.

[59] Adams, *Latin sexual vocabulary*, p. 151; Malcolm Jones, "Sex and sexuality in late medieval and early modern art," in Daniela Erlach, Markus Reisenleitner and Karl Vocelka (eds.), *Privatisierung der Triebe? Sexualität in der Frühen Neuzeit* (Frankfurt am Main: Peter Lang, 1994), pp. 197, 235 n. 53; Williams, *Dictionary*, p. 781; Malcolm Jones, *The secret middle ages* (Phoenix Mill: Sutton Publishing, 2002), pp. 257–58, 359 n. 47.

[60] Pietro Aretino, *Cortigiana*, ed. Angelo Romano (Milan: Biblioteca Universale Rizzoli, 1989), pp. 139–40 (the first version, of 1525); Aretino, *Ragionamento*, p. 34; Pietro Aretino, *Tutte le commedie*, ed. G. B. De Sanctis (Milan: Mursia, 1968), p. 423 (*La Talanta*); Riccardo Bruscagli

Matteo Bandello (d. 1561), a north Italian then French resident and Dominican monk, wrote in one of his stories about the character Cornelia bewailing her elderly husband's inadequacies, complaining that he rarely jousts with her. He "can barely break one lance (*romper una lancia*), and then he is so debilitated that he spends the next half hour gasping."[61] The masculine coding of the joust was mocked in Aretino's comedy *Il marescalco* (1533) when a braggart soldier boasted that at a wedding he tilted at a target and "I broke a hollow, painted lance filled with birds at six hits," which really meant that he had first failed five times, and that the lance was only a pretty, decorated fake.[62] That it released "birds," which in Italian meant the male genitals, accentuates the sexual (and homo-erotic) import of the buffoonish rupture performed at a wedding feast. In another of Aretino's comedies, a bawd's mission was to ensure that a man would soon "break two lances."[63] The multiplicity of the bursts, taken to extremes by the boasting soldier, is an indication that ideal virility consisted of more than one ejaculation per encounter, so bountiful was the production of semen.

Martinus Opifex depicted the metaphor when he illuminated the *Historia Troiana* for Emperor Frederick III's court around 1450 (fig. 3). Achilles lies in bed, having reached "his goal of love within a great tent whose labial lips spread open," as Michael Camille astutely noted.[64] Furthermore, however, female imagery is matched by visual symbols of masculine success within the chamber. His discarded helmet means his penile "head" is bared, and the nearby shield indicates that he has hit his "target." A board with three nails hammered through it is placed along an orthogonal that recedes into the tent's interior, referring to "nails" that signify the multiple unions of ejaculatory coitus. And a broken sword is prominent in the foreground, replacing a lance but again indicating Achilles' potency.[65] What we consider orgasm was pictured for men in terms of a bursting forth from a sinewy, rigid organ of missiles and nails, seeds and sound and fluids. A phalanx of lances, raised at various angles in all three panels of Paolo Uccello's series depicting the *Battle of San Romano* (fig. 4), suggests alert readiness, armed superiority and eager anticipation amongst the victorious

(ed.), *Trionfi e canti carnascialeschi del Rinascimento* (Rome: Salerno, 1986), p. 142. In verse on a German print of *Wedding dancers* attributed to Erhard Schoen the lady asks her swain why "you wish not to break a spear?" ("eyn sper züprechen"): Walter Strauss, *The illustrated Bartsch 13 (Commentary): German masters of the sixteenth century: Erhard Schoen, Niklas Stoer* (New York: Abaris Books, 1984), pp. 318, 322.

61 Matteo Bandello, *Le novelle*, ed. Delmo Maestri, 4 vols. (Alessandria: Edizioni dell'Orso, 1992), vol. I, p. 489 (first printed in 1554). In Bandello, *Novelle*, vol. II, p. 303, the sweetness of "la prima lancia che ruppe" is then augmented by four more breakages.

62 Aretino, *Commedie*, p. 36.

63 Pietro Aretino, *La cortigiana*, ed. Giuliano Innamorati (Turin: Giulio Einaudi, 1970), p. 114.

64 Michael Camille, *The medieval art of love* (New York: Harry N. Abrams, 1998), p. 155, with the illumination reproduced in color as fig. 142.

65 Williams, *Dictionary*, p. 781, points out that spear and lance are equally "broken" in English usage.

troops. The leader is surrounded by an eager cluster of jostling lances in the central panel, flanked on either side by scenes of profuse armour and broken lances abandoned on the ground. In conjunction with the dead body laid out on an orthogonal towards each outer edge of the two bracketing images, the splintered lances not only emphasize perspectival recession and violent warfare but remind viewers of the resounding noise, physical exhaustion and essential masculine ferocity of the conflict. The subtext of sexual, corporeal aggression subliminally accentuates the drama and the virility of the conquest that is vividly depicted in the life-size tableau.

Boys could learn the ejaculatory sense of the breaking lance whenever they had the opportunity to observe or, if members of the wealthy elite, participate in

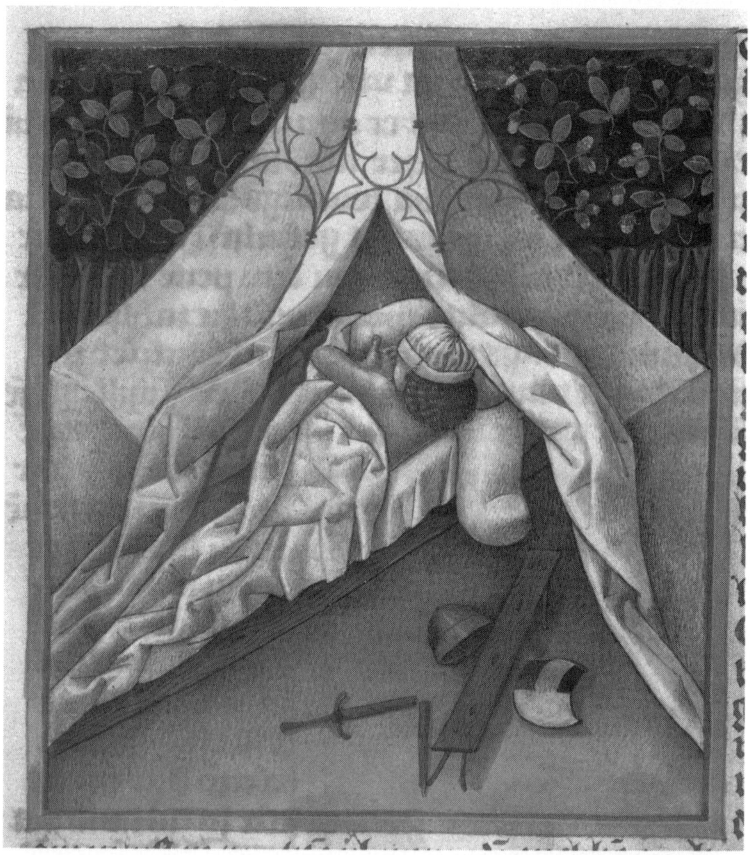

Figure 3 Martinus Opifex, Achilles the Lover, from *Historia Troiana*, *c*. 1450, Vienna, Österreichische Nationalbibliothek, Cod. 2773, fol. 164r

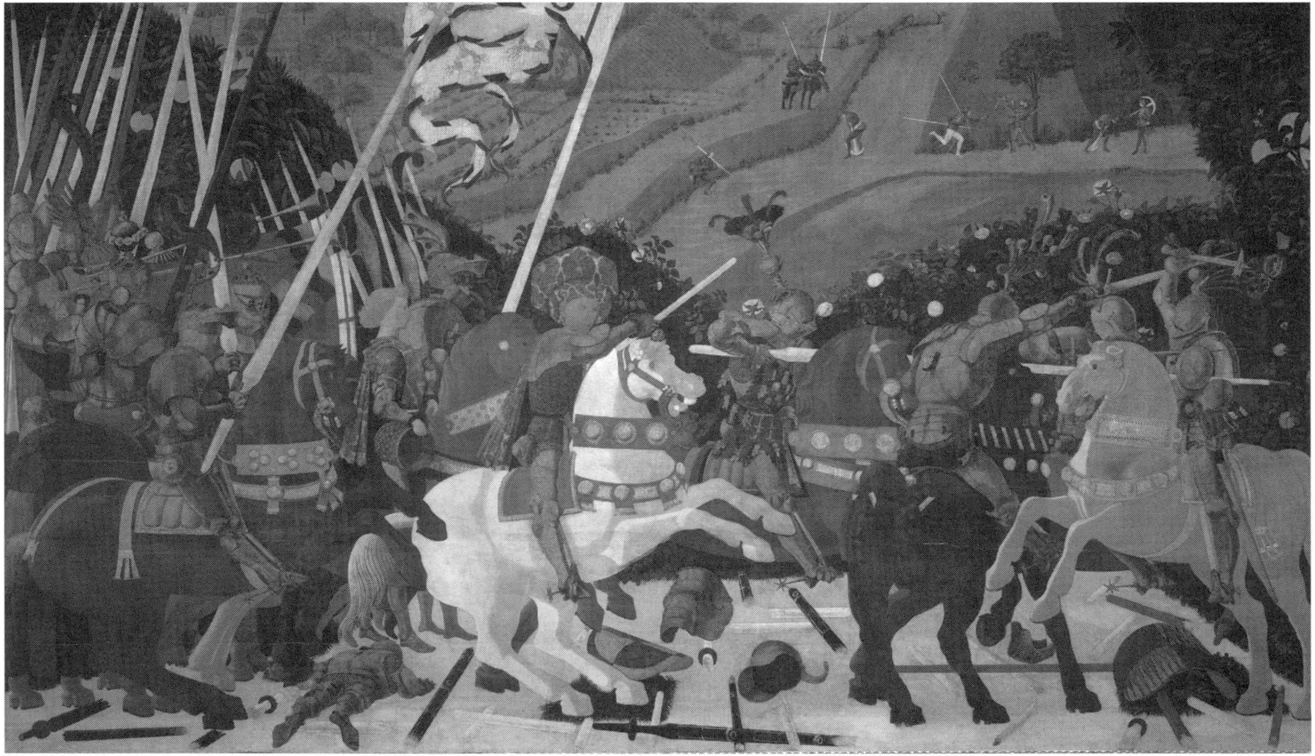

Figure 4 Paolo Uccello, *The battle of San Romano*, *c*. 1438–40, tempera on wood, 182 × 320 cm, London, National Gallery

a tournament or other chivalric games. As Ruth Karras has shown, in numerous courts and cities of France, Germany, Italy and England in particular, courtly and fictive nostalgia was instilled in the young and reinforced by older authorities.[66] Masculinity was conceptualized and performed according to a script of poetic metaphors, knightly ceremonies and aggressive acts, from throwing out challenges ostensibly in order to impress and woo a symbolic damsel, to intensive, sometimes erotic bonding between men as brothers-in-arms. Feminized castles, attacked by knights who are bestrewn with flowers and spices scattered by ladies from the castle's battlements, and which are then sexually breached by masculine entry, were common in texts like the *Roman de la rose*, popular through much of Europe, and were visually reiterated in ivory caskets and mirror cases from the fourteenth and fifteenth centuries, prints from the fifteenth century and tapestries or court games from the sixteenth century, to live on in the language and actions of a seventeenth-century gang manhandling a woman in a Somerset inn, as we will see below.[67] Another eroticized moment in the public theatrics of tournaments and chivalric play was the running of long lances at a suspended ring, clearly understood to have a sexual implication.[68]

A Florentine example of the *armeggeria*, a display of knightly prowess, demonstrates the erotic imagery and action of such events. One evening during the carnival season of February 1464, nine youths from leading families, surrounded by well over 400 attendants, torchbearers and musicians led by Bartolomeo Benci, traversed the city to perform beneath the windows of their fictive lady loves. Sources only record the first visitation in detail, Benci's spectacular social drama in the piazza of the Strozzi holdings, addressed to the young Marietta, renowned for her beauty.[69] The son from a pro-Medici clan

66 Ruth Mazo Karras, *From boys to men: formations of masculinity in late medieval Europe* (Philadelphia: University of Pennsylvania Press, 2003), pp. 20–66.

67 On the Castle of Love, in Italy, England, Germany and France, see Roger Sherman Loomis, "The allegorical siege in the art of the middle ages," *American Journal of Archaeology* 23 (1919), 255–69 (including Elizabeth I as "the Castle of Perfect Beauty" in 1581); Suzanne Lewis, "Images of opening, penetration and closure in the *Roman de la rose*," *Word and Image* 8 (1992), 215–42; Heather Arden, "The slings and arrows of outrageous love in the *Roman de la rose*," in Ivy Corfis and Michael Wolfe (eds.), *The medieval city under siege* (Woodbridge, Suffolk: Boydell Press, 1996), pp. 191–206; Peter Barnet (ed.), *Images in ivory: precious objects of the Gothic age* (Princeton University Press, 1997), pp. 72–74, 230–31, 245–48; Camille, *Medieval art of love*, pp. 35–36, 87–93; Charles Dempsey, *Inventing the Renaissance putto* (Chapel Hill: University of North Carolina Press, 2001), pp. 82–86.

68 Aretino, *Ragionamento*, pp. 34, 35, 52; Williams, *Dictionary*, p. 1182; Anglo, *Martial arts*, pp. 231, 246, 249, 251, 289, figs. 164–65.

69 Two contemporary descriptions survive, an anonymous account and a poem by Filippo di Lorenzo Lappaccini: see Isidoro del Lungo, *La donna fiorentina del buon tempo antico*, 2nd edn. (Florence: R. Bemporad & Figlio, 1926), pp. 207–10, for the first; Antonio Lanza (ed.), *Lirici toscana del Quattrocento*, vol. II (Rome: Bulzoni, 1975), pp. 1–6, for the second. On rituals of knighthood in fifteenth-century Florence see Richard Trexler, *Public life in Renaissance Florence* (New York: Academic Press, 1980), pp. 216–40, and 226, 230–32 for the political

was "playing the part of one enamored of the said damsel" when performing beneath the window of the unmarried, orphaned granddaughter of the prominent anti-Medicean exile Palla Strozzi.[70] Palla's rival Cosimo de' Medici had become, in Marco Parenti's shrewd assessment, "first citizen in the city of Florence, due to riches, prudence, authority and power," but he was currently ill and indeed died later that year.[71] In other words, political one-upmanship was at work, the virile vigor of scions of the Medicean faction was on display, and women's bodies, encased in the windows of "castles," were symbolic nodal points for rivalry and bonding between men.

The costumes of horses and participants were lavish and the entourage was accompanied by an elaborate cart representing the Triumph of Love, decked out with ornaments such as many *amoretti*, called "*spiritegli* of love with bows in their hands," coats of arms, greenery and silver bells, topped by "a bleeding heart, surrounded by flames of fire which continually burn." Cupid, usually present when castles were besieged, was absent on this occasion, but the conventional imagery of love was joined by Benci, called "Lord Love" (*Signore Amante*), adorned with "two wings at his shoulders, of gold and many other colors," resembling the renowned multicolored wings of Cupid. Then the show (*mostra*) began: each of the nine prominent youths rode in knightly fashion, "with a gilded dart in their hand, and then each ran with a blunted, gilded lance, and broke it at the foot of the window where the lady was displayed with much honorable graciousness in the middle of four lit torches."[72] Benci's wings were then removed and thrown upon the Triumphal cart, which was set ablaze and released noisy fireworks that seemed to come from the bows of the *spiritegli*. Several of these fiery "arrows" penetrated the lady's house, and they were said to have "entered also into her heart, [melting it with] compassion for the said lover."[73] Her surrender won, the large retinue departed, going on "to break the lances and demonstrate their skills at the house of the Lady of each of the men of the Company."[74]

The verb that described all the breaking of lances was *rompere*, the same as that used for sexual "lances." Notably, in 1464 the lances were not directed at male opponents, ensuring that homoerotic innuendo was downplayed in favor of a focus on distant damsels, framed within palaces that were symbolically possessed

meaning of the Benci-led events of February 1464. Two city proclamations of 13 February facilitated the event: Pietro Gori, *Le feste fiorentine attraverso i secoli* (Florence: R. Bemporad & Figlio, 1926), pp. 40–41. For the imagery see also Dempsey, *Renaissance putto*, pp. 77–86.

70 Del Lungo, *Donna fiorentina*, p. 207, translated in Trexler, *Public life*, p. 231.

71 Marco Parenti, *Ricordi storici 1464–1467*, ed. Manuela Doni Garfagnini (Rome: Edizioni di Storia e Letteratura, 2001), p. 57. Cosimo died on 1 August 1464.

72 Del Lungo, *Donna fiorentina*, p. 208.

73 Ibid., p. 209. Fireworks by the same designer, put on for an aristocratic wedding in Bologna in 1487, were described as shooting out, ejaculating: Dempsey, *Renaissance putto*, p. 243 n. 19.

74 Del Lungo, *Donna fiorentina*, p. 209.

or conquered. The extravagant event was about chivalric norms, masculine exhibition and the public display of honor and control. Both besieged households and the crowd of participants and onlookers all understood, or learned for the first time, the erotic meaning of breaking lances, bursting fireworks and arrows piercing the liminal plane of windows, memorably reinforced by music, noise, dazzling torchlight and splendid costumes. Earlier that month, a smaller-scale but still very public spectacle also focused on penetrating the palace façade where Marietta was on display through the aperture of a window. Benci and two other prominent Medicean men engaged in a snowball fight with her, accompanied by torches, trumpets, flutes and a cheering crowd.[75] The highlight was when one man "sprayed the face of the snow-white girl with snow," likened to an expert hitting the target with his arrow, which was again familiar sexual language. Even the projective act of throwing snow, especially through an open window, was taken suggestively in carnival songs, and in various romantic tales such as one written in 1444 by the man who later became Pope Pius II.[76]

Penetrative, bursting lances and sprayed snowballs were literary metaphors for sexual action but they were also publicly performed and political ones. For at least some of the participants in events like those of the 1464 carnival in Florence, they learned the language and vivid conceptualizations of bodily acts from seeing or engaging in spectacles and hearing the approbation of the crowd. Two of the most common times in the calendar for putting on jousts were during carnival and for weddings, both occasions when sexual implications were appropriate and rife.[77] In the 1430s, Matteo Palmieri's treatise on civil life complained that brides-to-be were publicly paraded on horseback "to the chosen field of jousting, circling the piazza and making an exhibition, to show that they were no longer going to be virgins."[78] The public visibility was shocking, exacerbated by trumpets preceding the woman (who was wearing ornate clothing and "lascivious" cosmetics), "calling the populace to see the unbridled audacity of meretricious passion." By such overt means, jousting was associated with the act of defloration, a demonstration clear to female as well as male spectators. Anticipation, heightened by parading virgins and thundering horses in their final run, would have made the ejaculatory release of the broken lances all the more stirring.

[75] A Latin letter from Filippo Corsini to Lorenzo de' Medici described the event: del Lungo, *Donna fiorentina*, p. 249 n. 51.

[76] Bruscagli (ed.), *Trionfi*, pp. 359–61, 481–82; Toscan, *Carnaval*, pp. 902, 1012, 1064 (straightforwardly read as penile, whereas I see it as semenotic); Enea Silvio Piccolomini, *Euryalus und Lucretia. Lateinisch/Deutsch*, ed. Herbert Rädle (Stuttgart: Philipp Reclam, 1993), p. 72.

[77] Richard Barber and Juliet Barker, *Tournaments* (Woodbridge: Boydell Press, 1989), esp. pp. 77–90, 169–76; Paola Ventrone (ed.), *Le tems revient, 'l tempo si rinuova: feste e spettacoli nella Firenze di Lorenzo il Magnifico* (Milan: Silvana, 1992).

[78] Matteo Palmieri, *Della vita civile*, ed. Gino Belloni (Florence: Sansoni, 1982), p. 114.

Rather than experiencing sexual sensation first and then applying or inventing language for it, people like Marietta or Benci's young pages were simultaneously learning from social, repeated words and deeds as well as corporeal responses. Chivalric verse and spectacle supplied husbands with the language to conceptualize and describe their sexual conquests in acceptably euphemistic, heroicizing, ever-vigilant terms. The newly married Leonardo Bruni, for example, boasted to another humanist after his wedding in 1411 that "the forts I'd come to conquer were invested and captured the first night; it was a bloody victory [that is, the bloodied sheets signified the bride's loss of virginity] . . . I return to camp at night and keep up my vigil."[79] Bruni's contemporary, the poet Domenico da Prato, decried that jousts and similar manly competitions were now being sponsored for the sake of lads (*garzoni*) rather than ladies.[80] In each case, athleticism, male bonding and sexual symbolism were explicitly located in the same erotic field, and desire was licensed on the part of spectators as well as participants.

Acting male: flinging liquids

Only an understanding of how charged male body acts and fluids could be helps us grasp the almost ritualized exploits of several gangs in early seventeenth-century Somerset. In 1609, a group of drunken men concocted an imaginative notion of how to consummate genital contact. At first, they gained satisfaction by forcing one of an inn's servants to let them "thrust their hands shamefully between her legs and feel her privities and look upon them."[81] Several physical and symbolic deeds of this kind climaxed in their final act of tossing beer at her genitals. The servant Edith was held fast as she endured the appearance of each besieger who "came forth with a glass of beer in his hand and taking up Edith's coat above her knees felt her privities and then threw the glass of beer at the same."

Their physical and optical aggression toward Edith was all the more direct because women rarely wore underpants until the eighteenth century. Numerous court records epitomize sexual access to female bodies as an act of lifting their skirts, reiterated in fictional tales, on the comedic stage, in songs, at carnival time and in images of eager men whose hands do sexual work.[82] Visual and verbal representations of men's hands burrowing into a bodice or under

79 James Hankins, "The Latin poetry of Leonardo Bruni," *Humanistica Lovaniensia* 39 (1990), 14.

80 Lanza, *Lirici toscana*, vol. I, pp. 570–71.

81 Quaife, *Wanton wenches*, p. 170, from which the following information, but not interpretation, is drawn. The case is also briefly mentioned in Gowing, *Common bodies*, p. 28.

82 See Gowing, *Common bodies*, p. 38 for the underwear, and pp. 35, 54–107 passim for pulling up skirts; also Quaife, *Wanton wenches*, pp. 54, 165–85 passim; Gowing, *Domestic dangers*, pp. 68, 75, 91. For visual representations and carnival, see Werner Mezger, *Narrenidee und Fastnachtsbrauch: Studien zum Fortleben des Mittelalters in der europäischen Festkultur* (Constance: Universitätsverlag, 1991), pp. 150–51, figs. 63–65; Jones, "Sex and sexuality," pp. 255–56 n. 230, figs. 42–43.

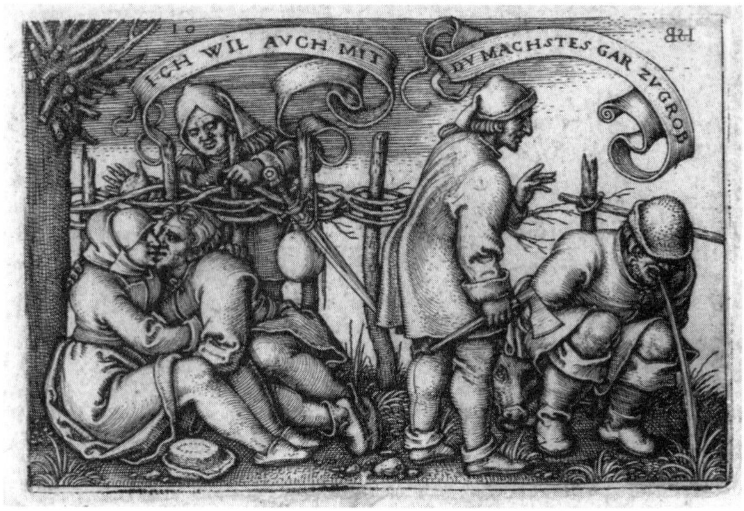

Figure 5 Hans Sebald Beham, *Behind the fence*, 1546–47, engraving, 51 × 74 mm, London, British Museum

women's skirts and thrusting an arm between a woman's bared legs (fig. 5) were both titillating representations of manual exploration *and* analogies for sexual intercourse in a visceral sense.[83] In various languages, including English, quips and literature presented the finger or hand as penile, the woman's petticoat or skirt (placket) as vaginal.[84] Only a few years before the Somerset gang's special night out, in 1605–06 mocking advice was offered on the London stage in William Shakespeare's *King Lear*: "keep thy foot out of brothels, thy hand out of plackets" (3.4.97). From capital city to rural taverns, fictive theater or daily life, masculine gestures of initiation, possession and intrusion were normalized, if improper when thought excessive.

The visual display and manual manipulation of genitals occupied a great deal of libidinal energy in a pre-penetrative regime of contraceptive denial or interruption. Pulling up a woman's clothing, more than the untying of male

[83] On Beham's engraving see Giulia Bartrum, *German Renaissance prints 1490–1550* (London: British Museum Press, 1995), pp. 111–12. The woman's inscription reads "I want to do it too," the man's, "You are too disgusting." Whereas the sober woodsman refuses excess, the older woman is eager to join in.

[84] Henderson, *Maculate muse*, pp. 114–15, 247; Adams, *Latin sexual vocabulary*, p. 209; and for English words such as finger, hand, placket, tickle and touch see Partridge, *Shakespeare's bawdy*, pp. 105, 108, 118, 138–39, 161–62, 165, 201, 203; Rubinstein, *Shakespeare's sexual puns*, pp. 101, 120; Williams, *Dictionary*, pp. 484–86, 1048–51, 1388–90, 1407–08; Williams, *Glossary*, pp. 30, 124–25, 150–51, 237–38, 308, 311.

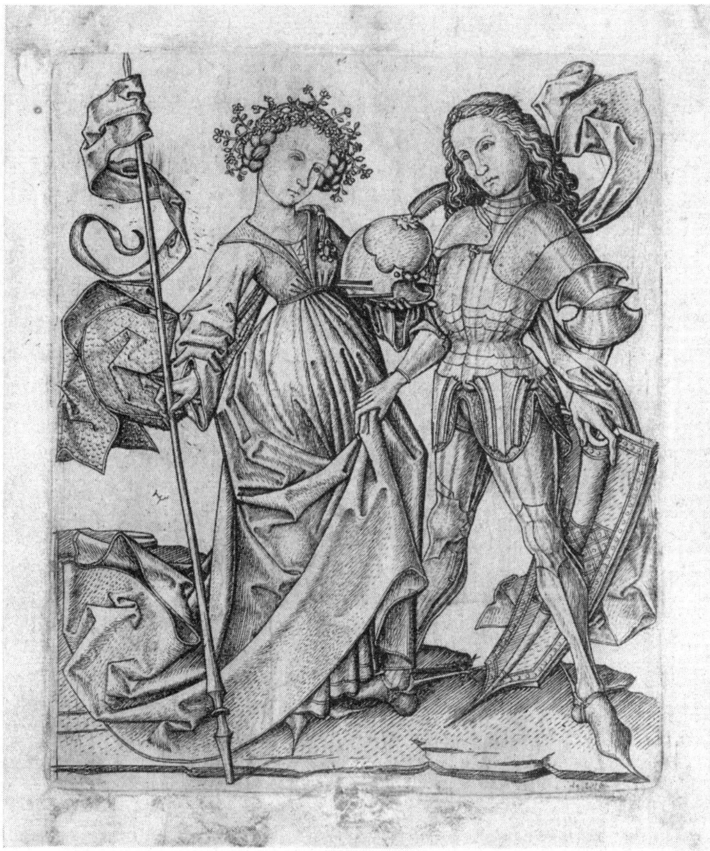

Figure 6 Master E.S., *Knight and lady*, 1460s, engraving, 137 (plate) × 114 mm, London, British Museum

breeches, signaled the commencement of genital contact. In both actual practice and in representational terms, an outer layer or veil is lifted and an active, initiating male member reaches beyond a barrier. Master E.S.'s engraving of the 1460s, depicting the seemingly genteel action of a young knight beginning to lift the outer garment of a besmitten, coy damsel thus takes on more erotically charged meaning (fig. 6).[85] She holds the helmet that is removed from his

[85] On the engraving, but not its eroticism see Alan Shestack, *Fifteenth century engravings of northern Europe from the National Gallery of Art, Washington DC* (Washington, DC: National Gallery of Art, 1967), no. 12.

"head" and delicately handles his symbolic lance, he fingers its target, the shield (a word used for a woman's genitals, and which is here suggestively furrowed) and inserts his penile foot beneath her garments. Future passion is foretold by the flurry of draperies flying from the downturned lance and out behind the knight.

The print also alludes to the erotic power of entering and plucking the flowery "rose" of virginity that was made famous in the conclusion of the medieval poetic epic the *Roman de la rose*. Other moments in the tale were illustrated with the penetration of architectural apertures, and the act of besieging or storming castles was a ubiquitous sexual metaphor (fig. 24).[86] Like jousts, the besieging of mock castles was a common entertainment during festive occasions like weddings, carnival or diplomatic receptions. Describing a married woman endlessly courted by suitors, Leon Battista Alberti used the metaphor of wooers "besieging her chastity like veteran soldiers," then portraying the husband vigorously repulsing "with manly strength the onslaughts of adversity," defending his possessions "with great industry, incredible diligence, immense labour, and countless vigils."[87] The wife's waywardness is presented in order to boost the husband's manly restraint and intelligence, and the literary construction of implied anxiety is obliterated by the successful defense of family honor. Secular romance had its complement, indeed probable origin, in Biblical exegesis. An erotic metaphor in the Song of Songs was illustrated with the lover thrusting his hand through a doorway, eagerly reaching in and penetrating her interior space.[88]

The Somerset men went on to borrow from the long-standing language and symbolism of courtly romance, having the key instigator name himself "knight of the castle." Laying down their "wicked rapiers" on a table, they made a homosocial oath together inviting anyone who "dareth to break down the walls of grimcunt castle." Disrespectful naming and mocking actions turned Edith's genitals into a metaphorical castle, rather like the fictive lady in the *Roman de la rose*, whose symbolic ramparts are finally breached at the end of many entertaining diversions and rising anticipation. However, the supposed restraint of chivalric codes did not avail Edith.

Firing up their passions, bonding together as an eroticized fraternity, and probably presuming they were rousing the woman too by means of manual contact, the men followed the model of the stages or "grades of love" advocated

86 For instance, Michael Camille, *The Gothic idol: ideology and image-making in medieval art* (Cambridge University Press, 1989), pp. 320–24; Camille, *Medieval art of love*, pp. 16, 87–93.

87 Leon Battista Alberti, *Dinner pieces: a translation of the "Intercenales,"* trans. David Marsh (Binghamton: Medieval and Renaissance Texts and Studies, 1987), pp. 141, 142.

88 Camille, *Medieval art of love*, fig. 8 (Bayeux Tapestry); Jeffrey Hamburger, *The visual and the visionary: art and female spirituality in late medieval Germany* (New York: Zone Books, 1998), pp. 409–10, figs. 8.4, 8.5.

by physicians and poets alike, graduating from tactile "foreplay" to more direct action.[89] Their final gesture was aggressive projection of beer at a woman's genitals. This act betrayed an understanding of a fundamental analogy for sexual intercourse first described in the influential Hippocratic treatise *On generation* from ancient Greece: "If, for example, you pour wine on a flame, first of all the flame flares up and increases for a short period when you pour the wine on, then it dies away. In the same way the woman's heat flares up in response to the man's sperm, and then dies away."[90] An orifice was not literally penetrated in Somerset but the final fluid moment of Hippocratic orgasm was blatantly performed. And the act was regarded as reprehensible, for the men were taken to court. They had enacted the mechanism of ejaculation, letting loose their symbolic, frothy fluid and at the same time dousing (with beer rather than wine) what they presumed was now a raging fire in the woman's nether region set ablaze by their fondling. One man acknowledged the nature of the intrusion and the sexual connotation of the thrown liquid by avowing that he was "the honest man in the company"; although groping her, he said he "would not break the walls of the castle but would drink a health unto it and so drunk up the glass of beer." Reiterating the metaphor of the castle showed him still a member of the homosocial gang; drinking the beer, symbolically, might have refused wasteful expenditure on a woman's body and made of him an "honest" man, but it did represent the imbibing of eroticized, masculine liquor. His lack of engagement with the woman's body, contrasted with his distinctive focus on masculine fluids and company, implies that his virtue was inflected with homoerotic commitment.

In another town, men also took their tossing of beer for an enactment of sex. They invaded a household where their activities included proclaiming that one woman, called "their bear [was] over heat, and must be cooled and therewith all threw a cup or glass of beer in her bare tail."[91] The medical model of dousing and temperature control led yet another group of Somerset villagers in 1650 to discipline a local woman, found in sexual concourse with a soldier, by throwing her in a stream, saying "if she was hot they would cool her."[92] So much was ejaculation valued alongside or even more than penetration, and so thoroughly was the inculcated model of sexual action about fluids, that two rowdy gangs were able to violate a woman by means of flung liquid. In such cases, physiological theory, literary metaphor, oral culture and physical practice are not easy to separate.

[89] John Baldwin, *The language of sex: five voices from northern France around 1200* (University of Chicago Press, 1994), pp. 161–69.

[90] *The Hippocratic treatises "On generation," "On the nature of the child," "Diseases IV,"* trans. and commentary Iain Lonie (Berlin: Walter de Gruyter, 1981), p. 2 (4.2).

[91] Quaife, *Wanton wenches*, p. 173.

[92] Ibid., p. 50; Gowing, *Common bodies*, p. 107.

Another act associated with excessive indulgence by men, the spurting, somewhat rhythmic ejections of vomiting, also had a sexual implication. Aristotelian notions of nutrients digested into vital spirit (that is, semen) informed a crude image of Pacifico Massimi's personified penis in homoerotic verse published in 1489: "you keep rising; you want to spew out (*vomeres*) your food."[93] Albertus Magnus had been explicit too, speaking first of ejaculation as pneumatic, then observing that "the situation is the same as in vomiting, which is caused by the force of what is vomited: the number of these spasms of vomiting corresponds to the number of climaxes experienced in coitus."[94] The eruptive purgations issuing from the mouths of over-indulgent male peasants in numerous early sixteenth-century prints by Nuremberg artists like Erhard Schön, Peter Flötner and the Beham brothers (fig. 5) probably alludes to that other kind of somatic ejaculation, as vomiting did in Massimi's Latin poem. In line with what German preachers and city councilors decried about behavior at local festivals and drunken gatherings, the printmakers show masculinity in its excessive, disruptive extreme. As summarized by Lyndal Roper, German moralists envisaged the male body as "a volcano of drives and fluids which constantly threaten to erupt, . . . through ejaculation, bloodshed, vomiting, defecation . . . Excessive eating and drinking led to an excess of semen, which had also then to run off."[95] Shameless gluttony and lust are thus coupled in Hans Sebald Beham's view of vomiting and illicit passion, yet the very display is visualized in the company of onlookers, an aging woman wanting some of the same and a woodsman rebuking the pig-like habits of the vomiting man. Social strictures are reinforced for those other onlookers, the viewers of the print, through humor, and medical notions about bodily release and sexual actions as projective more than penetrative are reinscribed.

Masculinity was a lived experience, behavioral and biological, defined in contexts and by others as well as selves. What most ties together the core features of masculinity is the capacity of projection, that is, to have external genitals (and beards) forced out by the male body's greater heat, to expel with some force the bodily fluids of urine and semen (and surrogates like beer or vomit), and to act in expansive, public, assertive and authoritative ways (including the ejaculatory rupture of lances or being on top of the sex partner). The

93 Pacifico Massimi, *Les cent élégies: Hecatelegium, Florence, 1489*, ed. and trans. Juliette Desjardins (Grenoble: Ellug, 1986), p. 346. I have used the English translation in James Wilhelm (ed.), *Gay and lesbian poetry* (New York: Garland, 1995), p. 299. For images see E. Bange, *Peter Flötner* (Leipzig: Klinkhardt & Biermann, 1926); Alison Stewart, *Before Bruegel: Sebald Beham and the origins of peasant festival imagery* (Aldershot: Ashgate, 2008); for words, Boggione and Casalegno, *Dizionario*, pp. 176, 347–48, 357 (*gettare* and *piumata*); Williams, *Dictionary*, pp. 1282–83 (spew).

94 Danielle Jacquart and Claude Thomasset, *Sexuality and medicine in the middle ages*, trans. Matthew Adamson (Cambridge: Polity Press, 1988), p. 79.

95 Roper, *Oedipus and the devil*, p. 112.

power of words, the influence of jokes, the allurement of poetry, the stirring rhythm of song, the efficacy of images and the ideological impact of medical theory and Church law, in tandem with social and kinetic experiences, together wove the fabric of male bodies into embodied, lived existence. It was material bodies as well as minds and wits that put knowledge to work, and that labor in turn forged further discourse, mediating, remaking, enhancing, augmenting, resisting it along the way.

2 The phallus: history and humor

Rethinking the relationship among masculinity, patriarchy and the male body necessitates a critical review of the history of the phallus as an artifact, term and symbol, especially in its psychoanalytic manifestation. To place the phallus in perspective, this chapter traces the vicissitudes of the phallus from use in antiquity to its current privilege as a Lacanian symbol of everything and nothing. The ancient image that was evident everywhere has developed into something not to be seen, the logocentric sign of patriarchal masculinity that must remain hidden and mysterious. In the Lacanian system it is also the impossible and non-existent object of desire. Ubiquitous in antiquity, it has become unattainable in modernity.

Taken during the Renaissance as one among many symbols of antiquity and its gods, the phallus swelled to universal proportions from the late eighteenth century as a syncretistic sign of all generativity, and thence it was later adopted by psychoanalysis as a somber, central emblem of the psyche. It was in premodern cultures an artifact more than an intellectual symbol, of talismanic, exuberant and even humorous use far more than remote majesty or hidden mystery. Its contingent, dependent nature makes it unsuitable as a bedrock on which to build a theory of masculinity.

Rather than continuing to afford the phallus either the authority of antiquity or the panreligious admiration of the late Enlightenment, this chapter especially points to its protective, humorous and celebratory functions. Word, object and effect, the phallus has its ups and downs, bobbing along in Greek processions, evoking awe or anxiety but having its funny side as well. The case of the disappearing phallus can never be solved, but clues point to its existence as a complex aggregate of elements and meanings.

The phallus as word, object and effect

The penile phallus has become the sign *par excellence* of masculinity, but phallus was an unfamiliar word for millennia and in early modern cultures the physical "sign" was more generic and inclusive. A telling range of words and images existed about male genitals, and these did not prioritize only one word or part. Thus, for instance, it was all the "membri genitali" of Benvenuto Cellini's life-size statue of *Jupiter* that were unveiled one night at Fontainebleau in January 1545.[1] Due to a dispute about court favor, the sculptor staged the insulting drama to belittle the French king's mistress Madame d'Étampes. The undifferentiated whole of male genitals was sometimes indicated by the semiotic word "segno" in Italian, the "segno de uomo" or "segno di maschio."[2] If a priority was assigned, the testicles often benefited, as they did in the case of the thirteenth-century French poetic epic *Roman de la rose* where the personification of Genius declared that men's "purse [scrota] and testicles" were "the signs (*signe*) that they are male."[3] To the extent that the "phallus" or core *segno* of masculinity was embedded in grammar and language, it was as much about a genital whole or just the testicles, as it was focused on the penis.

Phallos was the Greek word (φαλλοζ) for an object carried in procession, often by women or cross-dressed men, in celebration of Dionysus (god of wine, fertility and untamed excess). Usually made of wood, leather or clay, such artifacts do not survive; what remains are mainly phalli carved on stone herms, some small Greek pottery phalli and largely satirical images on drinking vessels.[4] Obscene humor, skits and dances in satyr costumes and eventually theatrical comedies were part of the religious festival of the Dionysia and, in general, phalli were often associated with the element of festive humor, put to comic use on stage and in vase paintings.[5] Testicles and glans were usually part of the *phallos*, in both two-dimensional representations and surviving three-dimensional examples, including the variety of male genital forms that served for amusement when holding fluids, such as perfume jars, oil flasks and

[1] Benvenuto Cellini, *Vita*, ed. Ettore Camesasca (Milan: Biblioteca Universale Rizzoli, 1985), p. 498; also, for example, Bandello, *Novelle*, vol. I, p. 487 ("tutti i membri miei"). Unless otherwise noted, I use Loeb editions and translations of ancient Greek and Latin texts.

[2] Sabadino degli Arienti, *Le Porretane*, ed. Bruno Basile (Rome: Salerno, 1981), p. 101 (first published 1483); Paolo Giovio, *Lettere*, ed. Giuseppe Guido Ferrero, 2 vols. (Rome: Istituto Poligrafico dello Stato, 1956–58), vol. II, pp. 38–39 (describing Vasari's covering of genitals in his fresco, *Paul III inspecting the rebuilding of St. Peter's* in 1546).

[3] Guillaume de Lorris and Jean de Meun, *Le roman de la rose*, ed. Félix Lecoy, 3 vols. (Paris: Honoré Champion, 1965), vol. I, lines 19637–38; Guillaune de Lorris and Jean de Meun, *The romance of the rose*, trans. Charles Dahlberg (Hanover: University Press of New England, 1986), p. 324.

[4] Early phallus vases (including perfume containers) and votives from Greek sites are noted in Anna Lemos, *Archaic pottery of Chios*, vol. I (Oxford: Oxford University Committee for Archaeology, 1991), pp. 24, 250.

[5] Herodotus, 2.48–49; Aristophanes, *Acharnians*, 243; Lucian, *De Syria Dea*, 16; Henderson, *Maculate muse*, pp. 112–13. A fragmentary list of stage props included "2 small phalluses": Jeffrey Rusten and I. C. Cunningham (eds. and trans.), *Theophrastus, 'Characters,' Herodas, 'Mimes,' Sophron and other mime fragments* (Cambridge, MA: Harvard University Press, 2002), pp. 420–21.

drinking cups.[6] Seeing and handling these objects generated and reinforced the important value of semen, even in the register of satire.

Frequent representations of the phallus as winged are confirmed by payment accounts from Delos after 200 BCE concerning the annual phallic procession by wagon of the object mounted on a little axle so that it could move.[7] While many were handheld, representations of the larger processional type tend to show it looking like a large log pulled on a cart or carried by a group of bearers (the phallic connotations of the May pole come to mind). On many occasions, a system of ropes or strings ensured that the *phallos* was a puppet, rising up and down in the parade, which would have accentuated the seasonal changes of the agricultural cycle but also provided a degree of levity, in both the literal and figurative senses.[8] Notably, the object had multiple connotations and uses but humor, festivity, agricultural abundance and protection are as much or more evident themes than the sole one of fertility, primarily human, that has more recently been ascribed to the phallus.

In the Roman empire, the object appeared everywhere, but the Latinized word *phallus* was rare, commonly replaced with *fascinum*, meaning fascination or enchantment. That latter word was used for protective, phallic amulets, for the exaggerated ithyphallic organ of Priapus (which was meant to avert threats from crops and gardens) and, occasionally, for shock value, it referred to human male genitals.[9] Although the artifact played some part in certain rituals, evidence about the apparently powerful moment of unveiling the supposedly mysterious object is relatively thin or late.[10] In antiquity the phallus was also a figure of amusement, and was not secretive but widely seen, from street signs to tableware, bath mosaics to bronze studs. Its very value as an object of apotropaic enchantment meant that it *had* to be seen.

Statues of well-endowed Priapus protected vineyards and gardens, forestalled envy and played a countervailing role in cult life. According to the first-century BCE Greek historian Diodorus Siculus, "in the sacred rites, not only of

6 Jean Ducat, *Les vases plastiques Rhodiens archaïques en terre cuite* (Paris: Éditions E. de Boccard, 1966), pp. 146–48, 158, Pl. XXII nos. 1–3; John Boardman, "A curious eye cup," *Archäologischer Anzeiger* 3 (1976), 281–90; Martin Kilmer, *Greek erotica on Attic red-figure vases* (London: Duckworth, 1993), pp. 87 n. 17, 192 n. 3.

7 Susan Guettel Cole, "Procession and celebration at the Dionysia," in Ruth Scodel (ed.), *Theater and society in the classical world* (Ann Arbor: University of Michigan Press, 1993), pp. 30–31.

8 Eric Csapo, "Riding the phallus for Dionysus: iconology, ritual, and gender-role de/construction," *Phoenix* 51 (1997), 253–95; Cole, "Procession and celebration," 25–38.

9 Adams, *Latin sexual vocabulary*, pp. 63–64, to which can be added Pliny, *Natural history* (NH), 19.19.50; *Priapea*, 83.8. The word was also used for a dildo (Petronius, 138.1) and for a prop in mimes (by the denigrating, Christian apologist Arnobius of Sicca, *Adversus Nationes*, 7.33.5).

10 Jacques Lacan, "The significance of the phallus," in Jacques Lacan, *Écrits: a selection*, trans. Alan Sheridan (London: Tavistock, 1977), p. 288, cites a scene in the Villa of the Mysteries in Pompeii, excavated in 1909, but the interpretation of a strange shape with a flat top as a phallus is dubious. I believe it is an altar table.

Dionysus but of practically all other gods as well, this god [Priapus] receives honor to some extent, being introduced in the sacrifices to the accompaniment of laughter and sport" (4.6.4). Laughter was preventive medicine as it were, prophylactic, dissipating melancholy and warding off ill will. Phallic amulets were displayed, especially by children, to protect wearers from malice, even from fathers or other relatives, according to Plutarch (d. 120), who explained that the charms worked through novelty and shock: "the strange look of [amulets] attracts the gaze, so that it [the Evil Eye] exerts less pressure upon its victim."[11] The unsettling yet fascinating appearance of the amulets was, I think, probably due to what Greeks and Romans would have considered their stark, ugly nature, stripped of the foreskin and exposed to view, made amusing by this combination of incongruous obscenity and deformity.[12] Another means of visual distraction was the common addition of eyes on either side of the glans, a motif apparently added for luck and safety as well as indicating the apotropaic function of the *phallos* against the Evil Eye.[13] To stop all sorts of harmful emanations, wind chimes were usually in phallic form, humorously hybrid, extravagant and animated (fig. 7). Literally oscillating in Roman mobiles, akin to phallic Greek puppets moving up and down, or phallic tongues floating in terracotta bird feeders, the phallus was both somber and amusing.

One of the few uses of the Latin word *phallus* in the ancient Roman world focused on a purely sexual, non-reproductive function. If a damaged graffito in Pompeii has been read correctly, its Latin writer understood the transliterated foreign word to mean penis: "Crescens' member (*Phallus*) is hard – and enormous," and the brag is witty because the name puns on enlargement (*crescare* meaning to grow).[14] The author was associating human flesh with the durability and scale of stony phalli, saying nothing about its capacity to father offspring. His raunchy tone echoes that of other ancient writers, including Aristophanes, the fifth-century BCE Greek writer of comedies, and the first-century CE Roman satirist Martial, as well as the sometimes excessive, explicit or parodic tone of imagery.

[11] Plutarch, *Quaestiones convivales*, 5.7.4. On emanations, see 5.7.2. On amulets, see also Pliny, *NH*, 28.7.39, and Varro, *De lingua Latina*, 7.97 (who noted that they were worn by boys); Adams, *Latin sexual vocabulary*, p. 63; Catherine Johns, *Sex or symbol? Erotic images of Greece and Rome* (London: British Museum Publications, 1982), pp. 62, 63–64, 73–74, 143–44, figs. 55–57, Pl. 10; Stefano De Caro, *Il Gabinetto Segreto del Museo Archeologico Nazionale di Napoli* (Naples: Electa, 2000), pp. 72, 74–75, 80, 86, with illustrations.

[12] See n. 32 below.

[13] On apotropea and the Evil Eye, see Johns, *Sex or Symbol?*, pp. 66–67; John R. Clarke, *Looking at laughter: humor, power, and transgression in Roman visual culture, 100 B.C.–A.D. 250* (Berkeley: University of California Press, 2007), pp. 19, 63–81, with further references.

[14] Adams, *Latin sexual vocabulary*, pp. 64, 228; Antonio Varone, *Erotica Pompeiana: love inscriptions on the walls of pompei*, trans. Ria P. Berg, David Harwood and Roger Ling (Rome: "L'Erma" di Bretschneider, 2002), pp. 87–88.

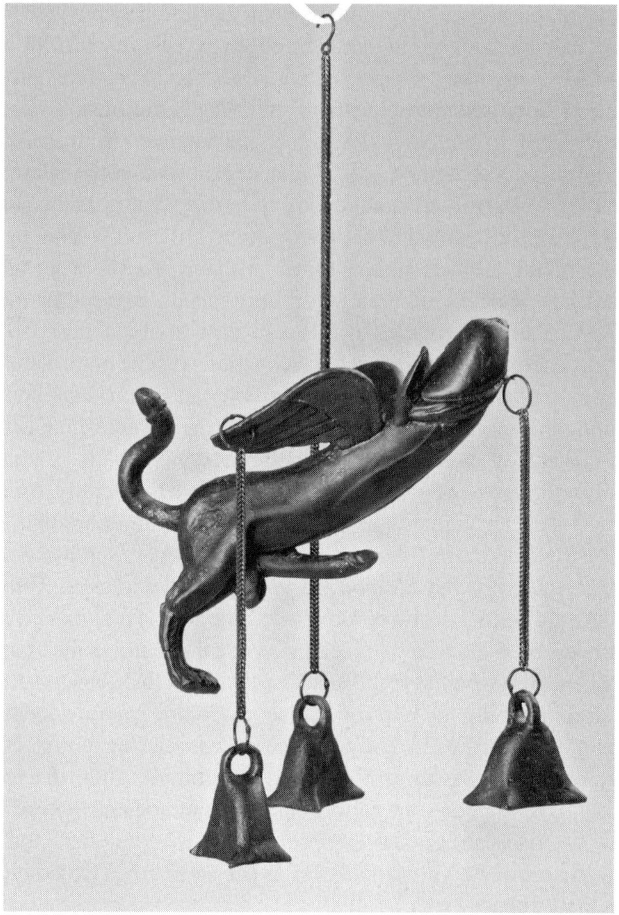

Figure 7 Roman, Tintinnabulum, *c.* first century CE, bronze, Trier, Rheinisches Landesmuseum

Yet, until the last few decades, the humorous role of the phallus has been underplayed, despite Diodorus' report of laughter. Aristotle believed that the very genre of comedy began with "the leaders of the phallic songs" accompanying processions of the sort exuberantly satirized in the previous century by Aristophanes' *Acharnians*, first performed on the Athenian stage in the year 425 BCE during the Dionysian festival.[15] Laughter itself was apotropaic, dispelling

[15] Aristotle, *Poetics*, 1449a11; Aristophanes, *Acharnians*, 241–79.

the Evil Eye; hence one vertical phallus carved on the wall plaque for a bakery in Pompeii merrily declared of the establishment that "here dwells happiness."[16] Danger from the ovens was averted, productivity encouraged, the suggestive rising and hence enlargement of dough – as well as the business enterprise – assured.

Befitting the marginalization of the idolatrous object in the Christian world (on stone capitals, graffiti, manuscript margins and badges, figs. 10–13, for instance), the rare Latin word *phallus* was adapted relatively late in vernacular languages. Even then it was only intermittently cited, as a foreign term referring to artifacts from the past. The first English appearance I am aware of occurred in a translation of Plutarch's essays published in 1603.[17] Italians adopted the habit of their Latin ancestry, paying the word scant attention. The earliest Italian use (*fallo*) is usually said to be 1728, but in 1554 a scholar aware of the Greek tradition cited *Fallon* as an ancient word for the object of Bacchic festivals.[18] Again it is a self-conscious importation, *Phallo*, in Vincenzo Cartari's iconographic manual of 1556, ostensibly written for artists.[19] It was correctly used for a processional object, *la figura del membo virile*, "the figure of the virile member," made of fig wood or red leather, though amulets were included in the woodcut illustration of 1647. The ithyphallic but veiled deities Priapus and Oro were illustrated, but their bodies were said to display the politely termed "membro" or, in the former's case *la insegna virile grande*, the great sign of virility. That the 1581 Latin edition has *Psallum* shows that it was not a familiar term. Instead, *priapus* was in many cases the substitute word for male genitals, used by Latin authors including the humanist Poggio Bracciolini in his joke book of the mid-fifteenth century. Emerging late as a word in the vernaculars, and referring to an ancient artifact rather than a contemporary symbol of corporeal body parts, the "phallus" was arcane and obscure for millennia after the Romans, occasionally entering discourse as an archaeological artifact or appearing in visual imagery as apotropaic, shocking and amusing.

Christian morality sidelined the pagan phallus. Roman rites devoted to Liber, deity of "liquid seeds . . . but also the seeds of animals," that is, semen, were particularly offensive to Bishop Augustine.[20] His early fifth-century *City of God* excoriated the "obscene license" with which the "pudenda virilim" were

16 Clarke, *Laughter*, pp. 72–73. Blacksmiths placed the *fascina* near their forges according to Pollux, *Onomasticon*, 8.118.

17 Plutarch, *The philosophie, commonlie called, the morals* . . . trans Philemon Holland (London: Arnold Hatfield, 1603), pp. 214 (*De cupiditate divitiarum*, 527d), 1294 (*De Iside et Osiride*, 358b, Isis' invention of the phallus).

18 Giambattista Giraldi Cintio, "Sopra il comporre le satire atte alle scene," in *Scritti estetici*, vol. II (Milan: Daelli, 1864), p. 131.

19 Vincenzo Cartari, *Imagini de i dei de gli antichi* (Venice: Presso Francesco Ziletti, 1580), p. 442.

20 Augustine, *City of God*, pp. 278–79.

publicly processed and then crowned by a matron in open view, to "ensure successful germination of seeds" and foil evil spells against the fields. Notably, the inclusion of testicles at the base of most representations of ancient phalli indicates that the generative component of the phallus necessarily entailed more than the shaft, just as Augustine's reference to Liber indicated. He also sarcastically reported that a "newly wedded bride used to be told to sit on [Priapus'] phallus (*fascinum*), that monstrous obscenity, following the most honorable and most religious custom of Roman matrons."[21]

Freud's sole citation of Augustine was to this latter passage, via a secondary source, in his paper on "The taboo of virginity" first published in 1918. There, the phallus was a symbolic example of the "father-surrogates entrusted with defloration," more often "an elder, priest or holy man" who performed "the privilege of the patriarch."[22] Constructing a woman's libido as focused on her father until she "matured" by directing desire toward having a male child instead, Freud regarded the priapic episode as one example of a universal practice, cited alongside folk custom and the Indian lingam. In this passage, Freud's sense of the phallus as more than a physical object or a mere representation of the penis is particularly clear, for it symbolically marks the assertion of patriarchal power while also physically performing the rite of passage of defloration. Meanwhile, Augustine's outrage did much to reinforce millennia of moral shame and official secrecy about the public sight of male genitals, of the repressive sort that Freud first defined and then began to overcome through his talking cure.

Alongside the titillating image of patriarchal defloration, the phallus came to be almost exclusively linked to fertility. Hence the OED first defines *phallus* as "an image of the male generative organ, symbolizing the generative power in nature," then associates it with religious veneration, especially the Dionysia. This shift from ritual prop mimicking male genitals described in the first English translations, to a symbol of generation that echoed a single, all-encompassing genital organ marks an emphasis which also occurs in Liddell and Scott's famous Greek lexicon and the Oxford classical dictionary.[23]

None of these reference works cites the illustrated, controversial book that nevertheless had a fundamental impact on the conceptualization of the phallus, two essays printed together in 1786: Sir William Hamilton's short *Account of the remains of the worship of Priapus* (written in 1781 by the British envoy to

21 Ibid., p. 246, also p. 285.

22 Sigmund Freud, "The taboo of virginity," in *Standard edition*, vol. XI (1957), p. 203.

23 H. G. Liddell and R. Scott, *Greek–English lexicon* (Oxford: Clarendon Press, 1996), p. 1914 (the first edition was published in 1843, the edition cited here is the ninth, of 1940); Herbert Jennings Rose, "Phallus," in *The Oxford classical dictionary* (Oxford: Clarendon Press, 1949), p. 674 (unchanged in the 2nd edn. of 1970).

Naples) and Richard Payne Knight's *A discourse on the worship of Priapus*.[24] Discussing material newly unearthed from ancient sites or contemporary wax votives in the shape of male genitals (again, with testicles) offered at a Catholic church in southern Italy, the antiquarians focused on Priapus. But the study also drew on examples like the Indian lingam and thence generalized about cultural and so-called "primitive" practices, divining deep allegorical significance and universal awe about the male organ.

James George Frazer's broad-ranging *Golden bough: a study in magic and religion*, first published in 1890 and enlarged considerably thereafter, took the comparativist approach further and thus, although genitals were not central to the argument, was even more important for establishing fertility as the paradigmatic purpose of a cult object like the phallus. Only very recently have modern gendered assumptions about the centrality of fertility begun to fade. Crucially, N. J. Lowe has pointed out that much of it rests on a single, problematic Greek document.[25]

The revised version of the Oxford classical dictionary issued in 1996 listed five rather than two contexts for the phallus, going beyond fertility rituals and permanent display on statues of Priapus or herms marking boundaries.[26] In particular, the comic element was recognized, as was the apotropaic effect of the phallus, capable of protecting infants and also averting various ill wishes from adults. The dictionary's overall conclusion is that the ancient phallus was "an expression of fertility and regeneration, but also of masculine strength," to which I would add the entertaining, healing and protective function of humor. Amusement and erotic bravura characterize medieval and early modern depictions of male genitalia too, which rarely seem focused on generation unless illustrated in an anatomical text. In linguistic presence and material reality, the phallus was neither invariable nor universal and it had multiple functions.

[24] The work is reprinted as *Sexual symbolism: a history of phallic worship* (New York: Julian Press, 1957), together with Thomas Wright's *The worship of the generative powers* (1866). On the eighteenth-century essays and the votives see Giancarlo Carabelli, *In the image of Priapus* (London: Duckworth, 1996); Ian Jenkins and Kim Sloan, *Vases & volcanoes: Sir William Hamilton and his collection* (London: British Museum Press, 1996), pp. 238–39.

[25] N. J. Lowe, "Thesmophoria and Haloa: myth, physics and mysteries," in Sue Blundell and Margaret Williamson (eds.), *The sacred and the feminine in ancient Greece* (New York: Routledge, 1998), pp. 149–73, which also offers a critique of the outmoded catch-all "fertility," and the single Greek textual source over-used in relation to such claims. It points out that the "daring new paradigm" which argued that "*all* religion was really about fertility magic" began to emerge in 1870 with the publication of Wilhelm Mannhardt's *Die Korndämonen* (pp. 151, 153).

[26] Richard A. S. Seaford, "Phallus," in Simon Hornblower and Antony Spawforth (eds.), *The Oxford classical dictionary* (Oxford University Press, 1996), p. 1153. The entry is unchanged in the 3rd edn., revised (2003). Citations are summarized but few conclusions drawn in Hubert Cancik and Helmuth Schneider (eds.), *Der neue Pauly: Enzyklopädie der Antike*, vol. IX (Stuttgart: J. B. Metzler, 2000), cols. 729–30.

The funny phallus

Scholars have exaggerated the somber persona of the phallus, yet humor and satire clearly regarded the ancient Greek *phallos* in less than awestruck terms. Irreverent fun was poked on stage, and somatic pleasures of food, wine and bawdiness characterized quite a few Greek rituals and festivities. Surviving paintings on wine vessels display the phallus for enjoyment during the convivial drinking party (symposium), at which elite men were entertained by male and female dancers, musicians and courtesans (*hetairai*). Amusing views of different kinds of phallic representations are presented on an early to mid-fifth-century BCE red-figure krater, used to mix wine with water at such parties. One side depicts a naked woman hurrying along with a large phallus under her arm (fig. 8). Attributed to the Pan Painter of Athens, the image has been associated with the December festival of Haloa, a woman's festival in honor of Demeter and Dionysus, especially observed by *hetairai*. Thereby, scholars linked the naked woman holding a phallus with an agrarian festival about fertility of the fields and vineyards. However, Matthew Dillon has recently

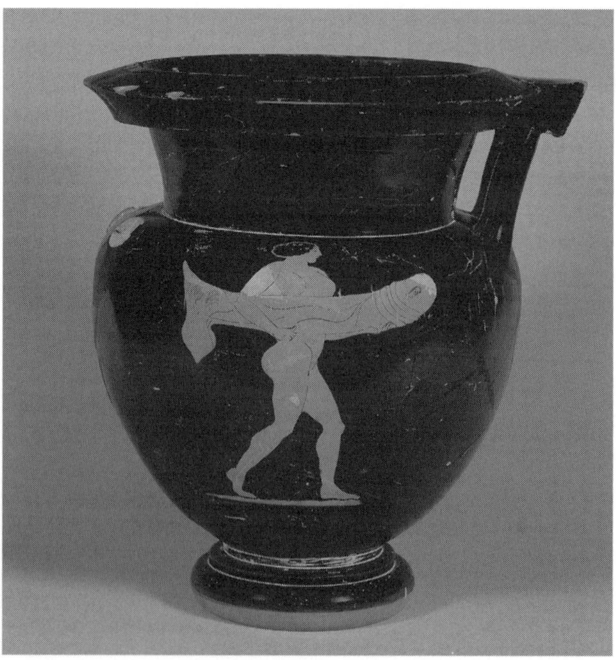

Figure 8 Pan Painter, *Woman carrying a large phallus*, Attic red-figure krater, side B, *c.* 470 BCE, Berlin, Staatliche Museen

pointed out that, although models and representations in dough of both male and female genitals were present at the Haloa (as they were at certain other rites too), "giant phalloi are not heard of in connection with this festival."[27]

The link first perceived in 1932 between the depicted phallus and female debauchery at a festival assumed that the painting was mere reportage. Belief in the transparency and deadpan nature of the image was also informed by the supposition that all women, even sex workers, were naturally desirous of the phallus. Going to the opposite extreme in 1985, but offering a valuable corrective regarding "sexual politics in ancient Athens," Eva Keuls believed the scene was "a caricature of a Dionysiac ritual in which women acted out phallic aggression against the male."[28] However, situating the image as either documentary reality or misogynist caricature in each polarized case conceptualizes the phallus as a detached object seen by artist and audience as exclusively, voraciously desired by women.

It is worth turning the issue over, literally, in that the krater has another side (fig. 9). There a cloaked youth hails an ithyphallic herm. Only related to the Haloa if that festival is misread as entirely about worship of the phallus (and also misreading herms as only about the *phallos*), the scene otherwise has attracted little comment. It contrasts a beardless youth with a bearded elder, but if it is understood to be an incidental view of ritual, as the other side once was believed to be, then the rite is not clear, nor is its relevance to symposia and wine drinking. Humor, rather, is the tone on both sides of the vessel, I suggest, and the phalli compel comparison.[29] Paintings on different facets of a pot sometimes present a connected narrative; if so here, the determined woman and her phallic projectile are about to collide with the youth's rear. The scale of the phallus is so large, however, that any homoerotic implication is deliberately rendered comic and ludicrous. If aggression is the story line, sheer hilarity is the denouement, so disproportionate is the woman's "weapon." She strides along, momentum stressed by the perky phallus, whereas on the other side movement comes to an emphatic halt, signaled by the clear, simple outline of the herm's back.

The youth's clasped stick rises up from the groin in answer to the herm's own. The delicacy of the handled item befits the ideal of Greek male genitals, having a "well-proportioned, sleek, tapered, protective, beautifying, and

27 Matthew Dillon, *Girls and women in classical Greek religion* (New York: Routledge, 2003), pp. 122–23. For the most important source on the Haloa, see Lowe, "Thesmophoria and Haloa," pp. 149–73. The older literature all depends on Ludwig Deubner, *Attische Feste* (Berlin: Verlag Heinrich Keller, 1932), pp. 60–69.

28 Eva Keuls, *The reign of the phallus: sexual politics in ancient Athens* (New York: Harper & Row, 1985), p. 371, not too different from saying that it is "a parody of the prostitute's substitute," that is, a dildo: Dillon, *Girls and women*, p. 124.

29 Alexandre Mitchell, *Greek vase-painting and the origins of visual humour* (Cambridge University Press, 2009), p. 79, makes a brief comment on side B only. For Greek obscene, ridiculing humor, see Henderson, *Maculate muse*, pp. 1–29.

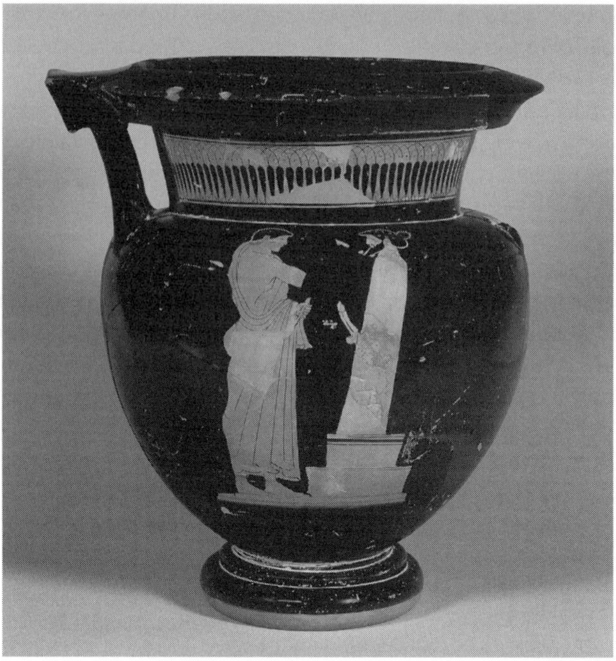

Figure 9 Pan Painter, *Youth standing before a herm*, Attic red-figure krater, side A, *c.* 470 BCE, Berlin, Staatliche Museen

propriety-preserving" foreskin.[30] The Pan Painter contrasts this metaphorical ideal with the adult, thick but still hooded shaft of the herm.[31] The youth's long "rod" only foreshadows adulthood, emerging from a coy body, so this "phallic symbol" is about modesty and potential rather than achieved authority. His desire is in check; hers, on the boil. Further, the adult organ of the herm is far too large to suit the Athenian ideal; this is a priapic herm, not an actual elder, and there is satire at work. The phallus on the other side of the krater has a retracted foreskin and the glaringly exposed glans signified to the audience ugly indecency, of the sort that characterized the genitals of bestial satyrs, barbarians (i.e.,

[30] Frederick Mansfield Hodges, "The ideal prepuce in ancient Greece and Rome: male genital aesthetics and their relation to *lipodermos*, circumcision, foreskin restoration, and the *kynodesme*," *Bulletin of the History of Medicine* 75 (2001), 405.

[31] On the idealized male genitals, with a small penis (often tied up with a leather thong, or infibulated with a clasp), ordinary scrotum and long prepuce, see K. J. Dover, *Greek homosexuality*, updated edn. (Cambridge, MA: Harvard University Press, 1989), pp. 124–35; Henderson, *Maculate muse*, p. 111 n. 17; Timothy McNiven, "The unheroic penis: otherness exposed," *Source* 15 no. 1 (1995), 10–16; Hodges, "Ideal prepuce," 375–405.

non-Greeks) and slaves.[32] Huge, unsightly, crude, it would have provoked laughter, as did other objects or people considered deformed by the standards of Graeco-Roman culture.[33]

Comedy, said Aristotle in the following century, was about imitating inferior, base or ugly characters, and "the ludicrous (*geloios*) is a species of the ugly (*aischros*)," alternatively translated as shameful.[34] Cicero later defined the province of the laughable as the "unseemly or ugly," including actual "deformity and physical defects."[35] Naked in public, the Pan Painter's woman is base and shameful; the phallus is amusingly ridiculous. In other words, both the female figure and the phallus are funny. Rounded shapes like breasts, glans, calves, backside and testicles resemble each other in form and firmness; the line of her mouth echoes those of the rolled back foreskin; the companions are smiling together, coupled in an embrace as though the phallus is a pet tucked under her arm as they briskly move along, joined in their single-eyed devotion to the cause of motion. This is a parody, so exaggerated that *hetairai* and other female entertainers would have laughed as well, in the context of a thoroughly phallocentric patriarchy.

The herm's general purpose was about stopping a person, declaring a boundary and protecting it with ithyphallic potency.[36] The four-cornered herm on the vase marks a crossroads, and the youth's raised hand properly acknowledges the boundary and territorial authority signified by the erect phallus. The youth is being incorporated into the body politic of patriarchal phallicism; she as a woman simply can never be.[37] He is charmingly coy, willingly learning about manly discipline. She is hilariously impertinent, self-indulgent and oblivious. The contrasted traits of control and excess were debated at the time in relation to different kinds of masculinity, and it is possible that the female figure is as much a personification as an exemplar of a woman's avid desire. She is a virtual allegory of over-eager motion, contrasted with the obedient halt depicted on the other side. In an ironic vein, one learns that moderation is best, that neither the

[32] Since the prepuce is rolled back rather than removed, the phallus is not circumcised, shockingly immodest to the Greeks, and to the Romans, to whom circumcision was disfigurement, even criminal: Hodges, "Ideal prepuce," 375–405.

[33] Robert Garland, "The mockery of the deformed and disabled in Graeco-Roman culture," in Siegfried Jäkel and Asko Timonen (eds.), *Laughter down the centuries*, vol. I (Turku: Turun Yliopisto, 1994), pp. 71–84; Clarke, *Laughter*, pp. 65–67 and passim.

[34] Aristotle, *Poetics*, 1449a33–34 (translation adjusted). *Aischros* can also be translated as shameful or dishonorable, *geloios* as ridiculous or amusing. For an example of laughter at burlesque, grotesque mimicry, see Xenophon, *Symposium*, 2.21–23.

[35] Cicero, *De oratore*, 2.236, 239 (my translation).

[36] On herms see Walter Burkert, *Structure and history in Greek mythology and ritual* (Berkeley: University of California Press, 1982), pp. 39–41; Robin Osborne, "The erection and mutilation of the hermae," *Proceedings of the Cambridge Philological Society* 23 (1985), 47–73.

[37] On the politics, though not this vase, see John Winkler, "Phallos politikos: representing the body politic in Athens," *Differences* 2 (1990), 29–45, esp. 35–36 on herms.

mixing of water and wine that takes place in the vessel nor the subsequent drinking (and, sometimes, sexual activity) should go to extremes.

On the other hand, while hilarious excess is depicted on one side, ideal control is not entirely the theme of the other, for the obedient youth is slightly mocked. His sign of phallic authority is too covered by cloth in the case of his actual genitals, too veiled by metaphor in the case of the stick. All the visible phalli on the vase are props, simulacra affirming, as Lacan would say much later, that the actual phallus does not exist. The painter appears to foreshadow Butler's insight about the "fundamental transferability" of phallic property, yet on the vase it takes place amongst secondary players.[38] Regulatory mechanisms like law (the herm) and laughter (the woman's pet) ensure that the phallic polity is maintained. The wit is that the phallus can precisely be shown in a variety of ways, and has a range of meanings, none of which betrays the partying symposiasts as filled with veneration, inner vulnerability or anxiety.

The angst of the phallus

In modern times, popularized psychoanalysis has brought the word "phallus" into common parlance; images, especially in advertising, are easily understood as phallic symbols, which are often humorous. In more theoretical terms, however, the phallus preoccupies psychoanalysis, much literary analysis and some historical interpretation, as an object of solemn grandeur, mystery and loss. Gloriously overt in a far distant past, then hidden and shameful under religious and State controls, the phallus was about the loss of innocence and the institutionalization of a patriarchal order of power and privilege in which not all men were equal and women were excluded due to their fundamental lack. Despite being complex and unresolved, the relationship between male bodies and this sign of a man's body part is elemental to the theory. Castration is a psychic trauma with explanatory potency, and physical vagaries of variability, susceptibility and impermanent erections are contrasted with the idealized, forever stable, coherent and univocal phallus that staves off otherwise ever-present vulnerability and anxiety. Yet, even in psychoanalysis the phallus does not have a fixed or stable meaning, though it is clearly about masculinity and power.[39]

Freud, "father" of psychoanalysis, used the word *phallus* relatively sparingly except as an adjective, despite the fact that it is today considered an essential

[38] Butler, *Bodies that matter*, p. 62.

[39] For the subsuming of the feminine and androgynous under the masculine, see the incisive comments of Daniel Boyarin, "Who wrote the dominant fiction? On the history of the early phallus," in Mieke Bal et al. (eds.), *Brief: intellectual traditions in movement* (Amsterdam: Amsterdam School for Cultural Analysis, Theory and Interpretation, 1998), pp. 41–83.

noun in psychoanalysis. He came to it as an object through his interest in ancient cultures, and many times that is what it remained in Freud's work, an artifact from antiquity, as it was in those rare early modern notices too. In his corpus the word in its various forms (including *phallisch-genitalen* and *Phallusprimats*) occurred less than half as much as "penis."[40] It first appeared in his study of Leonardo da Vinci (1910), referring to an attribute of an Egyptian mother-goddess, which denoted "the primal creative force of nature," just as Knight and others had believed in the late eighteenth century.[41] Later that decade, dreams contained a "phallic theme" or "phallic symbol," and the phallus was the tool used in antiquity to deflower a virgin (following Augustine).[42] During the 1920s, it was something far more important to the structuring of the psyche, becoming the primary element in the "infantile genital organization" of each sex.[43] Thereafter, the "phase of phallic primacy" was central to Freudian psychoanalysis, closely related to the Oedipus complex when children first fixate on the mother but then realize the traumatic fact of genital difference, girls wanting the phallus they cannot have, boys competing with the father who they think owns one, while adults understand that no one is able to possess the symbolic phallus.[44]

Psychoanalysis witnessed a fundamental, philosophical shift in the second half of the twentieth century, especially driven by the influence of Lacan, whose paper on "the signification of the phallus" was first delivered as a lecture in 1958. Whereas Freud wrote about a subconscious or unconscious level of significance attached to body parts, Lacan disembodied the psyche by situating it in the linguistic and symbolic rather than corporeal arena. The symbolic valence of the phallus and phallic power was linked with patriarchy and language (logos) more than copulation, and thence words like "phallocentric" and "phallologocentric" became common in late twentieth-century literary and cultural theory. To Lacan, the very formation of subjectivity was grounded in language; neither language nor the unconscious had any solid foundation (such

40 Samuel Guttman et al. (eds.), *Konkordanz zu den 'Gesammelten Werken' von Sigmund Freud*, vol. IV (Waterloo, Ontario: North Waterloo Academic Press, 1995), pp. xxxiii, 4098–101, 4135–36: used 90 times compared to 220 uses of *penis*, plus numerous variants including *Penissymbol*. See also J. Laplanche and J.-B. Pontalis, *The language of psycho-analysis*, trans. Donald Nicholson-Smith (New York: W. W. Norton, 1973), pp. 302–04, 312–14.

41 "Leonardo da Vinci and a memory of his childhood," in *Standard edition*, vol. XI (1957), pp. 94, 125. Although the *Konkordanz*, vol. IV, pp. 4135–36, lists seemingly earlier appearances, those citations were added in later editions and Freud's primary reference in most cases is to his 1920s work on the "phallic stage."

42 Sigmund Freud, "The interpretation of dreams," in *Standard edition*, vol. IV (1953), p. 375 (a passage added in 1914).

43 Sigmund Freud, "The infantile genital organization (an interpolation into the theory of sexuality)" (1923), in *Standard edition*, vol. XIX (1961), pp. 142, 144.

44 For example, "The dissolution of the Oedipus complex" (1924), in *Standard edition*, vol. XIX (1961), pp. 174–75, 177–78.

as referent or identity) to which it referred, and the phallus in particular was non-existent, yet it governed the structure of language because all desire was directed toward it. Desire was constructed through endless articulation and representation but never satiated, always trying to substitute for loss (of the mother's idealized love), forever engaged in an endless cycle of searching for itself. The phallus was both the cause of alienation and desire, and the end point of desire, standing for presence and for absence at once.

The Lacanian phallus marks sexual difference, but through the symbolic rather than somatic register. Sexual relations revolve around being or having the phallus.[45] Men have a cultural subjectivity because of it; they "have" the symbolic phallus because it is ascribed to them. In a problematic and hetero-centric conflation, women "be" the phallus because it is supposedly the object of all masculine desire.[46] The phallus is ineffable and non-material to Lacan, not only because he tries to avoid its connection to a body part but also because it has to stand for too much. He tries to slip it between meaning and meaninglessness, envisaging the phallus as the pivot between the two.

Psychoanalysis helps most in the understanding of repression, compulsion, trauma and personal anxiety, and an understanding of the psychic elements of individual subjectivity is currently impossible without the lens and vocabulary of psychoanalysis. Indeed, the very rise of modern subjectivity is historically imbricated with the formation and growth of psychoanalysis, alongside medical research into psychosomatics. But often the hermeneutic is almost tautological, the politics skewed in support of patriarchy, and the tone bleak. As one critic has wryly observed, Freud's work on *Jokes and their relation to the unconscious* (1905) is "one of the unfunniest jestbooks ever written."[47] In the end, I would agree with the assessment of philosopher Jacques Derrida, who pointed to the androcentric and idealized nature of the Lacanian phallus and its impossible "phallogocentristic transcendentalism."[48] What might be gaps in logic and the effects of Lacan's gnomic utterances contributes to the sense that the Lacanian phallus is about loss, about what never was or can be. Given Lacan's influence, the psychoanalytic import of the word "phallus" has come to stand for the impossible dream, the melancholic lack of fulfillment.

45 Lacan, "Significance of the phallus," p. 289. Lacan was influenced by mistranslations into French of Freud's "penis" as "phallus": David Macey, "Phallus: definitions," in Elizabeth Wright (ed.), *Feminism and psychoanalysis: a critical dictionary* (Cambridge, MA: Blackwell, 1992), p. 319.

46 The stereotypical "femme fatale" who supposedly has real power because she seduces hapless men is too evident. So too is the habit of using the empty female sign upon which to write allegorical meaning.

47 Pamela Allen Brown, "Jesting rights: women players in the manuscript jestbook of Sir Nicholas Le Strange," in P. A. Brown and Peter Parolin (eds.), *Women players in England, 1500–1600: beyond the all-male stage* (Aldershot: Ashgate, 2005), p. 308.

48 Jacques Derrida, "The purveyor of truth," *Yale French Studies* 52 (1975), 31–113, esp. 81ff.

Psychoanalysis was founded on the sense that it was rebellious, addressing the taboo, uncovering the hidden unconscious, remembering a long-ago mythic past of phallic overtness. It is presented as the unveiler of both the unconscious and the phallus. To justify his enterprise, Freud – a consummate bourgeois patriarch – proposed a nostalgic view of history and of repression, writing in 1910, that:

> the genitals have been for us the '*pudenda*', objects of shame, and even (as a result of further successful sexual repression) of disgust. ... It is only with reluctance that the majority of those alive to-day obey the command to propagate their kind ... What is to be found among us in the way of another view of sexual life is confined to the uncultivated lower strata of society; among the higher and more refined classes it is concealed ... In the primaeval days of the human race ... the genitals were the pride and hope of living beings; they were worshipped as gods and transmitted the divine nature of their functions to all newly learned human activities ... At the time when the connection between official religions and sexual activity was already hidden from the general consciousness, secret cults devoted themselves to keeping it alive among a number of initiates.[49]

Freud's grand sweep through history proposed that pride became disgust when State religion introduced repressive (but necessary) civilization. Only "secret cults" – like those classes beneath Freud's own who kept alive an "exhausted remnant" of "primitive forms of genital worship" – stood out against the State and against repressive standards of shame.

Nostalgia for some lost innocence evident in a "primitive," universal religion that worshiped the phallus characterized Freud's sole cited source as well (Knight). Psychoanalysis follows the cultural precepts appropriate to the class and gender of these men. The influential treatise *On love* written by the twelfth-century cleric Andreas Capellanus had already opined for the sake of his courtly readers that peasants were incapable of love, being too bestial for its refinements.[50] Lacan's "phallic *jouissance*" was conceptualized in disgusted, dismissive terms as transient, orgasmic satisfaction: "What is it? – other than this, sufficiently stressed by the importance of masturbation in our practice, the *jouissance* of the idiot."[51] Freud's distaste (and envy?) regarding the lower classes is in Lacan voiced as intellectual superiority in which what is most highly valued is the non-material (gendered masculine since Aristotle and Plato). Such judgements were predicated on philosophical, cultural and historical contingencies as well as socio-economic biases. Cultural and sociological histories of "civilizing" shame (and of surgical procedures, some of them

[49] Freud, "Leonardo," pp. 96–97.

[50] Andreas Capellanus, *On love*, ed. and trans. P. G. Walsh (London: Duckworth, 1982), pp. 222–23.

[51] Jacques Lacan, "God and the *jouissance* of The Woman: a love letter" (1972–73), in Jacques Lacan, *Feminine sexuality: Jacques Lacan and the "école freudienne,"* ed. Juliet Mitchell and Jacqueline Rose (London: Macmillan, 1982), p. 152.

punitive) may do as much to explain repression and anxieties like the "castration complex" as does psychoanalytic generalization.[52] Strikingly, Freud and Lacan shared traditional Judeo-Christian suspicions about corporeal materiality and were remarkably uneasy about physical sex. As a disembodied, abstract and classicized principle, the phallus operates to maintain a cloak over what is deemed smutty reality.

Freud's enterprise was the scholarly unveiling of the phallus in daring contradistinction to bourgeois propriety, while nevertheless claiming he kept to such values himself. Lacan too "was implicated in the phallocentrism he described, just as his own utterance constantly rejoins the mastery which he sought to undermine."[53] Each writer's dynamic, of being simultaneously outside and within the establishment, was quite conventional, as was their belief that desire was disruptive. Artemidorus, second-century Greek interpreter of dreams, understood that male genitalia were crucially related to semen and that their expansion and contraction were telling for dream interpretation.[54] Rather than regard the ancient dream diviner as a prescient forerunner to psychoanalysis, one could instead say that the modern system is the latest (and youngest, little more than one hundred years old) manifestation and refashioning of a long-lived European tradition. One could say that the ideas of the fifteenth-century Florentine philosopher Marsilio Ficino were "a startling prefigurement of Freud's own reading of the melancholic" or Ficino's discussion of the beloved is "bizarrely . . . similar to Lacan's" *not* because all hold to a joint, transhistorical truth but because they share a European legacy of androcentric theorizing about desire and its loss. If "Ficinian Neoplatonism describes an eros whose content was the nostalgic one of recapturing a lost ideal," so too does psychoanalysis, because it operates within intellectual tradition rather than *ex novo* discerning universal truths.[55] Biblical and mystical literature of longing, chivalric romance and Petrarchan poetry had already instilled in the European imagination the to-be-psychoanalytic model of desire as lack. Coming from another angle to the issue of the usefulness of psychoanalysis in historical studies, Stephen

[52] For instance, Jean Delumeau, *Sin and fear: the emergence of a western guilt culture, 13th–18th centuries* (New York: St. Martin's Press, 1990); Dympna Callaghan, "The castrator's song: female impersonation on the early modern stage," *Journal of Medieval and Early Modern Studies* 26 (1996), 321–53.

[53] Jacqueline Rose, "Introduction – II," in *Feminine sexuality*, p. 56.

[54] Artemidorus, *The interpretation of dreams: Oneirocritica*, trans. Robert White (Park Ridge, NJ: Noyes Press, 1975), pp. 38–39. The word *aidoion* is there translated as "penis" but is a euphemism for the male genitals in general ("private parts"): Henderson, *Maculate muse*, pp. 3–5, 113; Adams, *Latin sexual vocabulary*, pp. 51, 69.

[55] The quotation is from Juliana Schiesari, *The gendering of melancholia: feminism, psychoanalysis, and the symbolics of loss in Renaissance literature* (Ithaca: Cornell University Press, 1992), p. 115, previously quoted from p. 118 and n. 28. For Lacan's "Platonic idea of the penis," see Boyarin, "Dominant fiction," pp. 43–45, 48, 61, 63.

Greenblatt has suggested that "psychoanalytic interpretation seems to follow upon rather than to explain Renaissance texts."[56]

The "long, stiff objects and weapons" that bubbled up from the unconscious in the dreams Freud noticed were phallic, the stuff of shame, desire and secrecy, yet given paradoxical visibility by countless texts and images through the centuries, including Freud's own.[57] The phallic objects were also simplified renditions of a cultural icon, for Freud – and thence later psychoanalysts like Lacan – concentrated on only certain aspects of symbolized, masculine genitals. It was to Freud primarily a piercing, state-altering and patriarchal object that deflowered female virgins in solemn, almost cultic terms, and that obsessed everyone in their dreams while they lived repression.

In 1919, Freud accepted the work of colleagues published earlier that decade which indicated that "significant secretions, such as semen, are replaced in dreams by indifferent ones" like "mucus, tears, urine."[58] However, this was Freud's only reference to semen, and he also used the word "testikel" just once in all of his writings, simply to describe that body part in a drawing by Leonardo (fig. 29).[59] Thus, not much was made of bodily effluvia, still considered merely material by Lacan decades later. Modern medical assumptions led to the neglect of what had been in premodern cultures a crucial physical factor of masculinity, humoral heat; semen was incidental, perhaps because it was causal in the process of deflation; and the testicles were insignificant appendages.

But the system of what I have dubbed semenotics was central to earlier cultural moments, and not only within repressed libidos or on the obscene margins. Giovanni Boccaccio's fourteenth-century "Master Shaft" entering "the Obscure Valley" of women's bodies in his *Corbaccio* has a particular rather than immutable history.[60] *Messer Mazza* was going to venture back into that valley "from which he had been chased after many tears." Those liquid *lagrime* were a parodic, misogynist pun on supposed female suffering for they also referred to spermatic fluid, without which Boccaccio's adulterous lover had

[56] Stephen Greenblatt, "Psychoanalysis and Renaissance culture," rpt. in his *Learning to curse* (New York: Routledge, 1990), p. 142.

[57] Freud, "Interpretation of dreams," p. 359. Further: "All elongated objects, such as sticks, tree-trunks and umbrellas (the opening of these last being comparable to an erection) may stand for the male organ [1909]–as well as all long, sharp weapons, such as knives, daggers and pikes [1911]": p. 354. (Ejaculation seems as evident an association as erection in relation to umbrellas.)

[58] Freud, "Interpretation of dreams," p. 359.

[59] *Konkordanz*, vol. V, pp. 4891 (which lists solely this reference for *sperma* and otherwise has *spermatozoen* once and *spermatozoon* three times), 5119 for *testikel;* Freud, "Leonardo," p. 70 n. 3.

[60] Giovanni Boccaccio, *Elegia di Madonna Fiammetta. Corbaccio*, ed. Francesco Erbani (Milan: Garzanti, 1988), p. 256; Giovanni Boccaccio, *The corbaccio*, trans. and ed. Anthony Cassell (Urbana: University of Illinois Press, 1975), p. 42, with the ribald sense of *lagrime* noted on p. 127, for which also see Barbara C. Bowen, "Metaphorical obscenity in French farce, 1460–1560," *Comparative Drama* 11 (1977), 334; Boggione and Casalegno, *Dizionario*, p. 354.

no fun and could not assert his phallic mastery. When boasted about in a thirteenth-century burlesque Italian poem by Rustico di Filippo, the enormous size of a man's sodomitical penis was ultimately proven by its liquid output: "it'll seem that the Arno [river] is flowing out of your crack."[61]

Like hegemonic or dominant ideology, the phallus "can play its role only when veiled" according to Lacan.[62] Yet, the unveiling of a phallus or phallic symbol does not castrate or silence "speech" or immobilize the artist; rather, just the opposite results, at least in the premodern culture of people like Rustico or Boccaccio. Laughter and proliferation abound. Male genitals give rise to logorrhea, to countless slang terms, verbal jokes and insults, to written and visual metaphors, double or multiple entendres, allusions, euphemisms and visual signifiers of power, puns, and play. As the courtesan Tullia d'Aragona put it in her *Dialogue on the infinity of love* published in 1547, "this word 'love' . . . is a polyvalent noun."[63] Vignali's pseudo-academic discourse on cocks observed in a mocking key around 1525–26 that genitals "have so many names."[64] "Speaking of love," claimed Lacan, "is in itself a *jouissance*," but the French poet Louise Labé had already published the thought in 1555, summing up a long passage of hers by saying "in short, the greatest pleasure that there is, after love itself, is talking about it."[65] A veritable logorrhea or *copia*, the copious spillage of words, and also a stream of images (what one might call optikorrhea) celebrated "pissing" putti, for instance, or weighed the pros and cons of "spending" "coin." Male sexual action and the symbolism of its multiple aspects was public, spoken, read and visualized in a host of ways.

Another core dilemma in psychoanalytically informed thinking hinges on the relationship between body and unconscious. When mid-sixteenth-century Italian and early seventeenth-century English texts began to bring the word "phallus" into the vernacular, it referred to an artificial object, exaggerated in size and fashioned by pagans, but it was nevertheless interpreted as referring straightforwardly to penis or "yard," a conflation that frequently occurs in modern times too. Quite how the bodily genitals differ from the phallus is a problem particularly resistant to unraveling.

Feminist theorists and others have "disputed whether Freud's biological analogies [between penis and phallus] function as metaphors or whether they

[61] Christopher Kleinhenz, "Texts, naked and thinly veiled: erotic elements in medieval Italian literature," in Joyce Salisbury (ed.), *Sex in the middle ages* (New York: Garland, 1991), pp. 100–01.

[62] Lacan, "Significance of the phallus," p. 288.

[63] Tullia d'Aragona, *Dialogue on the infinity of love*, eds. and trans. Rinaldina Russell and Bruce Merry (University of Chicago Press, 1997), p. 89.

[64] Vignali, *Cazzaria*, p. 69.

[65] Lacan, "Love letter," p. 154; Louise Labé, *Œuvres complètes*, ed. Enzo Giudici (Geneva: Librairie Droz, 1981), p. 59.

imply a biological reality."[66] In his essay on the "signification of the phallus," Lacan was not able to distinguish clearly between the two, being profoundly anti-material at one point, then trying to ground signification in "the real" at another moment:

> The phallus is the privileged signifier of that mark in which the role of the logos is joined with the advent of desire. It can be said that this signifier is chosen [by whom?] because it is the most tangible element in the real (*le réel*) of sexual copulation, and also the most symbolic in the literal (typographical) sense of the term, since it is equivalent there to the (logical) copula. It might also be said that, by virtue of its turgidity, it is the image of the vital flow (*flux vital*) as it is transmitted in generation.[67]

Lacan "fails to prevent the collapse of the master signifier into the organ."[68] The feminist literary critic Jane Gallop has observed that

> for Lacanians ... the phallus is not a penis. Men are no more in possession of the phallus than are women ... *But* it *also* always refers to *penis* ... The Lacanians' desire clearly to separate *phallus* from *penis*, to control the meaning of the signifier *phallus*, is precisely symptomatic of their desire to have the phallus, that is, their desire to be at the center of language, at its origin ... As long as the attribute of power is a phallus which can only have meaning by referring to and being confused with a penis, this confusion will support a structure in which it seems reasonable that men have power and women do not.[69]

More forthrightly, separation is disavowed by Daniel Boyarin, who argues that "the phallus is pretending not to be the penis," when the two are really one.[70] The dissociation of the two serves to make the phallus appear transcendent and immaterial, thereby acting "to project masculinity as the universal – as the Logos." Although he does not discuss visual discourse, the argument elucidates the habit of visually representing the phallus as a severed organ, and virtually makes castration a *necessary* act of language and imagery under patriarchy.

By insisting that the phallic signifier was "the most tangible element in the real of sexual copulation," Lacan represented the partner's body – implicitly penetrated and receptive – as far less real, and virtually intangible or ethereal if that person was not endowed with a normative penis, that is, if they were female (to which must be added intersexed people, not yet recognized in standard psychoanalysis). He reiterated the sentimentalization common to many fertility cults and religions that emphasize reproduction: "it is the image of the vital flow

66 Nicola Diamond, "Biology," in Wright (ed.), *Feminism and psychoanalysis*, p. 22.

67 Lacan, "La signification du phallus" (1958), in *Écrits* (Paris: Éditions du Seuil, 1966), p. 692; Lacan, "Significance of the phallus," p. 287.

68 Biodun Iginla, "Black feminist critique of psychoanalysis," in Wright (ed.), *Feminism and psychoanalysis*, p. 32.

69 Jane Gallop, *Thinking through the body* (New York: Columbia University Press, 1988), pp. 126–27 (her emphases).

70 Boyarin, "Dominant fiction," p. 66, hereafter quoted from p. 57.

as it is transmitted in generation." Reproductive semen (the *flux vital*), linked to Aristotle's definition of it as "vital spirit," grounds the venerated phallus in the real for Lacan; indeed, it seems that semen is phallic, even though that again raises the question of the relationship between reality and symbol, as though he is falling back on Jungian archetypes. Although Lacan neatly slides over biological and psychic differences by tending to mark semen as merely material and the phallus as supra-material, in this instance he acknowledges the interdependence of two aspects of masculine apparati. Otherwise, however, semen is of no importance in Lacanian psychoanalysis, subsumed under the penis just as it was for Freud.

Given the centrality to psychoanalysis of the Oedipal complex and anxiety about castration, what constitutes the historical conceptualization of castration is an important matter, and that too has a crucial non-penile component. Castration actually involves the removal of testicles and Gary Taylor has pointed out that in many cultures and historical moments admired castrati singers and highly ranked Ottoman eunuchs were valued, even elite, figures.[71] Furthermore, the removal of certain body parts has sometimes been deliberate (as in the renowned case of Origen's self-administered castration) and can yield benefits. Abelard's infamous sexual mutilation in the early twelfth century, argues Yves Ferroul, actually consisted of the standard, less painful removal of the testicles alone, and it provided the philosopher and theologian with a justification for turning away from Heloise and focusing on his intellectual career.[72] Or consider the way in which bloodletting and scarification of the penis was a marker of royal distinction in Mayan culture.[73]

In Foucauldian terms, attempts to police, contain and classify sexuality instead led to "the incitement to discourse," a polymorphous proliferation of voices and approaches.[74] From the late nineteenth century, psychoanalysis has been the most important of new methodologies striving to explain and discipline sex and sexuality. Given the degree to which discourse can effect corporeal experiences, one could suggest that the focus on male genitals brought about by psychoanalysis has not only made everyone a ready expert in identifying "phallic symbols" but fundamentally contributed to and exacerbated fears and delicacies about those body parts.

[71] Taylor, *Castration*, passim. Stephens, *Demon lovers*, pp. 302–14 argues that the most influential witch-hunting manual, the *Malleus maleficarum*, did *not* evince a fear of castration.

[72] Yves Ferroul, "Abelard's blissful castration," in Jeffrey Jerome Cohen and Bonnie Wheeler (eds.), *Becoming male in the middle ages* (New York: Garland, 1997), pp. 129–49.

[73] Traci Ardren and David Hixson, "The unusual sculptures of Telantunich, Yucatan: phalli and the concept of masculinity among the ancient Maya," *Cambridge Archaeological Journal* 16 (2006), 7–25.

[74] Foucault, *History of sexuality*, vol. I, pp. 17–35.

Anxiety, crisis and *cui bono*

The influence of psychoanalysis on cultural studies is especially evident in the concept of anxiety; the Oedipal complex, "castration anxiety" and other troubles supposedly make of masculinity a constantly fearful, fraught, threatened, vulnerable state. The deflated penis haunts the modern phallus. When from the 1990s, men joined women as subjects of the history of gender, books began to proliferate with words like "crisis," "anxiety" and "problem" in the title.[75] This basic principle of explanation has resonated in cultural and historical studies because, I suggest, the notion accords with elementary habits and traditions of Euro-American patriarchy (which can be defined as the system of adult male domination, from the household to the State). Analyzing literary evidence from early modern England, Mark Breitenberg has gone so far as to argue that "masculine anxiety is a *necessary and inevitable* condition," enabling the continuation of patriarchy and simultaneously revealing the contradictions of such a system.[76] In that regard, the principles of patriarchy operate like any other ideology, continually constructing enemies and oppositions against which to define and clarify itself. What distinguishes patriarchy, by definition, is the centrality of masculinity to its crises and challenges. Since ideologies can change over the *longue durée* for a host of reasons, I would focus attention on ways in which anxiety is *not* inherent or ubiquitous in either historical or present circumstances. Whereas it has been claimed that "ejaculation represents the supreme moment of masculine disempowerment *and* vulnerability," that weakened state does not adequately characterize the pleased viewers of Opifex's Achilles (fig. 3), for example, or the participants and spectators who were stirred by the breaking of jousting lances.[77] Nor does it try to take into account whether or how female orgasm is or was different. Temporary lassitude after physical activity is not a sufficient basis on which to build the theoretical edifice of always-already vulnerable masculinity.

"Anxiety," having provided insights as a core hermeneutic principle in the 1990s, has come to offer too easy, trite and superficial an explanation for complex social processes, one that tends to avoid issues of responsibility and

75 Judith Allen, "Men interminably in crisis? Historians on masculinity, sexual boundaries, and manhood," *Radical History Review* 82 (2002), 191–207. See also Toby Ditz, "The new men's history and the peculiar absence of gendered power: some remedies from early American gender history," *Gender and History* 16 (2004), 1–35, for the tendency "to see the masculine subject as everywhere fragile and endangered, and even in constant crisis . . . [which] elides the operations of power and creates false equivalencies" (5–6).

76 Breitenberg, *Anxious masculinity*, p. 2 (my emphases), which also points to "the profound costs of maintaining [patriarchal] superiority," as does, for example, Scott Hendrix, "Masculinity and patriarchy in Reformation Germany," in S. Hendrix and Susan Karant-Nunn (eds.), *Masculinity in the Reformation era* (Kirksville: Truman State University Press, 2008), pp. 71–91.

77 The quotation is from Breitenberg, *Anxious masculinity*, p. 50.

inequalities of power. Whereas Breitenberg and others focus on the "costs," "burdens," "encumbrances" and "vulnerability" endured by men living in patriarchy, we need to remember the social, political and economic advantage accrued through the mechanisms of differentiation, between various kinds of men and also from those considered lesser according to factors such as gender, rank, age, marital status and wealth. Valuable recent studies on young men are investigating both their excesses and ultimate incorporation into the social order as they learned to govern themselves, evident in the use of chivalric nostalgia at tournament time, for instance, or the "camaraderie of misrule" that Alexandra Shepard identifies amongst early modern students at Cambridge which sometimes entailed appropriation and mock performance of regulatory authority.[78] To construct historical argumentation on the basis of an ahistorical, idyllic, prelapsarian origin is deeply flawed, as is Freud's reliance on the once-upon-a-time unfettered phallus. The core question needs to be what we may learn by applying the general lens of "anxiety" to a particular historical moment.

To my mind, the condition of having to be alert and erect constantly, ever battling foes and overcoming challenges, from Hercules to superheroes, from one-party States to market capitalists, is a social and cultural convention whereby masculinity is defined in a way that *serves* patriarchal privilege. The supremely macho hero Hercules is forever laboring, yet always victorious in the face of demons and crises.[79] Justifications about control and hierarchical orders of power require the elaborate identification of dangers. Tania Modleski has pointed out that "we need to consider the extent to which male power is actually consolidated through cycles of crisis and resolution, whereby men ultimately deal with the threat of female power by incorporating it."[80]

In 1995, the sociologist R. W. Connell influentially characterized masculinity in terms of the benefits reaped from the "patriarchal dividend" by multiple types of men within a hierarchy of hegemonic power.[81] Subsequent studies elaborated upon differentiations between men, often based on the model of crisis and anxiety. Historiographically, an early round of feminist history that named core exclusions, gender inequities and women's victimization was answered by work showing that men too suffered under patriarchy. Power effectively seemed to be owned at all times by someone *other* than one's subject of study. Hence, in a recent review of three books treating modern Euro-American history, Judith Allen summarized their joint sense that: "inherently unstable, masculinity is always in process, under negotiation, needing to be 'shored up,'

78 Shepard, *Meanings of manhood*, pp. 96–113. On tournaments see Ch. 1 above.

79 Patricia Simons, "Hercules in Italian Renaissance art: masculine labour and homoerotic libido," *Art History* 31 (2008), 632–64.

80 Tania Modleski, *Feminism without women: culture and criticism in a "postfeminist" age* (New York: Routledge, 1991), p. 7.

81 R. W. Connell, *Masculinities* (1995), 2nd edn. (Berkeley: University of California Press, 2005).

reinforced, buttressed against its many enemies."[82] From a broader perspective, Laura Gowing has astutely observed that "gender is *always* in contest: gender relations seem to be continually renegotiated around certain familiar points."[83] The details of those points matter if one wants to make them less familiar and harder to reiterate.

Phenomena such as extreme misogyny and witch-hunting certainly bespeak personal and institutionalized fears, largely acted out upon women; other externalizing, angry accusations were at particular historical moments hurled against, say, foreigners or people of other races or national groups, or practitioners of same-sex acts who were mostly male.[84] But, to the age-old question *cui bono* (who benefits), the answer would have to note that crises over the centuries did not decimate patriarchy but instead resulted in centralization and the institutionalization of power and resources in the hands of the patriarchal elite. If a book's cover blurb can declare that "masculinity is *unavoidably* anxious and volatile in cultures that distribute power and authority according to patriarchal prerogatives," then anxiety is of little historical value and not a particularly useful heuristic tool.[85]

Undeniably, the early modern period witnessed numerous articulations of male "crisis" and concern, amongst them trials to ascertain the evidence regarding attempts by wives and families to end marriage by charging husbands with impotence.[86] Yet the canon law was not new, trials were relatively rare, and variations in medico-legal opinions provided room for argumentation, victory and appeal.[87] Some men were judged to have permanent defects, such as castration (though sterility was not grounds for dissolution of a marriage), immature genitals or an impaired quality of humoral heat, assessments that reinforced the normative status of those virile traits. In other cases male impotence was regarded as temporary or due to enchantment, which could be countered by other magic. Men with overly large genitals could find a wife better suited to their dimensions, men considered too young to be potent would

[82] Allen, "Men interminably in crisis?" p. 199.

[83] Gowing, *Domestic dangers*, p. 28.

[84] For the debate on the relationship between psychoanalysis and history, especially in relation to struggles to understand individual subjects while also explaining historical change, see Roper, *Oedipus and the devil*, pp. 1–34, 226–48; Roper, *Witch craze*, pp. ix–xii.

[85] The quotation, with my emphasis added, is from the back cover of the paperback edition of Breitenberg, *Anxious masculinity*.

[86] Darmon, *Tribunal de l'impuissance*; Brundage, *Law, sex and Christian society*; Bajada, *Sexual impotence*; Angus McLaren, *Impotence: a cultural history* (University of Chicago Press, 2007); Edward Behrend-Martínez, *Unfit for marriage: impotent spouses on trial in the Basque region of Spain, 1650–1750* (Reno: University of Nevada Press, 2007), esp. pp. 85–89, 100–5.

[87] Regional variation is important. The chapter on impotence in Daniela Hacke, *Women, sex and marriage in early modern Venice* (Aldershot: Ashgate, 2004) is based on thirteen cases, one female, drawn from the period 1570–1700 (p. 146 n. 8). In the Spanish diocese of Calahorra, eighty-three cases survive for 1650–1750: Behrend-Martínez, *Unfit for marriage*, p. x.

simply develop over time, men too old could sometimes transform themselves by changes in diet and other Galenic non-naturals. Impotence, then, was not always and everywhere a dire fear. Nor did it necessarily function in today's psychic terms, for concerns instead centered on the diminution of masculine honor, the loss of marital authority and social standing and on economic factors such as access to dowry funds.

The historical images and words in this book are chiefly about the making of an assuring definition of manliness and the celebration of both masculine excess and its control under patriarchy. In Freudian terms, obscene and sexual humor functions to legitimize and enable spurts of release against regimes of sexual repression.[88] Joke-work was tellingly described by Freud in 1905 as a "discharge" of pleasure, and thus the semen-centric humor analyzed in my study is particularly effective in its manliness, naming and visualizing of the forbidden with glee. Freud's "discharge" was literally a burst of laughter, and Renaissance jokes precisely likened that sudden release to ejaculation.[89] Political and psychic subversion and macho bonding are evident in much of the material, but the same sorts of words, concepts and metaphors also appear in mainstream textbooks of anatomy and popular health compendia. Instead of focusing on the unconscious and individualized psyche, this study joins that of other scholars who are interested in embedding bodily experience in historical contexts.[90]

The phallus can be disaggregated through focusing on physiological components. If anxiety is at work in the profusion of phalli and genital jokes, it is so successfully laughed away by apotropaic explicitness and aggressive obscenity that the anxiety is marked as much by its absence as by its presence. Concerns about privilege were multiple, about such matters as personal or national manliness or reproduction (to be fostered within marriage, avoided and condemned if likely elsewhere). These gave rise to many forms of discourse, including humor and sex manuals alongside sober medical treatises, learned

88 Sigmund Freud, *Jokes and their relation to the unconscious* (1905), in *Standard edition*, vol. VIII (London: Hogarth Press, 1960).

89 Ibid., *Jokes*, pp. 146–58, 176 and passim on "discharge"; Toscan, *Carnaval*, pp. 1127–28, 1179–81, 1389, 1704. In one of the anecdotes about Donatello's erotic relations with apprentices, sculptor and assistant reconciled by "laughing," a tale glossed in the sixteenth century as "licenzioso": Angelo Poliziano, *Detti piacevoli*, ed. Tiziano Zanato (Rome: Istituto della Enciclopedia Italiana, 1983), p. 84; Lodovico Domenichi, *Detti, et fatti de diversi signori et persone private* (Venice: Francesco Lorenzini, 1562), 127v. In 1628 a London woman's description of another woman's orgasm noted that she "did laughe or cry aloud hah hah hah": Gowing, *Domestic dangers*, p. 81. For "coughing," see Ch. 7 below.

90 See, for instance, Ulinka Rublack, "Fluxes: the early modern body and the emotions," *History Workshop Journal* 53 (2002), 1–16; Anne Jacobson Schutte, "Suffering from the stone: the accounts of Michel de Montaigne and Cecilia Ferrazzi," *Bibliothèque d'humanisme et renaissance* 64 (2002), 21–36; Gowing, *Common bodies*; Canning, *Gender history*; and Roper's work cited below.

political philosophies and criminalizing statutes, but they are not very usefully gathered together under one conglomerate or overarching rubric like anxiety.

Models of desire can be built around the armature of plenitude instead of absence, production rather than lack.[91] That alternative archetype is characteristic of semen-centric metaphor, especially as used in humor. Renaissance sexual humor from the pens of male authors like Poggio Bracciolini, Pietro Aretino, François Rabelais and Thomas Nashe was marked by logorrhea, an endless profusion of word plays and metaphors spilling forth. Images too were patriarchal propaganda, exuberantly outshining "anxiety" and busily, assuringly overcoming absence. Essential tools of patriarchy like superiority, confidence and prerogatives were constructed and reinforced in jokes, medical ideology and behavioral patterns. The language of medicine and humor alike represented women being fired up then doused, hammered, churned, grated, ground, ploughed, watered, lanced and brushed. Sexual women were usually figured as excessive and out of control; when applied to men, such traits were about pleasurable release and virile youth.

Anxiety operates in many historical studies as a core explanatory factor for change. On the practical level, however, it is noticeable that male-dominated ideological structures like patriarchy and capitalism remain strong. Instruments of power distract and mollify, appropriate and recuperate, and on the theoretical level it can be argued that authoritative ideologies need transgression in order to reconfigure and entrench their dominance.[92] Norms are clarified and reinforced by such means as policing institutions (like those examining Eleno/a's case, in Chapter 1), and by numerous other elements, some studied in later chapters here, such as cultural metaphors and artifacts, epistemological systems (including medical knowledge) and assertive, distinguishing strategies like humor. Anxiety is a contributing but not necessarily determining factor; concerns about the proof of paternity or the denial of impotence, for instance, were not always widespread and they were overcome or balanced by strategies such as legal categorization, satire and exclusion from the normative body politic.

Corporeal instability evident in Elena/o's body need not be read as automatically giving rise to widespread personal or social anxiety, especially when medico-legal institutions arrived at a determination. Not all kinds of instability or multi-layered identities need be conflated with anxiety and vulnerability. Such phenomena as psychic anxiety, the defense of self-interest or the regulation of norms by institutional authorities are not all the same, so our vocabulary

[91] See Elizabeth Grosz, "Refiguring lesbian desire," in Laura Doan (ed.), *The lesbian postmodern* (New York: Columbia University Press, 1994), pp. 67–84.

[92] See, for instance, Louis Althusser, "Ideology and ideological State apparatuses," in *Lenin and philosophy and other essays*, trans. Ben Brewster (New York: Monthly Review Press, 1971), pp. 127–86. I thank Heather Vinson for discussions on this issue.

and analytical models need to recognize the overlap but also the differences. A degree of tautological reasoning undergirds models of change based on anxiety, for sometimes the change that results from the vulnerability of certain men leads to the installment of other men who quickly develop susceptibilities, many of them remarkably similar to those of the previous rulers. *Cui bono*? At one and the same time, men could be anxious and victorious, impotent at home and assertive in office for example, but in relation to ideological patterns of power and change I suggest that anxiety is a symptom more than a determining cause. While not losing sight of systemic inequities, one can disavow Freud's disgust and Lacan's unease regarding the pleasurable facets of sexual physiology and erotic culture when seeking to interweave the traces of materiality and language in relation to the study of male bodies.

3 Material culture in late medieval and early modern Europe

From major sculptural monuments to small, cheap badges, from graffiti to codpieces, signs of male genitals were a central part of the material culture of early modern Europe. A virtual personification of the genitals was, in one sense, a sign of man's alienation from his body part, but more often those genitals were animated in gestures of ever-virile, energetic and often humorous defiance and aggression.

Beasts and badges

Studies with no psychoanalytic bent can also endow the phallus with solemn majesty, yet humor well beyond the ancient world remains a central component of phallic display. Traditional awe is summed up in the title of a recent mass-market book by the journalist David Friedman: *A mind of its own: a cultural history of the penis*.[1] There it is conceded that "phallus" is a "perfectly apt word for the erect organ and all the symbolic meanings that attach to that state," but a history of the actual genital organ is purportedly kept apart, despite the fact that the penis is envisaged in the book as "an idea," always "mysterious," and as "the organ with whom [sic] man has his most awesome and mysterious relationship."[2] In the opposite corner, a professor of film studies Peter Lehman has examined "the over-importance our culture places on the penis by maintaining an extraordinary awe and mystique about it."[3] The tendency to anthropomorphize male genitals is revealing, indicative of what Lehman notes is the degree to which men under patriarchy are simultaneously empowered by "the penis-phallus" and yet "profoundly alienated from their own bodies." It is significant that any psychic causes for the sense of alienation from a part of one's body are exacerbated by physical actions, by the occurrence of nocturnal emissions and initially involuntary arousal. These used to be explained primarily in terms of

1 Friedman, *Mind of its own*.
2 Ibid., pp. 5, 6, 13, and see 4–17, 24 ("awesome and mysterious"), 51, 54, 60, 62, 63, 74, 76, 80, 164, 306 and passim for the frequent use of "mystery."
3 Lehman, *Running scared*, p. xi, hereafter quoted from p. 39.

imagination, sometimes in conjunction with sin, though night-time "pollution" was usually regarded as unconscious and thence forgiven.[4] The latest form of engagement with the ever-challenging relationship between apparently only two aspects of selfhood, "mind" and "body," is modern psychoanalysis, which offers another form of expiation and attempts to tame the beast by means of analysis and renaming.

The beast with a mind of its own has a stellar pedigree. The sixteenth-century French essayist Michel de Montaigne was aware of the description written around 360 BCE by the Greek philosopher Plato, of the male genitals as "disobedient and self-willed, like a creature that is deaf to reason, and it attempts to dominate all because of its frenzied lusts."[5] Involuntary movements that made the genitals similar to "a separate vital organism" also struck Plato's pupil Aristotle, and "the seminal force [that] comes forth from it" was akin to "a living thing."[6] The notion lived on in Augustine's doctrinal insight around 750 years after Plato that the "novel disturbance of their disobedient flesh" was the consequence of the Fall of Adam and Eve.[7] Centered on genital response, the human body was now alienated from the control of the will, conscious of shame and mired in concupiscence and lust. Amidst his anatomical observations drawn around 1506–13, Leonardo da Vinci mused about the obstinacy of the organ, evident in nocturnal emissions or moments of impotence. In the tradition of the ancient Greeks and Augustine, "this animal" acted as though it "often has a soul and intellect separate from a man."[8]

In a sense, the psychoanalytic and modern attempt to separate penis and phallus is one more strategy in the ongoing cultural habit of alienating the male organ from its wider corporeal and human context. Displacing irrational, unruly genital action onto phallic animals or ithyphallic satyrs, for instance, reinstated the presumption that masculine self-control and rationality were possible for human men. In Boyarin's terms, the phallus "as a representation consists precisely of the separation of masculinity from the embodied male body."[9] However, the dissociation might better be said to

[4] For a sampling of the ecclesiastical and medical debates about nocturnal emissions see Crooke, *Mikrokosmographia*, pp. 247–48, 288; Dyan Elliott, "Pollution, illusion, and masculine disarray: nocturnal emissions and the sexuality of the clergy," in Karma Lochrie, Peggy McCracken, and James Schultz (eds.), *Constructing medieval sexuality* (Minneapolis: University of Minnesota Press, 1997), pp. 1–23; James Brundage, "Obscene and lascivious: behavioral obscenity in Canon Law," in Jan Ziolkowski (ed.), *Obscenity: social control and artistic creation in the European middle ages* (Leiden: Brill, 1998), pp. 251–58.

[5] Plato, *Timaeus*, 91b; Michel de Montaigne, *Les essais*, 3 vols. 2nd edn., ed. Pierre Villey (Paris: Quadrige/ PUF, 1992), vol. III, p. 859.

[6] Aristotle, *Movement of animals*, 703b. [7] Augustine, *City of God*, p. 522, see also p. 582.

[8] Kenneth D.Keele, *Leonardo da Vinci's elements of the science of man* (New York: Academic Press, 1983), p. 350.

[9] Boyarin, "Dominant fiction," pp. 52, see also pp. 55, 63, 86 and passim on the separation.

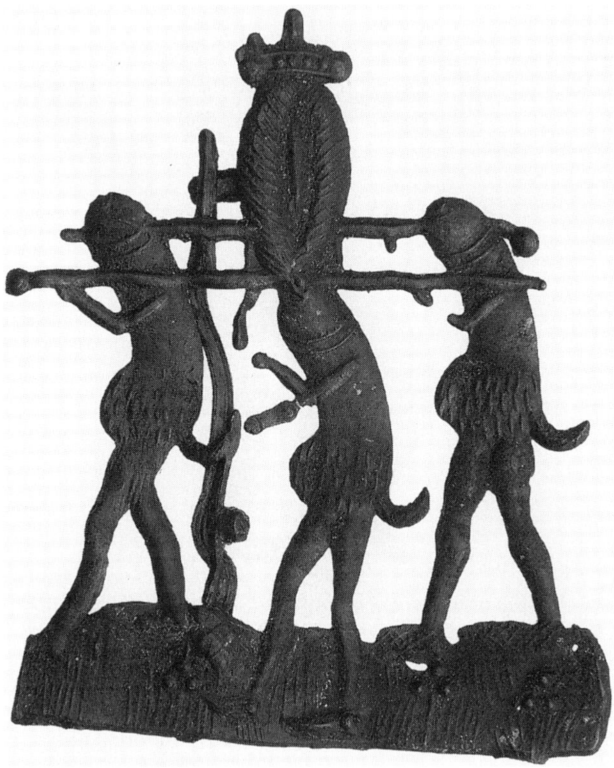

Figure 10 *Three phalli process a crowned vulva*, 1375–1425, lead tin alloy, 56 × 45 mm, found in Bruges, Family van Beuningen Collection

work in reverse when animalistic imagery is under consideration. In those cases, it is the strategy of bestializing the phallus that makes the subject of the representation particular, material and embodied, and thus it is the human male who becomes universal and idealized by contrast.

On the one hand, figural forms reinforced the seeming alienation; on the other hand, they were often appropriated for purposes like amusement and defensive protection, whether in antiquity's phallos-birds or the animal forms of wind chimes, badges and graffiti (figs. 7, 10–13). Many vernacular languages preserved the relationship between birds and male genitals ("uccello," bird, along with particular species like "passerotto," sparrow, in Italian, for instance, "pájaro" in Spanish, "Vogel" in Dutch and German, or "cock" in English), and the creature caught in sexual hunts was frequently a phallic "bird," though it was sometimes a generic, lusty

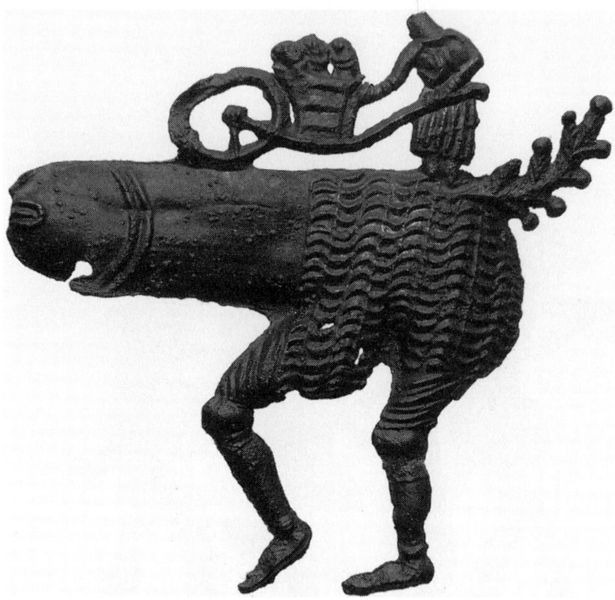

Figure 11 *Woman with a barrow of phalli atop a walking phallus*, 1400–50, lead tin alloy, 56 × 55 mm, found in Nieuwlande, Family van Beuningen Collection

"animal."[10] The beast is an inventive winged hybrid on one side of a fifteenth-century engraving plate associated with Ferrara (fig. 14), with lion's paws and haunches.[11] The rolled back hood of the foreskin, to which a bell is attached, reveals a head and mouth that anthropomorphize the being into an eager voyeur. Various quips and medical comments indicate that its small bell referred to semen but also to testicles, though the lion, commonly understood as a virile beast, has contributed strikingly testicular haunches to the crossbreed.

The engraved beast has a tail somewhat like that of a horse. "Tail" was the very meaning of the Latin word *penis*, and the genital sense lived on in numerous vernacular languages.[12] In general, the tail also sometimes signified

[10] Toscan, *Carnaval*, pp. 274, 456–57, 1282–83, 1661. On the genital bird, see Ruggiero, *Machiavelli in love*, pp. 98–103 and passim; Allen Grieco, "From roosters to cocks: Italian Renaissance fowl and sexuality," in Matthews-Grieco (ed.), *Erotic cultures*, pp. 89–140.

[11] See Mark Zucker, *The illustrated Bartsch 24 Commentary part 3: early Italian masters* (New York: Abaris Books, 2000), pp. 198–200. For the recto, see fig. 55 here.

[12] Italian *coda*, French *queue*, English *tail*, German *Schwanz*, and so on for that part of the male genitals. "Tail" also came to refer to the backside.

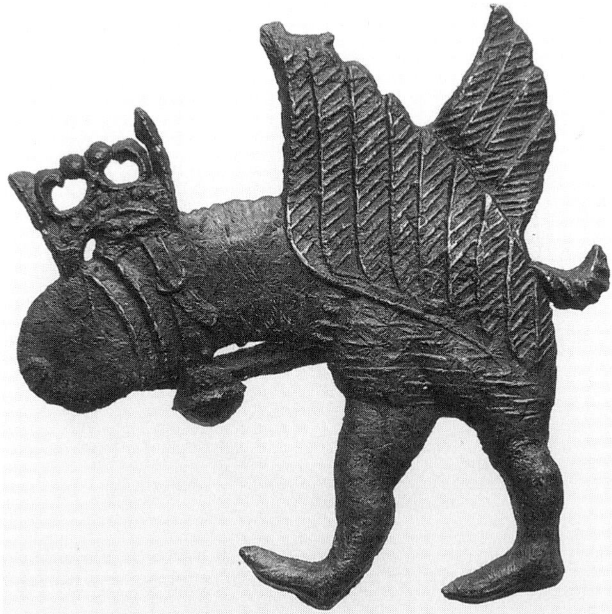

Figure 12 *Crowned phallus with wings and a bell*, 1375–1425, lead tin alloy, 29 × 28 mm, found in Nieuwlande, Family van Beuningen Collection

a horse, and that animal was notoriously associated with lust, having a hot, sanguine nature and unrestrained sexual appetite if unbridled.[13] "Horse" simply meant the male genitals to ribald authors like Aretino, who devised a mixed metaphor similar to the engraved plate when he imagined a parodic St. Nafissa depicted on a convent's walls "consoling" the afflicted. She uncovered a man's "young Turtle Dove" (*tortorino*), which she admired so much that it puffed up with pride "and plunged between her legs with the fury of a stallion that breaks his halter and hurls himself on a mare."[14]

Most often, Renaissance Italian writers associated horses with sexual avidity and the movements of sexual congress, especially "mounting" or the rhythmic motion of "riding." The hybrid beast of the engraving plate is an overly

[13] Erwin Panofsky, *Problems in Titian, mostly iconographic* (London: Phaidon, 1969), p. 118; James Marrow and Alan Shestack, *Hans Baldung Grien: prints and drawings* (Washington, DC: National Gallery of Art, 1981), pp. 264–69; Rubinstein, *Dictionary*, pp. 851–52, 914–15, 1154–55, 1304–05; Boggione and Casalegno, *Dizionario*, pp. 176–82, 277–80, 283–85, 450–51.

[14] Aretino, *Ragionamento*, pp. 22, 146; Aretino, *Aretino's "Dialogues,"* p. 23. "*Tortorino*, a yongue Turtle Dove. Used also for a mans pillicocke": Florio, *Queen Anna's new world of words*, p. 570.

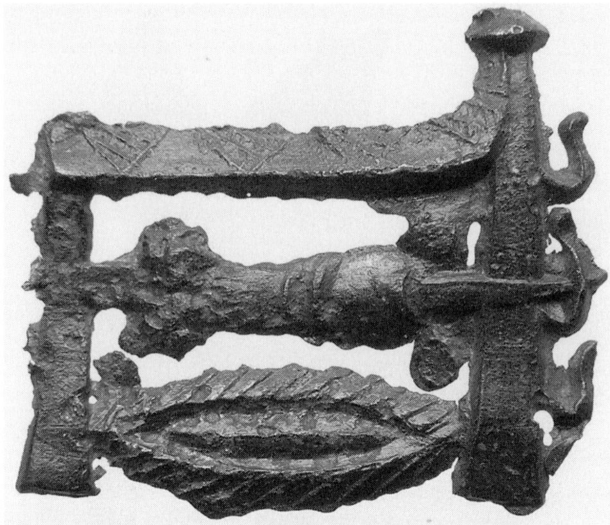

Figure 13 *Phallus roasting on a spit over a vulva as a grease trap*, 1375–1425, lead tin alloy, 20 × 22 mm, found in Nieuwlande, Family van Beuningen Collection

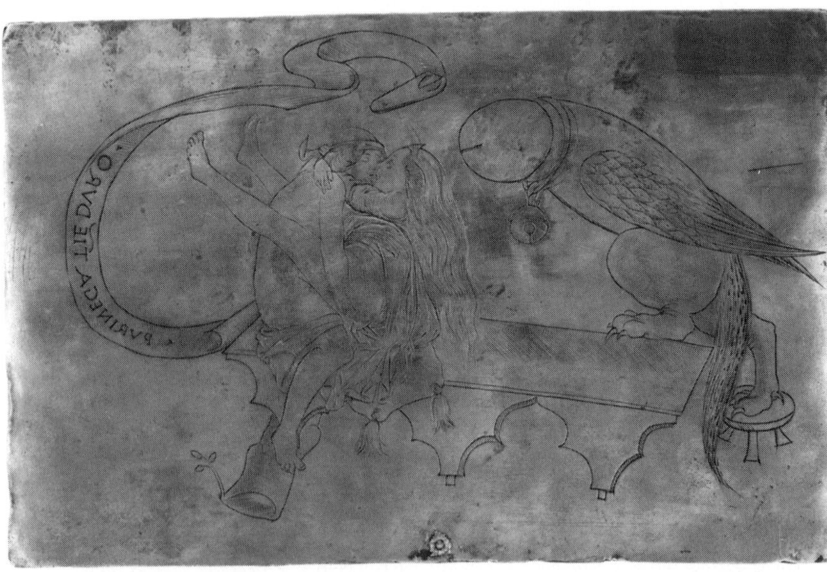

Figure 14 Anonymous northeast Italian, *Copulating couple with phallus bird*, last quarter of the fifteenth century, verso, engraved copper plate, 150 × 224 mm, Washington DC, National Gallery of Art, Rosenwald Collection

endowed creature whose core action is that of clambering onto the bench, mounting it and rising up as if to guarantee the rocking couple's success as they "ride" the bench. The apotropaic creature of ancient amulets and other objects like wind chimes (fig. 7) is here too a protector resembling Aretino's patron saint, eagerly rearing up on one leg (*gamba* being a common Italian metaphor for the penis). Indeed, he gets a leg up with the aid of a three-legged stool, another of Aretino's many metaphors for the penis (*piedi-di-trespolo*).[15] An amusingly ironic inscription reads: "Even though I try to resist, it stays hard" (*Pur i' nega, tien duro*), pressure and friction precisely producing genital rigidity.[16]

Personification was widespread, evident in everyday speech and medical terminology, and often attributing to the organ lordly authority well before Lacan. In an Italian song surviving in a collection of 1508, a wife attempting to arouse her husband begins by pulling out "my little lord."[17] When a married woman from Devon complained in 1666 about a man chasing her with "his foreman in his hand," it is not clear whether she meant that the organ signified the man's phallic power in general or its particular control over him, or both, but the personification certainly signified distance as well as authority.[18] The testicles were, in the words of a London gossip sheet in 1660, a man's "masters."[19] Meaning penis, the word "Fore-man" appeared a few years later in the first vernacular midwifery written by an Englishwoman, Jane Sharp; in 1615 the anatomist Crooke had used "yeoman" when translating the straightforward Latin term *pene* for penis.[20] Both English words grant some authority to the anthropomorphized penis, as overseer, land freeholder or officer, but it does not reign as king or general over all. Ultimately, the word stems from ancient agricultural metaphors, and the sower of seed, ploughman or yeoman farmer has come to personify the penis.

15 Aretino, *Ragionamento*, pp. 91, 437. For *gamba* see Boggione and Casalegno, *Dizionario*, p. 309.

16 The image is instead read as a moralizing warning against lust in Anthony Colantuono, "The penis possessed: phallic birds, erotic magic, and sins of the body, ca. 1470–1500," in Julia Hairston and Walter Stephens (eds.), *The body in early modern Italy* (Baltimore: Johns Hopkins University Press, 2010), pp. 92–108. That interpretation does not sufficiently explain the purpose or popularity of such a print (issued in more than 1,000 copies judging by the worn state of the plate). I thank Nerida Newbigin for her assistance with reading the north Italian phrase.

17 William Prizer, "Games of Venus: secular vocal music in the late quattrocento and early cinquecento," *Journal of Musicology* 9 (1991), 32.

18 The phrase is in Gowing, *Common bodies*, p. 55. 19 Ibid., p. 83.

20 Jane Sharp, *The midwives book or the whole art of midwifry discovered* (1671), ed. Elaine Hobby (Oxford University Press, 1999), p. 20; Crooke, *Mikrokosmographia*, p. 212, translating Gaspard Bauhin, *Theatrum anatomicum* (Frankfurt: Matthäus Becker, 1605), p. 204. For another example see Levinus Lemnius, *The secret miracles of nature* (London: Jo. Streater, 1658), p. 19 (first published as *Occulta naturae miracula* [Antwerp: G. Simonem, 1559]). See Ch. 7 below.

The tinge of deprecation for purposes of amusement is instead evident in a less polite characterization made by a fifteenth-century carnival play from Nuremberg. An indicative mix of intimacy, cross-gender personalization yet distance marked the "proud little dolly" that a man nightly dressed up in "skirts" when his fingers enfolded the organ while masturbating.[21] More often, metaphors for male genitals associate them with beasts or inanimate objects like weapons, but the personifications most strikingly indicate the imaginary distance that could be placed between body part and its action. The Lacanian tenet that the phallus is so all-powerful that no one can attain the ultimate desire to "have" or "be" the phallus, is the nihilistic end point of the cultural habit of separation. Overall, the social result is the excuse that "boys will be boys." Men are apparently disconnected and alien from themselves because that vital body part is too awesome and disobedient. Yet, that astounding grandeur redounds to the benefit of those closest to it, bestowing and enforcing patriarchal privilege. Either way, the phallus is a hard taskmaster, taking control, asserting differences between men as well as between men and women.

Humor, on the other hand, can bring the "phallus" down to size as it were, making it an object of manipulation, mockery and braggadocio. Paradoxically, enlarging the organ to ludicrous proportions as did the Pan Painter on a Greek vase (fig. 8), or the north Italian engraver (fig. 14) induces mirth more than awe. Since the male genitals are often the object of comedy, it is worth considering key theories of genital humor. Freud's famous function of "joke-work," that of "liberating pleasure by getting rid of inhibitions," relies on a contrast between the hidden and the exposed.[22] To unveil, to reveal the repressed (which is exemplified in psychoanalysis by the phallus), is the work of the obscene joke in particular, though the dynamic is one that is fundamental to psychoanalytic work in general and that labor is usually a rather sober affair. Freud's gendered model of obscene joking is that of an early twentieth-century Viennese gentleman: two men bond over the joke but only because a woman has been the conduit, pivot or foil, excluded from the club.[23]

An alternative theory of humor posited by Mikhail Bakhtin, of carnivalesque and excessive, often scatological release, importantly does not rely on a policy of secrecy, since the carnival was given institutionalized license.[24] The

[21] Anonymous, "Ein Vasnachtspil," in Adelbert von Keller, *Fastnachtspiele*, vol. I (Stuttgart: Gedruckt auf Kosten des Litterarischen Vereins, 1853), p. 96.

[22] Freud, *Jokes*, p. 134, see also pp. 41, 97, 221 and passim. For Lacan too, revelation was central, precisely because no secure "reality" existed behind the curtain.

[23] See especially Freud, *Jokes*, pp. 97, 99, 101, 133.

[24] Mikhail Bakhtin, *Rabelais and his world*, trans. Helene Iswolsky (Bloomington: Indiana University Press, 1984). For a critique from the historian's point of view see Aaron Gurevich, "Bakhtin and his theory of Carnival," in Jan Bremmer and Herman Roodenburg (eds.), *A cultural history of humour from antiquity to the present day* (Cambridge: Polity Press, 1997), pp. 54–60.

"grotesque body" of Bakhtin's carnival – which arose in the late medieval period and continued through much of the Renaissance – is robust, untroubled, guiltless and irreverent, quite a contrast to the anxious psyche. Scholars have since critiqued yet broadened his insights, for the opposition he posited between a dour, learned elite and the "culture of laughter" only evident at the "popular" level was too simplistic and sentimentally favorable to "the people," whereas his characterization of key elements of release through excess remains attractive. Furthermore, he was crucially aware of the ambivalence of festive laughter: "it is gay, triumphant, and at the same time mocking, deriding. It asserts and denies, it buries and revives."[25]

A combination of psychoanalytic release and carnivalesque lack of embarrassment is evident in the "grotesque body" on the engraving plate and in some inexpensive tin/lead alloy badges, preserved chiefly in riverbeds and dating from the late fourteenth and fifteenth centuries. Pins and loops indicate that the badges were attached to clothing and hats or worn as pendants.[26] The majority are pilgrims' religious mementos, but some are secular in theme, serving various purposes like cheap jewellery and love tokens, or declaring membership in organizations like confraternities and guilds, similar to what the Italian architect Filarete referred to as a *segno* (sign) when embroidered and sewn on to outer garments.[27]

Many of the surviving secular badges depict humorous, caricatured genitals; some are vulvas, most are male organs personified (figs. 10–13). Presumably, due to their cheap material and mass manufacture, badges are artifacts of the middling and lower ranks, made for short-term display. Somewhat like other badges that signified membership in a lord's household or a guild, the rude ones may have been a kind of profane livery, marking the wearer as a member of a

[25] Bakhtin, *Rabelais*, pp. 11–12.

[26] H. J. E. van Beuningen and A. M. Koldeweij (eds.), *Heilig en Profaan: 1000 Laatmiddeleeuwse insigne suit de collectie H. J. E. van Beuningen* (Cothen, Netherlands: Stichting Middeleeuwse Religieuze en Profane Insignes, 1993); A. M. Koldeweij, "A barefaced *Roman de la rose* (Paris, B.N. ms. Fr. 25526) and some late medieval mass-produced badges of a sexual nature," in Maurits Smeyers and Bert Cardon (eds.), *Flanders in a European perspective: manuscript illumination around 1400 in Flanders and abroad* (Leuven: Peeters, 1995), pp. 499–516; Denis Bruna, *Enseignes de pèlerinage et enseignes profanes* (Paris: Réunion des Musées Nationaux, 1996), esp. pp. 317–21; Brian Spencer, *Pilgrim souvenirs and secular badges* (London: Stationery Office, 1998); H. J. E. van Beuningen, A. M. Koldeweij and D. Kicken (eds.), *Heilig en Profaan 2: 1200 Laatmiddeleeuwse insigne suit openbarae en particuliere collecties* (Cothen, Netherlands: Stichting Middeleeuwse Religieuze en Profane Insignes, 2001); Jos Koldeweij, "'Shameless and naked images': obscene badges as parodies of popular devotion," in Sarah Blick and Rita Tekippe (eds.), *Art and architecture of late medieval pilgrimage in northern Europe and the British Isles: texts* (Leiden: Brill, 2005), pp. 493–510; Jos Koldeweij, *Geloof & Geluk: Sieraad en devotie in middeleeuws Vlaanderen* (Brughes: Bruggenmuseum, 2006).

[27] Antonio Averlino detto il Filarete, *Trattato di architettura*, ed. Anna Maria Finoli and Liliana Grassi (Milan: Edizioni il Polifilo, 1972), vol. II, p. 524.

gang, brigade, "mock kingdom" or company that put on rousing performances during carnival and events of charivari. While some of the societies and groups were of peasants and middling folk, people from all levels of society could have worn these bawdy badges during events of temporary misrule and role reversal.[28] The rustic play that was "very lascivious with very dirty words" staged by Ruzante before many Venetian senators and ladies during carnival 1525 may be an example of the kind of occasion that suited the badge wearers.[29] The six hours of performances included intermezzi in which the instrumentalists and singers were dressed in various costumes, including "eight dressed as crazy women with distaffs" dancing to the rustic, rude bagpipe. Some Venetian players appeared to be pilgrims, a persona adopted by certain figures on the genital badges, which were mocking the usual, pious wearer of the cheap, religious version of such accoutrements. Another Ruzante comedy, performed in the Paduan residence of Alvise Cornaro in February 1533, promised women that the rascal Truffo would use a little "anemaleto" (animal-like) amulet attached to their belts to satisfy them while their philandering husbands were away, an allusion to dildoes used during the absence of men but also to phallic badges and pendants.[30] The social echelon attending such a play during carnival would have already understood the allusions or learned of them by means of the humor, which may well have been heightened by stage props.

On occasion, the cheap religious badges were definitely owned by members of the elite. The French king Louis XI wore pilgrim badges of lead in 1481 and 1483, and collected over forty of them sewn on to hats and prayer books, devoutly treating them like amulets.[31] Bakhtin's "culture of laughter" crosses the very lines he drew between "high" and "low" groups, evident in the licentious margins of manuscripts illuminated by monks, for instance, or present in vernacular after-dinner speeches delivered by the elite literati during carnival. To take one example: the motif of the bagpipe-playing pig appears on badges, misericords and other church furnishings, and in the margin of a 1486 manuscript of scientific writings by Aristotle in Latin, adjacent to a jester

[28] For "abbeys," societies of fools and other organizations largely of unmarried men, see Natalie Zemon Davis, *Society and culture in early modern France*, rev. edn. (Cambridge: Polity Press, 1987), pp. 97–123; for plebeian festive brigades in Florence, David Rosenthal, "The spaces of plebeian ritual and the boundaries of transgression," in Roger Crum and John Paoletti (eds.), *Renaissance Florence: a social history* (Cambridge University Press, 2006), pp. 161–81. An excellent overview of carnival, and of charivari, is available in Edward Muir, *Ritual in early modern Europe* (Cambridge University Press, 1997), pp. 85–116.

[29] Marino Sanuto, *I diarii*, ed. Rinaldo Fulin et al., 59 vols. (Venice: F. Visenti, 1879–1903), vol. XXXVII, col. 560; trans. in *Venice: cità excelentissima, Selections from the Renaissance diaries of Marin Sanudo*, ed. Patricia Labalme and Laura Sanguineti White, trans. Linda L. Carroll (Baltimore: Johns Hopkins University Press, 2008), pp. 523–24.

[30] Ruzante, *La vaccària*, Prologue 2, in *Teatro*, ed. Ludovico Zorzi (Turin: Einaudi, 1967), p. 1047.

[31] Yvonne Hackenbroch, *Enseignes. Renaissance hat jewels* (Florence: SPES, 1996), pp. 2–3.

"fiddling" on his genitals.[32] Young noblemen in Venice and courtesans in Rome were amongst the street performers during carnival time.[33] Commonly masked and often cross-dressed or garbed as peasants and artisans, the carnival entertainers and others in the crowd presented imaginary class or erotic personas, staging multiple theatrics of homoerotic and cross-sex desire. But for those with wealth and privilege the temporary nature of the reversals enabled a license that was all the more enjoyable because boundaries were not traversed with much risk.

Although find spots for secular badges have so far been restricted to northern Europe (chiefly embedded in the deep, moist soil of the Seine and Thames rivers and in various Netherlandish sites), there is good reason to believe that they were evident or at least known in Italy, especially northern cities like Venice. Lead was a material for cheap religious artifacts in Italy too, such as a fifteenth-century medal or badge showing the Virgin and Child from Loreto.[34] Badges of greater expense were certainly familiar to Aretino, who sardonically described affected, wooing noblemen wearing them, yet he happily received one from the Duke of Mantua in 1527 and mentioned the prestigious objects in several letters.[35] Aretino's elegant attire in Marcantonio Raimondi's engraved portrait of him includes a badge of indeterminate subject on his cap.[36] He cited raunchy examples of badges as a justification for the open representation of sexual material, especially in the *Modi* engravings of sexual positions, for which he had written explicit verse. In the spirit of libertine excess and boundary crossing, and employing bountifully fluid metaphors, Aretino asked:

32 Kathleen Scott, "Sow-and-bagpipe imagery in the Miller's portrait," *Review of English Studies* 18 (1967), 287–90, esp. 289 n. 1 for the British Library's Sloane MS 748 fol. 82v; van Beuningen and Koldeweij (eds.), *Heilig en Profaan*, p. 268; Jones, *Secret middle ages*, p. 109, fig. 6.6. The musical pig features in the margin of the *Visitation* scene in the Duc de Berry's *Très riches heures* (fol. 38v), probably to contrast its rude sound with that of the Magnificat. For the sexual meaning of bagpipes see Ch. 8 below.

33 Ruzante, *Teatro*, pp. 1246–49, esp. 1249; William Prizer, "*Facciamo pure noi carnevale*: non-Florentine carnival songs of the late fifteenth and early sixteenth centuries," in Irene Alm, Alyson McLamore and Colleen Reardon (eds.), *Musica franca: essays in honor of Frank A. D'Accone* (Stuyvesant, NY: Pendragon, 1996), pp. 191, 195, 205 and passim; Eckehard Simon, "Carnival obscenities in German towns," in Ziolkowski (ed.), *Obscenity*, p. 203.

34 Floriano Grimaldi, *Loreto: Palazzo apostolico* (Bologna: Calderini, 1977), p. 122 (5.5 cm in height).

35 Aretino, *Ragionamento*, pp. 139, 236, 250; Hackenbroch, *Enseignes*, pp. 135–38. For luxurious hat badges made by goldsmiths, usually with mythological subject matter, and displayed in men's portraits (e.g. fig. 17 here) see, for example, Cellini, *Vita*, pp. 135, 155, 185; Benvenuto Cellini, *Autobiography*, trans, George Bull (Harmondsworth: Penguin, 1956), pp. 50, 63, 83; *The treatises of Benvenuto Cellini on goldsmithing and sculpture*, trans. C. R. Ashbee (New York: Dover, 1967), pp. 45–50; Hackenbroch, *Enseignes*, esp. pp. 2–3, 283–87 on the derivation from pilgrim badges and military signs.

36 Innis Shoemaker and Elizabeth Broun, *The engravings of Marcantonio Raimondi* (The Spencer Museum of Art, University of Kansas, Lawrence, 1981), pp. 150–52.

> what harm is there in seeing a man mount a woman [on the back or the front is implied]? Should beasts, then, be freer than we? It would seem to me that such a thing, given to us by nature to preserve the species, should be worn around the neck as a pendant and as a medallion (*medaglia*) on berets, since it is the spring from which gushes rivers of people and the ambrosia that the world drinks on feast days.[37]

He is probably being sarcastic here, precisely aware that such obscene badges already existed. The Italian copper plate (fig. 14) depicts an habitué of such badges, Ruzante's "anemaleto" alludes to them, and so does an anonymous Italian song of the sixteenth century warning women against a womanizer who "wears your genitals as his device (*baschiera*)."[38]

Like Aretino, Leonardo's notes on the male organ called for forthright visibility: "a man who is ashamed to name or show it is in the wrong, always being anxious to cover it up and hide what he ought to adorn and show with solemnity like a minister of the human species."[39] He may, however, be as satirical as Aretino, because he noted on another occasion that "the act of coitus and the parts employed in it are so repulsive that if it were not for the beauty of the faces and adornments of the participants and their frenetic disposition, nature would lose the human species."[40] The thought was voiced in professional anatomy too, though Leonardo's emphasis on beauty and ornamentation is novel, revealing an artist's interest in such enticements as codpieces and attractive faces.

Aretino's mention of feast days points to the importance of the calendar that regulated sexual actions. Giordano Bruno's comedy *Candelaio* referred to numerous limitations on sexual freedom and regulations (*legge*) on time and place, which must mean all the feast days, Sunday (and sometimes several other days of the week too), and other occasions on which the Church prohibited married couples from engaging in sexual intercourse.[41] In the weeks or days leading up to the taking of the Eucharist at communion, one was not to have sex, nor immediately after; widespread unease about the harmful effects of menses was bolstered by the Church's insistence on abstinence during menstruation. After carnival, for the Lenten span of forty days leading up to Easter, abstinence was advised (as it was before Christmas and after Pentecost), and in some areas

37 Pietro Aretino, *Lettere*, ed. Paolo Procaccioli, 6 vols. (Rome: Salerno, 1997–2002), vol. I, p. 425 (no. 308, 19 December 1537), translation adapted from Bette Talvacchia, *Taking positions: on the erotic in Renaissance culture* (Princeton: Princeton University Press, 1999), p. 85.

38 Prizer, "Games of Venus," 47. 39 Keele, *Leonardo*, p. 350.

40 Martin Kemp, entry in *Leonardo da Vinci* (London: South Bank Centre, 1989), p. 80.

41 Bruno, "Candelaio," pp. 285–86; Bruno, *Candlebearer*, p. 75; Thomas N. Tentler, *Sin and confession on the eve of the Reformation* (Princeton University Press, 1977), pp. 213–19; Pierre Payer, *Sex and the penitentials: the development of sexual code 550–1150* (University of Toronto Press, 1984), pp. 24–27, 127–28, and passim; Leah Otis, *Prostitution in medieval society: the history of an urban institution in Languedoc* (University of Chicago Press, 1985), pp. 85–88; Brundage, *Law, sex, and Christian society*, pp. 91–92, 155–61, 198–99, 242, 283, 451–52, 508, 601, 604; Pierre Payer, *The bridling of desire: views of sex in the later middle ages* (University of Toronto Press, 1993), pp. 98–101.

brothels shut down during Holy Week. Boccaccio's *Decameron* had an adulterous wife accuse her husband of caring too much about observing a host of holy days and thus neglecting her sexual "service," during Sabbath, Fridays, vigils, the Ember Days and the drawn-out period of Lent.[42] At carnival, then, the coming Lenten period of denial and self-control was the catalyst for license in the here and now.

Aretino's comment about feast days seems to me to allude to the subversive, unrestrained and anti-clerical nature of such raunchy tinwear. Sometimes said to be akin to ancient phallic amulets by having an apotropaic function, the secular badges might be equally warding off the alternative "Evil Eye" of Church surveillance and moral codes.[43] At times of carnival and holiday, the badges marked a relaxed calendar, during which Aretino's ostensible focus only on licit, reproductive sex would have been all the more tongue-in-cheek. Of course, the "carnivalesque" connotations of the badges made them entertaining and edgy at any time of the year, though there were probably peak periods of sales during festivals and fairs.

Satirical critique of moral restraints and anti-clerical mockery of practices like processions and pilgrimage are evident in the imagery of the badges, and the element of humor and carnivalesque "world-upside-down" audacity cannot be denied. Some phalli are being roasted on spits, carnal flesh prepared for sinful feasting (fig. 13). Since certain foods like meat, cheese, milk and eggs were banned during Lent, dining on protein-rich phalli during carnival or other periods of prohibition was deliciously subversive, all the more so when the visual joke also contravened the widespread taboo against oral sex.[44] Other genitals are crowned, a few hold scepters or are processed, like pre-Lenten kings and queens elected by their drinking clubs and merry gangs (fig. 10); jesters with penile noses wear hoods dangling genital "tails"; couples copulate out of doors; figures convey containers of dildoes, usually atop a phallic mount (fig. 11); acrobatic genitals perform on stilts or ladders; female figures are sometimes on top, controlling the breeches, which was a mark of carnival time. Quite a few genitalia masquerade as pilgrims, satirizing the impure reputation of pilgrimage (as Chaucer did in his *Canterbury tales*) while also pointing to the deliberate reversal of pious behavior performed by badge, wearer and producer alike. Many are just jaunty phalli, some

42 Giovanni Boccaccio, *Decameron*, ed. Cesare Segre (Milan: Mursia, 1966), p. 174.

43 The argument that badges were exclusively apotropaic is especially made in Ruth Mellinkoff, *Averting demons: the protecting power of medieval visual motifs and themes* (Los Angeles: Ruth Mellinkoff Publications, 2004), vol. I, pp. 141–43 and passim, on which see the acute review by Louise Marshall, *Speculum* 81 (2006), 891–93.

44 The diet of a sixteenth-century Friulian miller deliberately disobeyed the Lenten fasts and was a serious count against him in his trials before the Inquisition: Andrea Del Col, *Domenico Scandella known as Menocchio: his trials before the Inquisition (1583–1599)*, trans. John and Anne Tedeschi (Binghamton: Medieval and Renaissance Texts and Studies, 1996), pp. 14, 16, 37, 42, 63, 85, 158–59.

winged, trotting along on testicular, hairy haunches, wagging their perky and multi-penile tails, a bell often announcing their coming (fig. 12).

Notably, many of the genital creatures are on a journey, wings accentuating their speed on occasion (fig. 12) and suggesting the potential for further erection and future ejaculation. Determined on their projective path as though they have a particular place to reach (uterus or anus?), as was true too of the Pan Painter's phallus (fig. 8), they perform their public nature through open spaces, emphatically visible at the task of pilgrimage, procession, conveyance or busyness. Narrative is usually implied, and dynamic, outward, unrestricted purpose appears central to their existence. Details like open mouths or shod feet clinch the personifications. The beasts are elaborate, extroverted, active images of all-inclusive male genitalia, present also on objects like maiolica jars and letters and frequently the subject of graffiti. The shock value of much rude language and imagery – including Roman amulets and marginalia in manuscripts both medieval and early modern – simultaneously involves a moralizing intake of breath and an expulsion of laughter, averting demonic influences and melancholia, perking up the viewer's attention, reawakening one to the embodied materiality of the world. Many wearers probably hoped their badges would attract sexual good fortune while averting bad luck, Evil Eye, impotence and other dire fates.

The Bakhtinian model of a unified carnivalesque community, however, is not proven either way by the badges; cruelty, violence and exclusion were also properties of both humor and holidays. The Freudian notion of triangulation pivoting around a woman also seems unlikely. Women could wear badges, phallic or vulval, to advertise their sexual wares or take delight in temporarily licit boldness; for other women, and on other days, the badges are openly insulting. Weary pilgrims might wear the badges to entertain themselves and leaven their burdens; thugs would signal their bravado; carnival celebrants on the margins could mock others whose everyday badges declared them integrated members of organizations; temporary visitors to the marginal realm could indulgently bond with strangers precisely because the normative rules of exclusion remained unchallenged elsewhere. Overall, the functions and effects of sexual material were multiple, sometimes superficially anxious, oftentimes exultant or at least parodic, satirical and amused, and always historically conditioned.

Phallic display of Bakhtin's "grotesque body" was occasionally overt at the highest levels of power too, despite his notion of a repressive elite. A notable example is Giulio Romano's fresco from the late 1520s for the ducal apartments of the Palazzo del Te in Mantua depicting an aroused Jupiter about to enter Olympias (fig. 15), in which the god's features are possibly those of Duke Federico II Gonzaga, shown with his mistress.[45] According to legend, Jupiter in

[45] Bertelli, *King's body*, pp. 162, 164; Talvacchia, *Taking positions*, pp. 45, 47.

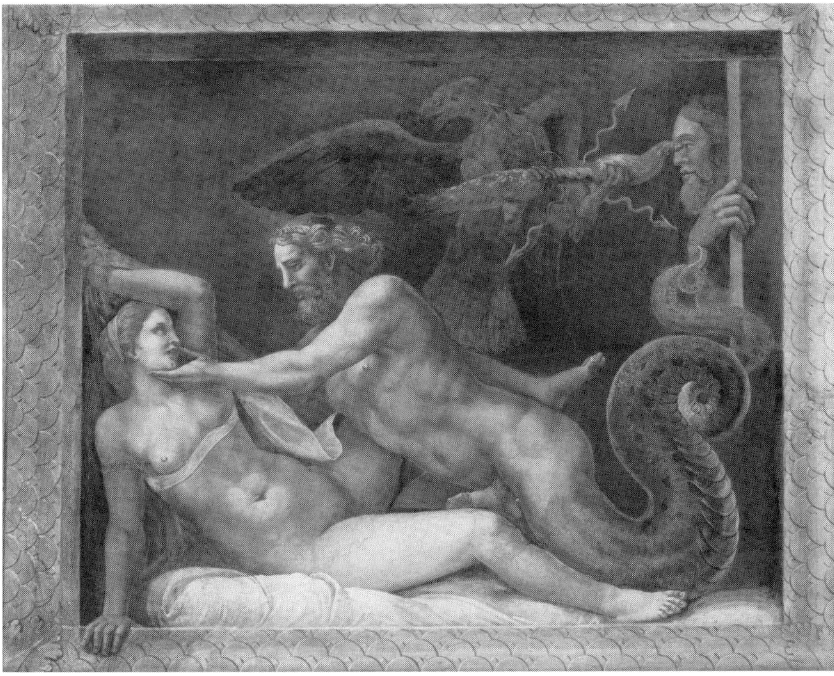

Figure 15 Giulio Romano, *Jupiter and Olympias*, 1527–28, fresco, Mantua, Palazzo del Te, Camera di Psiche

the guise of a huge serpent and in a blaze set off by his powerful thunderbolt fathered Alexander the Great, for his mother Olympias dreamt that "a thunderbolt fell upon her womb" on the night before her marriage to a mortal man was consummated.[46] Jupiter's tactic of metamorphosing into a variety of beasts in order to satisfy his lust is appropriated to the service of Gonzagan power, in a tale of assertive virility, patriarchal paternity and imperial possession. Giulio adds at the margin the element of voyeuristic inspection by the husband, Philip of Macedon (probably the artist's self-portrait), and invites the gaze of viewers below, placing Olympias' lower hand on the fictive frame's border to imply a connection with their courtly affairs. The thunderbolt, central to the tale and prominently represented in Giuilio's view of the god's imperial eagle, was both an attribute of the supreme god and an emblem of the Gonzaga, furthering the link of phallic potency between god and duke.[47] Whether or not Federico is

[46] Plutarch, *Alexander*, 2.2; Marcus Junianus Justinus, *Epitome of the Philippic history of Pompeius Trogus*, vol. I (Books 11–12), trans. J. C. Yardley (Oxford University Press, 1997), pp. 51, 69.

[47] For the thunderbolt see David Chambers and Jane Martineau (eds.), *Splendours of the Gonzaga* (London: Victoria and Albert Museum, 1981), p. 180, and no. 183.

portrayed specifically, his potency is on display, with the naturalistic details of an erect penis, testicles and pubic hair all attesting to the worldly reality of erotic power. The foreskin is not retracted, however, and the area is shaded in Giovanni Battista Scultori's reproductive engraving of the scene, tactics that only slightly mute the audacious, even amusing display of sexual power.

Fantasies of divine conquest captivated the literate elite, in visual and poetic language that featured animal elements like serpents (a common "phallic symbol"). The hybridity on display in Mantua is voiced in a more "vernacular" mode on the badges, but in both cases the genitally explicit material is thereby licensed, and derives from classical antecedents. Patriarchal propaganda in the form of fresco and print, or anti-authoritarian pewter each demonstrate not so much anxiety as creative ways in which to situate phalli on the public stage in support of claims to power. As in any historical period, men were "vulnerable" in a host of ways, but so too did groups band together to regulate, overcome and solidify power differentials. Men but also women, for instance, spoke words and enacted rituals of ridicule about cuckoldry, effectively reinforcing notions that neither honorable men nor respectable women should commit disruptive adultery.[48] The instructive fun mocked a husband's inability to control his wife and manage his household; the biting humor was engineered around the body of a woman, à la Freud, and created a community in Bakhtinian terms.

While attempts to theorize humor disagree about a great deal, three key threads tend to form a pattern in the weave.[49] The first is that humor is about release, not necessarily sexual but certainly a physical and emotional sense of immediate yet temporary relief from tension, inhibition, rationality, restrictions and norms. Whether exercised by those in the elite or at the margins, humor is often ugly, obscene, absurd, excessive and transgressive. Such ugliness was the fundamental cause of laughter according to Cicero and hence Quintilian. The Renaissance courtier learned from Castiglione's popular manual that "the laughable consists in a certain deformity (*deformità*), for we laugh only at those things that have incongruity in them and that seem to be amiss and yet are not."[50] The idea was developed by Laurent Joubert, renowned chancellor of the medical school of Montpellier and royal physician, whose *Treatise on laughter*

48 Gowing, *Common bodies*, pp. 86–87, 177–81; Pamela Allen Brown, *Better a shrew than a sheep: women, drama, and the culture of jest in early modern England* (Ithaca: Cornell University Press, 2003), pp. 83–117; Fissell, *Vernacular bodies*, pp. 197, 214–20 (for the later seventeenth century).

49 The following is largely drawn from Freud, *Jokes*; Susan Purdie, *Comedy: the mastery of discourse* (University of Toronto Press, 1993); Jerry Palmer, *Taking humour seriously* (London: Routledge, 1994); Bremmer and Roodenburg (eds.), *Cultural history of humour*; Clarke, *Laughter*, esp. pp. 2–9, 229–34.

50 Castiglione, *Courtier*, p. 106. First published in 1528.

was first printed in 1579. His chapter on the causes of laughter opened with the observation that "what we see that is ugly, deformed, improper, indecent, unfitting, and indecorous excites laughter in us, provided we are not moved to compassion. Example: if perchance one uncovers the shameful parts which by nature or public decency we are accustomed to keeping hidden, since this is ugly and yet unworthy of pity, it moves the onlookers to laughter."[51] In a sense, Joubert provides the missing link between ancient theorists, who stressed physical properties and social proprieties, and Freud's emphasis on sexual inhibition.

At the very least, as Aristotle and Cicero recognized when theorizing about Greek and Latin rhetoric respectively, humor entails the unexpected.[52] Incongruity (*disconvenienzia*) and the unexpected (*fuor d'opinione*) were the foundations of humor according to Castiglione too.[53] Having observed his compatriots amused by the unfamiliar garb and conduct of the Russian ambassador's retinue in November 1662, Pepys was dismayed that "Englishmen . . . cannot forbear laughing and jeering at everything that looks strange."[54] Something deemed physically or socially ugly or deformed, as we have seen in the previous chapter, belongs in this constellation of the laughably surprising and different. Turning the tables or invoking a double take might result from mere word play, such as the excess or doubling of a pun or incongruous imagery like hybrids (figs. 7, 10–14), or it can involve subversive aggression and exposure.

The second and related element is that jokers stick together, that is, humor is about group bonding. Others must thus be excluded and the humor often attacks perceived opponents, satirizing those who police the central rules, for instance, or ridiculing those considered lesser and marginal (women and peasants are common butts). Laughter can also forge links across groups, even over a power divide, charming the elite or disarming those positioned as inferior.

The third element follows, that humor is about power and "its operation is always political."[55] The individual maker or teller is empowered, usually at someone else's expense, and those who laugh share in the potent mastery.[56] Even when norms and rules seem to be broken or reversed, the very apprehension that the expected has been interrupted reinforces the notion of what those

51 Joubert, *Treatise on laughter*, trans. Gregory David de Rocher (Tuscaloosa: University of Alabama Press, 1980), p. 20. See also Aristotle, *Poetics*, 5 ("the shameful . . . ugly and twisted"); Cicero, *De oratore*, 2.216–89, esp. 236 on the "unseemly or ugly"; Quintilian, 6.3.8 ("a certain deformity and ugliness").

52 Aristotle, *Art of rhetoric*, 3.11.6; Cicero, *De oratore*, 2.235, 255, 289; Quintilian, 6.3.24, 84.

53 Castiglione, *Courtier*, pp. 102–40, esp. 106, 115.

54 Samuel Pepys, *The diary of Samuel Pepys*, ed. Robert Latham and William Matthews, 3 vols. (London: G. Bell and Sons, 1970–83), vol. III, p. 268.

55 Purdie, *Comedy*, p. 127. 56 Ibid., pp. 120–21.

expected norms really are. As the joke about the boundary-marking herm indicates (fig. 9), the attempt to cross a border simultaneously demarcates that line, establishing its existence and importance. Hercules unmanned by Omphale is a mythic tale about love conquering a manly hero so much that he willingly submits to womanish gossip, female labor (spinning) and feminine attire.[57] To laugh at the joke is to indicate that, of course, this is unexpected because the world is upside down. The temporarily disruptive laugh is also tinged with the reassuring sense that the object of fun is ridiculous, and that all is still actually right with the world, the normative world. Such tales affirm the parameters of proper gender behavior.

Indeed, the very circumstances and theorization of humor, by figures like Castiglione and Freud, entailed clear gender differentiations, and situated women in particular as receivers or butts of jokes rather than as producers, even though historical evidence points to women's lively contribution to humorous discourse despite strictures against it.[58] In the fifteenth-century court of Isabella d'Este or the court of sixteenth-century France, parties in seventeenth-century Netherlands or the household of a powerful family in Norfolk during several decades of the early to mid-seventeenth century, women were in on the joke, indeed telling many of them, learning and reiterating the language in letters, taverns, streets, markets, lyings-in, law courts, brothels, libertine parties and evening gatherings.[59] Secular badges blatantly personified vulvas as well as male genitals, and the male characters are often subservient, indicating that stock, clear gender divides do not always illuminate how laughter is evoked.

Not all three of these elements of humor are necessarily present, or weigh in equally, and the functions and venues of humor can vary considerably, but each factor contributes to the pleasure one gets. The wit or absurdity has often escaped scholars, in relation to images such as the Greek krater (fig. 8–9) or the fifteenth-century engraving plate (fig. 14), though less so in the case of material more easily identified as "popular" like the badges. Rather than assume

[57] According to Sidney in 1595, the subject "breeds both delight and laughter: for the representing of so straunge a power in Love, procures delight, and the scornefulnesse of the action, stirreth laughter": *Defense of poesy*, quoted in David Brumble, *Classical myths and legends in the middle ages and Renaissance: a dictionary of allegorical meanings* (Westport, CT: Greenwood Press, 1998), p. 162, with further examples.

[58] Castiglione, *Courtier*, pp. 122, 138; Freud, *Jokes*. Hence, the stereotype that women, especially feminists, do not have a sense of humor. See Purdie, *Comedy*, pp. 128–49.

[59] Brantôme, *Les dames galantes*, ed. Maurice Rat (Paris: Éditions Garnier Frères, 1965); Rudolf Dekker, *Humour in Dutch culture of the Golden Age* (New York: Palgrave, 2001), pp. 96–98; Brown, *Better a shrew*, esp. ch. 1; Fissell, *Vernacular bodies*, p. 70; Brown, "Jesting rights," pp. 305–14; Cipolla and Malacarne (eds.), *El più soave*, pp. 391–93; Molly Bourne, "Mail humour and male sociability: sexual innuendo in the epistolary domain of Francesco II Gonzaga," in Matthews-Grieco (ed.), *Erotic cultures*, pp. 211–14.

an aura of mystery or gravity about the pictorial phallus, an understanding of what is normative or expected in a particular historical and cultural context often helps us get the joke.

Testicular signs

The hairy haunches of many phallic creatures allude to testicles. In word and image, testicles were significant in early modern culture, mocked as mere baubles on the one hand, proudly displayed as part of a codpiece or on a family's coat of arms on the other. Unlike *phallus*, the two predominant Latin words for scrotal stores of seed, *testiculus* (testicles) and *coleus* (balls), were readily adapted into the vernacular.[60] Early modern English terms are compiled in Randle Cotgrave's definition of the French *couillon* in 1611: "a cod, stone, testicle, cullion." Sometimes the testicles were regarded in the same syndecdochal way as the penile shaft, for a scrotal word could mean a man's entire genital apparatus. Thus, Florio's Italian dictionary recorded that *scroto* was "the outward skin of the cods wherein are the stones of a man," and that *coglioni* meant "stones or testicles," but *coglia* referred to "a mans whole privities" and a *cogliuto* was "a man well tooled."[61]

On their own, obscene balls were the subject of insults when snidely thought of as small or as body parts that were toyed with and fingered. Thus sixteenth-century goldsmiths hurled abuse at each other in Rome by speaking of wares as "pimping little trash" (*bordellerie piccole*) or dismissive baubles (*coglionerie*).[62] In the same city, "Messer Coglione" was a satirized pedant in an Italian pasquinade of 1510, reducing the whole man to one ignoble body part, and alluding to the reputation of tutors for pederasty.[63] Having learned his trade as a bawdy wordsmith in the same environment, Aretino resorted several times to belittling words about the balls, joining anti-Petrarchan critics, for instance, in referring to flowery poetic discourse as *coglionerie* (mere trifles and trickeries).[64] *Coglione* was an easy insult for the painter

[60] For the Latin see Adams, *Latin sexual vocabulary*, pp. 66–67.

[61] Florio, *Queen Anna's new world of words*, pp. 107–08, 484. Also Williams, *Glossary*, pp. 72–73; Williams, *Dictionary*, pp. 266–67. Balls did, of course, give rise to sexual language: Williams, *Dictionary*, pp. 61–63; Williams, *Glossary*, pp. 34–35.

[62] Cellini, *Vita*, pp. 125, 130; Cellini, *Autobiography*, pp. 44, 47.

[63] Anne Reynolds, "Cardinal Oliviero Carafa and the early cinquecento tradition of the Feast of Pasquino," *Humanistica Lovaniensia* 34A (1985), 197.

[64] Aretino, *Cortigiana*, ed. Romano, p. 61 (*c.* 1525); also Aretino's letter to Titian of September 1547 (*Lettere*, vol. IV, no. 222), and *I modi*, 8.1. *Coglionare* meant "to play with ones stones. Also to cogge or deceive one": Florio, *Queen Anna's new world of words*, p. 107. For English, chiefly referring to the penis, see "bauble" and "toy" in Partridge, *Shakespeare's bawdy*, pp. 62, 203; Williams, *Dictionary*, pp. 77–79, 1412–13; Williams, *Glossary*, pp. 36–37, 311–12.

Caravaggio to hurl in August 1603 at a rival artist named Giovanni Baglione, again in the competitive setting of Rome.[65]

Amongst the elite, those baubles or "family jewels" were during much of the sixteenth century encased in eye-catching, padded codpieces, though more ordinary cloth gussets and flaps had already been devised after tight-fitting hose and shorter doublets came into fashion in the course of the fourteenth and early fifteenth centuries. The function was primarily to enable ease of access and unlacing for urination, though the embellished variety also perhaps protected the genitals from swords, purses and other items suspended from a man's waist. Evidence from surviving costumes indicates that the fancy codpiece did not house the genitals and was instead constructed around a frame made of material like leather or tightly pleated cloth, and was either empty or filled with cloth or straw.[66] Some of these adornments became so elaborate and awkward, at least in the pictorialized form, that if actually worn they may have impeded bodily functions; their purpose, in other words, went beyond the utilitarian or the decorous. As the English name implies, it was not so much a "penis sheath" as simultaneously a means to store, protect and accentuate the cods, that is, the scrotum.[67] In the Romance languages, variants on the Italian *braghetta* stemmed from the Latin *bracae*, for breeches, and thus the name was about an item of clothing, as it was in German (*latz*, for flap), but writers and artists drew overt genital inferences.

The codpiece was "the first piece of harness in the arming of a warrior" according to Rabelais' satire of 1532, derived from fig-leaves which were specially suited to "covering and arming the ballocks," that is, the testicles. Men were imitating Nature's cunning coverage of all "germs and seeds" in husks and other shells which were "fine, strong natural codpieces." The fanciful costume addition protected the site of stored seed, called "profitable ball-bags" whose load had to be spent before the Judgement Day because "such precious stuff should not be foolishly wasted."[68] When Shakespeare inverted the word codpiece to coin "peascod," he made more overt the testicular reference apparently already present in the "rustic custom of using a pea-pod as a love token."[69] In 1580, at a time when the codpiece was at the height of its ornate elaboration,

65 Walter Friedlaender, *Caravaggio studies* (Princeton University Press, 1955), p. 271.

66 Janet Arnold, *Patterns of fashion: the cut and construction of clothes for men and women c1560–1620* (London: Macmillan, 1985), pp. 53–55, 58–59, 61, 62, 63.

67 The phrase frequently occurs in Grace Vicary, "Visual art as social data: the Renaissance codpiece," *Cultural Anthropology* 4 (1989), 3–25.

68 Rabelais, *Gargantua*, pp. 307–09, 361, 362. See also J. C. Persels, "Bragueta humanistica, or humanism's codpiece," *Sixteenth Century Journal* 28 (1997), 79–99.

69 Williams, *Glossary*, p. 231; see also Partridge, *Shakespeare's bawdy*, pp. 77–78, 80–81, and Williams, *Glossary*, pp. 72–73. For the codpiece in England, see Fisher, *Materializing gender*, pp. 59–82. "Pea" (pisello) was used for the male genitals in Italian: Toscan, *Carnaval*, pp. 355, 538–39, 812–13, 914, 968–69, 1416.

Michel de Montaigne disdainfully characterized it as "that vain and useless model of a member that we cannot even decently mention by name, which however, we show off and parade in public."[70] The *membre* was a polite term for the entire genitals, and the *modelle* shows there was no doubt about the bodily referent that was simultaneously concealed yet exhibited in *parade en public*.

As Montaigne understood, the codpiece both revealed and concealed, exhibiting a hollow model. Contradiction is fundamental to the codpiece, alluding to body parts and masculinity but intensely artificial (*vain* and *inutile* for Montaigne) and hence, according to the principles of the day, inherently feminine. Attacked as lewd on the one hand, codpieces were overt signs of exhibitionism on the other; in either case, contemporaries regarded them as noteworthy and symbolic of a cocky, youthful manliness. In response to the shortening of doublets and the abandonment of long tunics, the consequent sight of male genitals and rear views concerned preachers and legislators during the fifteenth and sixteenth centuries, especially when it was of youths whose display was interpreted as coquettish and arousing. In 1425, the preacher Bernardino of Siena told Florentines that parents were pimping their sons, letting them wear short doublets and "stockings with a little piece in front and one in the back, so that they show a lot of flesh for the sodomites." The Sienese heard his similar worries in 1427, and he also told them that such enticing youths were always "having the sodomite on his tail."[71] I suspect that one reason for the development of ornate codpieces was that they drew attention away from the buttocks and thence implied that the wearer was never a "passive," effeminate sodomite but only an "active," virile man (whether his sexual partner were to be male or female). The implications of reckless or indecorous youth might then only appeal all the more to certain male sitters of any age who chose to portray themselves wearing outrageous, extravagant codpieces as though forever young, rebellious and virile.

The elaborate codpieces evident in portraits, which advance the image's overall purpose of attracting attention and offering declarative statements about the sitter, are protruding, conspicuous, usually colorful and decorative items of fashion. Modern scholars speak of the "conspicuous resemblance between certain forms of the cod-piece and the erect penis" but the codpiece

70 Montaigne, *Essais*, vol. I, p. 118, translation adapted from *The complete works of Montaigne: essays, travel journal, letters*, trans. Donald Frame (Stanford University Press, 1958), p. 86.

71 Michael Rocke, "Sodomites in fifteenth-century Tuscany: the views of Bernardino of Siena," in Kent Gerard and Gert Hekma (eds.), *The pursuit of sodomy: male homosexuality in Renaissance and Enlightenment Europe* (New York: Harrington Park Press, 1989), pp. 12–15. For unease about codpieces, primarily German, but not for the explicit mention of sodomy, see Thomas Lüttenberg, "The cod-piece – a Renaissance fashion between sign and artefact," *Medieval History Journal* 8 no. 1 (2005), 59–67; Lyndal Roper, "Blood and codpieces: masculinity in the early modern German town," in Roper, *Oedipus and the devil*, pp. 117–20.

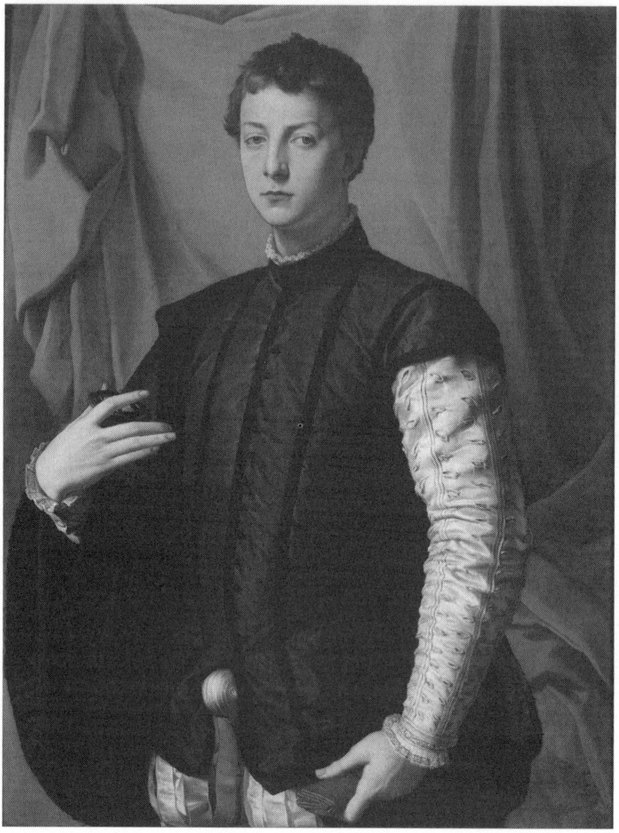

Figure 16 Agnolo Bronzino, *Portrait of Lodovico Capponi*, 1550s, oil on panel, 116 × 85 cm, New York, The Frick Collection

did not literally mirror genital forms and the shapes observed in contemporary images do not include a rigid, erect pole.[72] Rather, there are three basic types, one of which rises up (not out) with a slight curve (but not erectile rigidity) or, often, it begins to push aside clothing of another color which emphasizes its animation and potential for projection (fig. 16). Another form is an undifferentiated, ovoid bulge that is not distinctly penile, worn by Emperor Charles V in

[72] The quotation is from Lüttenberg, "Cod-piece," 49–81, at 53, and see also 66, where another scholar's word "phallus" becomes "penis." The elaborate codpieces "assumed the shape of a permanent erection" according to Aileen Ribeiro, *Dress and morality*, 2nd edn. (Oxford: Berg, 2003), p. 62. Fisher, on the other hand, rightly notes that "many of them were distinctly non-phallic": *Materializing gender*, p. 68.

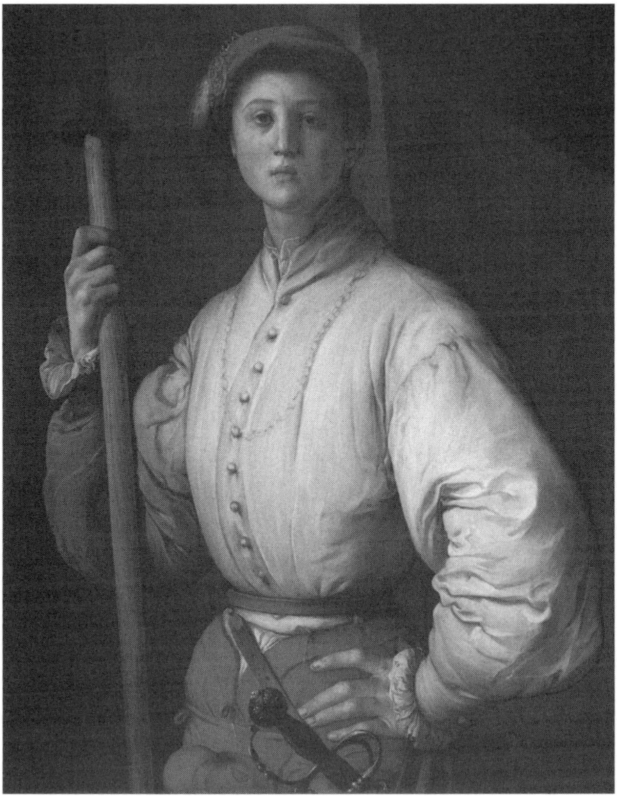

Figure 17 Pontormo, *Portrait of a halberdier*, 1529–30, oil on panel transferred to canvas, 92 × 72 cm, Los Angeles, California, J. Paul Getty Museum

Jakob Seisenegger's portrait of 1532, for instance, or Cranach's good thief (fig. 61). A third sort is comprised of inventive adaptations of the bulge, curving in one or two circles (fig. 17) or decorated so that it appears to be about to spring or gush forth (fig. 18).[73] Don Garzia, son of Eleanora of Toledo and Cosimo I de' Medici, was buried upon his death at the age of fifteen in 1562 wearing a suit decorated with "a velvet cod-piece, made like a folded

[73] For this range, see the illustrations in Loren Campbell, *Renaissance portraits* (New Haven: Yale University Press, 1990), including Pl. 255 for the Seisenegger portrait; Gundula Wolter, *Die Verpackung des männlichen Geschlechts: Eine illusrierte Kulturgeschichte der Hose* (Marburg: Jonas Verlag, 1991).

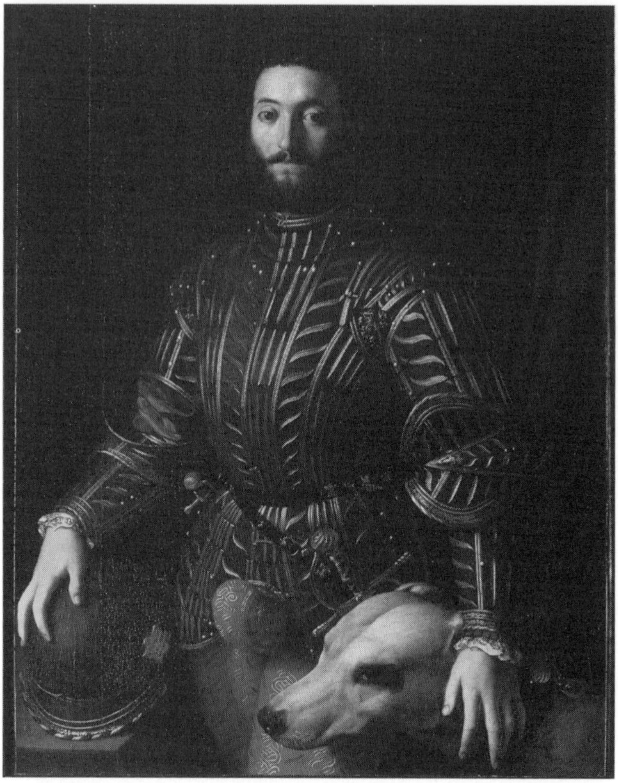

Figure 18 Agnolo Bronzino, *Portrait of Guidobaldo della Rovere*, 1531–32, oil on canvas, 114 × 86 cm, Florence, Palazzo Pitti, Galleria Palatina

pouch, decorated with couched gold cord and cut to reveal the crimson satin lining which pads it out."[74] The common ovoid shape in this case was dramatized by the red slashes, hinting at the hidden, heated flesh underneath and suggesting the potential for blood-derived semen to burst forth.

What is most shared by all these varieties is a non-flaccid, outwardly directed, enlarged mass, implying a degree of tumescence. A load of semen was thus signified because, according to medical theory, swelling and erection were caused by the accumulation of semen, composed of air (*pneuma*) and blood. The codpiece creates the impression of future release, as Aretino had imagined. His letter of justification for *I modi*, dated late in 1537, argued that the generative organ – hence implicitly one endowed with testicles – should be granted

[74] Arnold, *Patterns of fashion*, p. 53.

a special feast day "rather than shutting it away in a bit of cloth or silk."[75] He thus wanted the male genitals to be imagined bursting out of their codpiece, a defiant extension he also pictured in a letter of November that same year, when he boasted that, unlike impotent Titian, the sculptor Jacopo Sansovino and himself swore they would face death still feeling the sap rising and lust pricking in their codpieces.[76]

The punch packed by codpieces consisted of Aretino's "sap," blood and *pneuma*, beginning to swell up and project beyond its casing. When "knots" in the ties of a codpiece were thought to cause impotence, they were regarded as obstructing the entire genitals, impeding the proper production and flow of semen that led to an erection. According to the etiology of impotence outlined in the witch-hunting manual *Malleus maleficarum* (1486), it had two main causes, "suppressing the hardness of the member" and "halting the sending of spirits to the limbs in which the virtue of motion resides, as if closing off the seed's path."[77] Codpieces were not mentioned, but as their use grew they became the material focus of rumors and rituals. Perhaps spurred by practical difficulties with the complex arrangement of cloth and bindings, numerous male writers attributed impotence to ligatures in codpieces caused by magic (usually cast by women or the occasional jealous male suitor). Italian prostitutes were said furtively to remove and knot the fastenings of codpieces in order to render a man impotent, then restoring them in order to free him from that condition, a tale that hints at ways in which sex workers might assuage as well as control their clients.[78] Friars and love magicians, amongst others, undid binding spells that notoriously befell the codpiece ties of newly wed husbands.[79] To read codpieces as literally and simply penile is to mistake their broader genital reference and miss their allusion to virility that went beyond the merely physical to encompass familial, political, misogynist and amorous assertion.

While the codpiece actually contained very little except padding, it could be deployed for a variety of strategic, representational purposes. Red leggings and a codpiece suit the determined halberdier (fig. 17) painted by Pontormo, firmly holding his weapon in front of a fortress's prominent edge and jutting one elbow into the viewer's space.[80] This Florentine patriot seduces all to his noble, manly cause. The sword's dark pommel, ornamented with a white flourish at its top,

75 Talvacchia, *Taking positions*, pp. 86, 256 n. 1.

76 Aretino, *Lettere*, vol. I, p. 341 no. 244 (23 November 1537 letter to Luigi Anichini).

77 Kramer and Sprenger, *Hammer of witches*, p. 188, repeated on pp. 321, 422.

78 Ioannis Wieri (d. 1588), *Opera omnia* (Amsterdam: Peter van den Berge, 1660), p. 328.

79 For example, Cotgrave, *Dictionarie*, s.v. *Esguillette*; Emmanuel Le Roy Ladurie, "The aiguillette: castration by magic" (1974), in Siân Reynolds and Ben Reynolds (trans.), *The mind and method of the historian* (University of Chicago Press, 1981), pp. 84–96; Darmon, *Tribunal*, pp. 27, 40–42; Williams, *Dictionary*, pp. 769–70 (knot); Ruggiero, *Machiavelli in love*, pp. 23–24.

80 Elizabeth Cropper, *Pontormo: portrait of a halberdier* (Los Angeles: Getty Museum Studies on Art, 1997).

acts as a symbol of erection and perhaps hints at ejaculation, whereas the large codpiece consists of two swollen balls notably without a central anchor. These enlarged testicular signifiers virtually act like "apples," a metaphor for male buttocks as well as female breasts, and a key component of the painting's enduring appeal is that its erotic enticement remains ambiguous, open and inviting without settling into a definitive penile or sexual identity.

Pontormo's younger associate Bronzino often portrayed aristocratic youths with distinctive, telling codpieces. Guidobaldo della Rovere sports a fiery red, gold-embroidered confection in a portrait that declares his independence by means of inscription and visual assertion (fig. 18).[81] Eighteen years of age and locked in a dispute with his father about marrying for dynastic rather than personal reasons, the sitter displays his manliness through new armour, codpiece, stance and alert dog, complemented by a more coded avowal, an inscription in Greek on the helmet that states "It will certainly be as I have decided." Bulging forward in a package that appears to be curled up into one large ball but able to spring forth forcefully, the codpiece promises projection, of a kind that unites penile and scrotal components.

Family honor and personal virility are also evident in Bronzino's portrait of a man from the Capponi clan (fig. 16).[82] *Capponi* (capons, cocks castrated so they would fatten), were commonly invoked in references to castration and cruel jokes must often have assailed men of the noble Florentine family. All the more reason for Lodovico Capponi to have himself portrayed with a codpiece thrust forward from his breeches, its white stark against the jerkin's surrounding black, a determined reiteration of his family's heraldic colors of black and white. Young enough to still be beardless, Lodovico nevertheless holds a cameo of a beloved in one hand, asserting his right to engage in poetic games of love. Here, the aggressive codpiece asserts, is no castrated or sexless man, but a courtly member of a clan with a proud history and a sexual and manly as well as reproductive future.

The codpiece is a false simulacrum, but it is going too far to say that it matches uterine images because the outward male genitals supposedly resembled the interior female reproductive system. Nothing in the texts or depictions of codpieces suggests that the accoutrement was "transformed into the womb," or that it bears "a remarkable resemblance not just to a prolapsed uterus but to a swaddled child."[83] The codpiece can approximate a flask because of the seed it holds and which will be poured into a predetermining uterine

[81] See Patricia Simons, "Alert and erect: masculinity in some Italian Renaissance portraits of fathers and sons," in Richard Trexler (ed.), *Gender rhetorics: postures of dominance and submission in history* (Binghamton: Medieval and Renaissance Texts and Studies, 1994), pp. 163–86, repeated in Lüttenberg, "Cod-piece," pp. 73–76. See also Maurice Brock, *Bronzino* (Paris: Flammarion, 2002), pp. 48–52.

[82] Brock, *Bronzino*, pp. 140–43.

[83] Laqueur, *Making sex*, p. 94 and caption to fig. 40.

vessel. It can indeed look "often decidedly unphallic, . . . broader at the end than at the base, blunt not sharp, decorated with ribbonlike braids," as Laqueur observed, but this is because it is not a "bundle for the penis" alone. The ribbons, or dandy's feathers on their caps (fig. 17), or projective apparati evident in portraits all suggest a cocky spraying forth on to the world. And to contrast the "phallic and scrotal" or the "penetrative and reproductive" elements is not only to separate the phallus from the testicles (a true castration), but also to reduce the functions of each to modern notions.[84] Like Rabelais' natural husks covering seeds, the pea-pod protecting and storing its contents alluded to a man's entire genital package of semen along with its delivery system. While the codpiece was rarely evident by the late sixteenth century, another kind of spermatic container began to be more widely distributed during the mid-seventeenth century: the condom.[85] The codpiece's outward flaunting of genital health, vigorously denying the ravages of injury or the new disease of syphilis, was in a sense replaced by another spermatic container. Technological ingenuity devised the less visible, protective sheath, denoting suspicion of sexual partners and the need for manly self-management, at a time when male semen was coming to be understood as less essential to female pleasure and thus could be withheld.[86]

The visual efficacy of the codpiece relies on the knowledge that testicles were signifiers of male sexual potency, as they had been since the ancient Greeks and Romans.[87] When criticizing Michelangelo for the depiction of male genitals in the *Last judgement* fresco of the Sistine Chapel, Aretino used a common euphemism, "virili," for the testicles.[88] Testicular power was legal as well as medical. The Latin *testis* was primarily an anatomical term (along with *testiculus*) for the obscene *coleus* (balls) but *testis* literally meant a witness, a testifier, and hence the anatomist Vesling was punning on the Latin when he observed that testicles "witness strength and man-hood."[89] Several decades earlier but from the same University of

84 The quotations are from Fisher, *Materializing gender*, p. 74.

85 Jeannette Parisot, *Johnny come lately: a short history of the condom* (1985), trans. and enlarged Bill McCann, rev. Geraldine Rudge (London: Journeyman, 1987), pp. 10–17.

86 See Chs. 6 and 7 below for women needing male semen.

87 Henderson, *Maculate muse*, pp. 113, 118, 124–26; Adams, *Latin sexual vocabulary*, 66–71.

88 Aretino's letter addressed to Michelangelo, dated in a confused manner but probably of November 1545, survives in handwritten form ("i membri genitali"). It was altered when printed in 1550, and there dated to July 1547 ("i membri genitali et virili"). Both versions are in Paola Barocchi and Renzo Ristori (eds.), *Il carteggio di Michelangelo*, 5 vols. (Florence: SPES, 1965–83),vol. IV, pp. 215–19.

89 Vesling, *Anatomy*, p. 23; Adams, *Latin sexual vocabulary*, pp. 67–68, 212, and passim; *Isidore of Seville: the medical writings*, trans. William Sharpe, *Transactions of the American Philosophical Society*, n.s., 54 no. 2 (1964), 45; Partridge, *Shakespeare's bawdy*, pp. 24, 63 (bawl); Rubinstein, *Dictionary*, pp. 174–75 (oaths), 205 (proof), 308 (witness); Williams, *Dictionary*, pp. 1376–77; Williams, *Glossary*, pp. 34–35 (ball).

Padua, Alessandro Massaria's gynecological book drew a misogynist analogy: "*Testes* signifies properly, witnesses; and a man without such witnesses will have bad success in his cause, if women be of the Jury."[90] Other medical authorities also pointed out that "the Stones are called Testes because they are witnesses of virilitie," as the English surgeon and anatomist Helkiah Crooke put it in 1615.[91] The double meaning of potency informed the oath-taking gesture in Genesis (24.2, 47.29) of placing a hand under the senior man's "thigh," or genitals. It underpinned the ritual of papal inspection when a tactile witness had to affirm the man's right to hold high office, and it informs today's notion of what it means to be truly "a man with balls." "Without *testes*, one could not 'bear witness,'" that is, have the legal authority and social rank to testify.[92]

The Biblical tradition joined with classical heritage, for puns were common in such antique texts as the raunchy *Priapea*, in which *magnis testibus* connoted both trustworthy witnesses and large testicles in the phrase "I've got balls enough to spill it."[93] On the other hand, around 45 CE the Roman orator Cicero tried to keep the senses apart, observing a contextual difference: "*Testes*, in place of judgment [a court of law], is a very honest word; in another place it is not so."[94] But the play with the legal sense of testifying to a man's virility was too good an allusion to pass up. The lengthy mock *Testament* of the French poet François Villon (*c.* 1461) came to a close with the note that "this he swore on his testicle (*couillon*)."[95] In the mid-fifteenth-century curia and papal court of Rome, anecdotes and bawdy jokes collected by the humanist Poggio Bracciolini included a joke that relied on awareness of the Latin word's legalistic sense. A maligned young husband proves his

90 Alessandro Massaria (d. 1598), *Praelectiones de morbis mulierum* ... (Leipzig: Abraham Lamberg, 1600), republished in *Practica medica* (Frankfurt: Nicolai Bassaei, 1601), translated by R. Turner as *De morbis foemineis: the woman's counsellour* (London: John Streater, 1657), reissued in 1686. Here quoted from the first English translation, p. 12.

91 Crooke, *Mikrokosmographia*, p. 204. Other examples include André du Laurens, *Opera anatomica* (Lyon: Ioannis Baptistae Buysson, 1593), pp. 230–31, repeated in du Laurens, *Historica anatomica*, p. 340; Bauhin, *Theatrum anatomicum*, p. 180; Duval, *Hermaphrodits*, p. 19; Caspar Bartholin, *Anatomicae institutiones corporis humani* (Oxford: William Turner, 1633), pp. 99, 103; John Bulwer, *Anthropometamorphosis* (London: J. Hardesty, 1650), p. 208; [Thomas Bartholin], *Bartholinus anatomy: Made from the precepts of his father, and from the observations of all modern anatomists, together with his own* (London: John Streater, 1668), pp. 54–55, 57; Nicholas Culpeper, *A directory for midwives* (London: Peter Cole, 1651), pp. 11–13; Sharp, *Midwives book*, p. 71.

92 Scarborough, *Medical terminologies*, p. 211.

93 *Priapus poems*, 15.7, and another usage probably occurs at 2.1. See also, for example, Petronius, *Satyricon*, 44.14; Martial, 2.72.8, 7.62.5–6.

94 *The familiar epistles of M. T. Cicero* (London: Edward Griffin, 1620), p. 471; Cicero, *Epistularum ad Familiares*, 9.22.4.

95 François Villon, *The poems of François Villon*, new edn., trans. Galway Kinnell (Hanover: University Press of New England, 1977), pp. 152–53.

manhood by calling on relatives to be visual witnesses (*vos testes*) of his *egregiae priapo*, a distinguished priapic organ (with *testes*).[96] Female readers also knew the term. Writing stories that were dedicated to a duchess in 1525, the Florentine litterateur Agnolo Firenzuola used a simple euphemism for the balls of a priest caught in adultery and threatened with their excision: "i testimoni."[97]

Since the testicles were a potent symbol of manhood, verbal attacks against them could be aimed at a man's core honor and social identity. Aretino, ever adept at sharp critique, singled out the condottiere Bartolomeo Colleoni, who served Venice for more than twenty years until he died in 1475, but whose memory lived on in that city because a life-size equestrian monument was dedicated to the general. From a long line of renowned soldiers with the family name that was often written as *coglioni* or variants, all with the same telling sound as the Italian word for "balls," Bartolomeo and his kin must have been used to endless jokes amongst the troops. Aretino's quips were particularly biting, and occurred over a span of more than a decade, indicating that play on the proper noun was always good for a laugh. The anonymous "Captain with a bad name" mentioned in his comedy *Il marescalco* (published in 1533) was surely Colleoni.[98] The following year, Aretino's *Ragionamento* opened with an orgy in a nunnery, overseen by the ecclesiastical "father General" pretentiously dressed up and strutting like a military commander called "Bortolameo Coglioni."[99] From Aretino's references, the impression is that, rather than ballsy, the man was full of bollocks (*coglioneria*).

In military camps, taverns, streets and palaces, the only thing for the family to do was face down the jibes by self-confidently proclaiming the testicles as a public, overt sign of pride and virility. A family boast from the Florentine Martelli involved threatening their opponents with overwhelming numbers, symbolized by the fact that "we have in our house thirty two pairs

96 Poggio Bracciolini, *Facezie*, ed. Marcello Ciccuto (Milan: Biblioteca Universale Rizzoli, 1983), p. 164.

97 Agnolo Firenzuola, *Opere*, ed. Adriano Seroni (Florence: Sansoni, 1958), pp. 128, 130. Around the same time, *coglioni* were "witnesses (*testimoni*)" "of every fucking pleasure" in Aretino's *I modi*: Talvacchia, *Taking positions*, p. 199; see also Boggione and Casalegno, *Dizionario*, p. 374.

98 Aretino, *Commedie*, p. 36, also 79. During carnival in 1532, Bartolomeo was ironically mentioned in a Sienese play amongst "the good men of old": Accademici Intronati di Siena, *Gl'ingannati* (Bologna: Arnaldo Forni, 1984), B vii verso.

99 Aretino, *Ragionamento*, p. 28. He is also disparaging about "Bartolomeo Coglioni" in the *Cortigiana*, a comedy he wrote in Rome in 1524–25, and in a letter of 25 June 1537: Aretino, *Cortigiana*, ed. Romano, p. 126; *Lettere*, vol. I, p. 230. Even the biography by a poet in Colleoni's employ during the 1470s implied that his claim of descent from Hercules was unfounded: Antonio Cornazzano, *Vita del Bartolomeo Colleoni*, trans. and ed. G. Crevatin (Rome: Vecchiarelli, 1990), pp. 8–9.

of balls (*coglioni*)."[100] Few dared make derogatory jokes about the balls (*palle*) on the Medici coat of arms, and it was probably only in a later century that someone quipped about Cosimo il Vecchio's placement of *palle* all over the refurbished monastery of S. Marco that "he has emblazoned even the monks' privies with his balls."[101] Although *palle* was not a common term for testicles, playing ball games was a euphemism for copulating, and at least one sixteenth-century comment caught the overlap between the Medici emblem and an allusion to testicles. During the siege of their city by Medicean forces in 1530 some Florentines noted that the Medici could either sweetly accept the city's submission or they would turn nasty because they had the "balls" (*palle*) to inflict great pain on the citizens' testicles.[102] Portrayed in reference to that very siege, Pontormo's sitter (fig. 17) is probably the Republican Francesco Guardi and the prominence of the balls of his hot red codpiece may well answer the Medicean threat.

As described by a document in June 1454, the Colleoni coat of arms consisted of two white pairs of testicles against a red ground and below that one red pair against a white background, the color ensuring absolute, declarative clarity although some surviving examples are carved in marble (fig. 19).[103] Well paid by the Venetian government in order not to defect (as he had done twice in the 1440s), Bartolomeo was one of the richest men in Italy, and his patronage of various castles as well as an elaborate funerary chapel in Bergamo designed by Giovanni Antonio Amadeo ensured that the *coglioni* were liberally spread throughout his domain on coats of arms.

Disappointed by his lack of actual battle experience and hence glory earned under Venetian employ, Bartolomeo provided in his will for a monument that resulted in his longed-for eternal fame. Andrea del Verrocchio's bronze equestrian statue was eventually unveiled in a prominent Venetian square in March 1496, but only after a complicated history that included local opposition to the individualistic celebration in a public square (fig. 20).[104] Not long after his death, Bartolomeo was rumored to be "the greatest usurer and the most

[100] Poliziano, *Detti*, p. 85.

[101] Christopher Hibbert, *The rise and fall of the house of Medici* (London: Allen Lane, 1974), p. 42, without attribution or date.

[102] Giovio, *Lettere*, vol. I, p. 128 (letter to Marco Contarini, 9 August 1530). See Toscan, *Carnaval*, pp. 468, 693, 1123, 1249, 1342–43 for ball games, where balls are read as penile.

[103] For the early family history, including names, and the document of 1 June 1454 describing the coat of arms, see Bortolo Belotti, *La vita di Bartolomeo Colleoni* (Bergamo: Istituto Italiano dArti Grafiche Editore, 1923), pp. 37–41, 597. Numerous illustrations of the stemma are available there, and also Gianmario Petrò, "Stemmi colleoneschi a Bergamo e nel territorio: per una geografia delle presenze," in Lelio Pagani (ed.), *Bartolomeo Colleoni e il territorio bergamasco* (Bergamo: Edizioni dell'Ateneo, 2000), pp. 13–35.

[104] Andrew Butterfield, *The sculptures of Andrea del Verrocchio* (New Haven: Yale University Press, 1997), pp. 158–83, 232–36; Dario Covi, *Andrea del Verrocchio: life and work* (Florence:

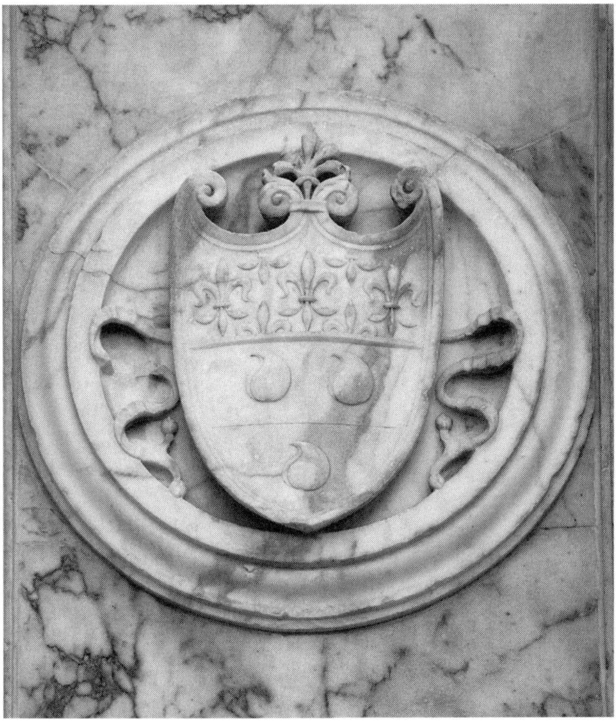

Figure 19 Colleoni stemma, detail of pedestal of fig. 20, *c.* 1495, marble, Venice, Campo di SS. Giovanni e Paolo

avaricious and least liberal man the world has ever had," presumably because more than 200,000 unspent ducat coins were discovered in his castle at Malpaga.[105] Decades later, the fame-seeking mercenary was represented by Aretino as vain and over-reaching. An anonymous late fifteenth- or early sixteenth-century poem in Latin, written on a sheet of sketches by Verrocchio, also implied ongoing disquiet about such matters as the non-Venetian origin of the sculptor.[106] Its description of the sculptor as *crassus* (stout, stupid, "dense") is unexpected in seemingly solemn, laudatory verse. *Crassus* also means rude or

Leo Olschki, 2005), pp. 151–63, 346–49. For a satirical reference to the gilded and high/haughty statue see Vittorio Rossi, "Il canzoniere inedito di Andrea Michieli detto Squarzòla or Strazzòla," *Giornale storico della letteratura italiana* 26 (1895), 11.

105 Evelyn Welch, *Art in Italy 1350–1500* (Oxford University Press, 1997), p. 272, quoting a report of the Milanese ambassador of 17 November. Colleoni died on 2 November. Some contemporary comments suggest he virtually bought his right to construct a monument by paying the Venetian State some of his fortune: Butterfield, *Verrocchio*, pp. 164–66.

106 Charles Seymour, Jr., *The sculpture of Verrocchio* (London: Studio Vista, 1971), p. 173.

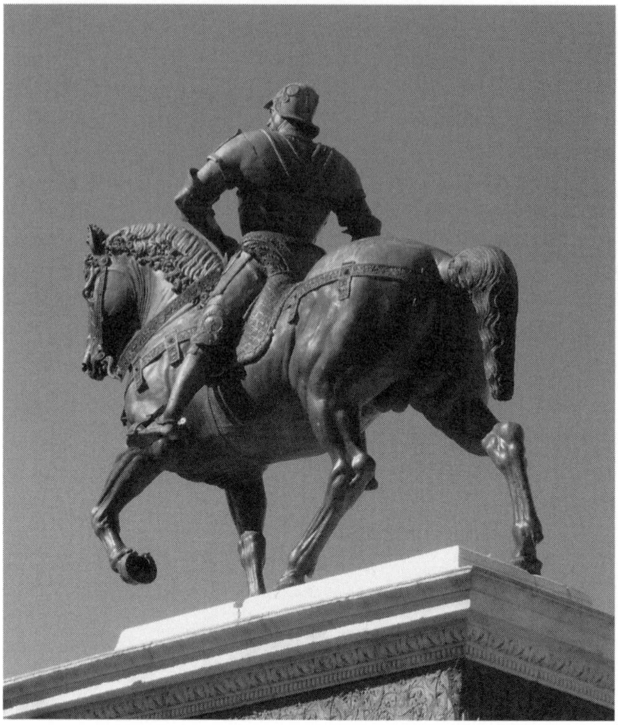

Figure 20 Andrea del Verrocchio and Alessandro Leopardi, *Colleoni monument*, dated by inscription 1495, Venice, Campo di SS. Giovanni e Paolo

uncouth ("crass"), and the poem may be making a sly reference to contemporary inside-jokes about *coglioni*.

Testicles appeared in multiple ways on the sculpture. Colleoni's *arme* were displayed prominently on the pedestal: his personal stemma (two bands held at each end by open lions' mouths) was under the figure's left, and the family's coat of arms (three testicles beneath Angevin fleur-de-lis) was exhibited on the other side, visible to all those entering the prestigious *scuola* of S. Marco or the important church of SS. Giovanni e Paolo nearby. Furthermore, Verrocchio's striding horse ensured the exhibition of *coglioni* in punning bronze, for nearly all views of the three-dimensional work reveal that it is a well-endowed stallion (figs. 20–21). Colleoni's namesakes were thus fully on public view, and would have been even more visible before the original gilding was eroded, glistening in the sunlight.[107] Horses were infamously lusty and "horse" (*cavallo*) was a

[107] On the gilding see Covi, *Verrocchio*, pp. 151 n. 1, 156 n. 30.

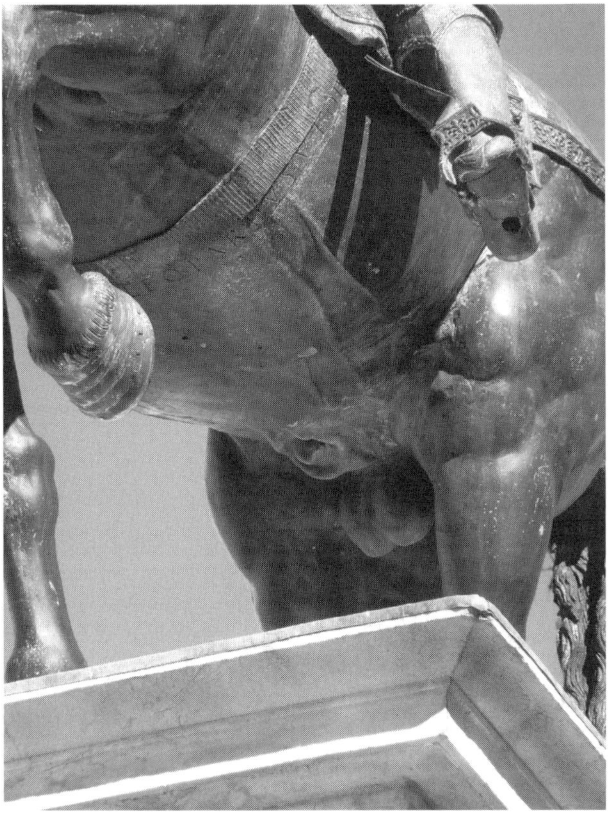

Figure 21 Andrea del Verrocchio, *Colleoni monument*, detail of fig. 20

metaphor for the male genitals, so Colleoni's placement "riding" a huge "horse" between his legs may also have engendered jokes, including homoerotic ones. Pomponio Gauricus' treatise on sculpture cited Verrocchio's bronze horse in 1504 as an instance of crude realism that must be avoided, for he reported that it was commonly said to resemble nothing more than a flayed horse. Denuded of its very skin according to many, that loss of what Gauricus pointedly called "delicacy" probably alludes to the anatomical exaggeration not only of flaring nostrils and rippling flanks but also the penis and prominent testicles.[108]

Other grand steeds seating commanders and rulers in their commemorative monuments, like the Roman Emperor Marcus Aurelius (d. 180), the Milanese

[108] Pomponio Gaurico, *De sculptura*, ed. Paolo Cutolo (Naples: Edizioni Scientifiche Italiane, 1999), pp. 222–24.

ruler Bernarbò Visconti (*c.* 1363) or the equestrian portrait of the Holy Roman Emperor Charles V painted by Titian (*c.* 1548), are usually conspicuously male too, befitting the rider's authority and potency. The mercenary John Hawkwood sits astride a stallion in Uccello's frescoed version of an equestrian monument executed in Florence's Cathedral in 1435, though the consciously similar honor bestowed on the condottiere Niccolò da Tolentino by Andrea Castagno in the same place in 1456 entailed a far more explicit view. The virility of their mounts crucially affirmed and redounded upon that of such honored, powerful men. Yet, the *coglioni* of Colleoni's mount are especially noticeable, visible even in silhouette, and they accompany inscribed names and sculpted emblems that declare publicly the distinctive masculinity of this military commander, who hungered for fame and honored the Venetian state while also giving rise to misgivings and jokes.

"Phallic symbols," and more

The sexual association of masculinity with penetration and violence in the European tradition is incontrovertible. However, even some of these most obvious penetrative metaphors are inflected with semenotic implications. The penis is a detached, solitary, sufficient, piercing element in plentiful references that conceptualize sexual intercourse as a joust or battle. Following on from the tradition of medieval romance and the ongoing practice of public spectacles, sex was likened to the conquest of a castle when Ludovico Ariosto imagined the fulfillment of desire in *Orlando furioso*, his immensely popular epic poem of the sixteenth century. Richardet fell upon an eager Fiordispina: he "leapt onto the battlements and planted my standard there at one jab, and thrust my enemy beneath me."[109] Freud acknowledged the ubiquity and proverbial nature of the symbolism: "whips, sticks, lances and similar objects are familiar to us as phallic symbols."[110] Popular writers including Boccaccio, Aretino and Bandello, to name a few Italian examples, all used words like "joust" or "lance" to make sexual references, and similar ploys worked in other vernaculars.[111]

109 Ludovico Ariosto, *Orlando furioso*, ed. Lanfranco Caretti, 2 vols. (Turin: Einaudi, 1966), vol. II, p. 751; trans. Guido Waldman (Oxford University Press, 1974), p. 303. The third, final edition was issued in 1532. For innuendo about war, battles and jousts see Boggione and Casalegno, *Dizionario*, pp. 100–16.

110 Freud, "Interpretation of dreams," in *Standard edition*, vol. IV (1953), p. 380.

111 Boccaccio, *Corbacacio*, pp. 264–65; Boccaccio, *Decameron*, p. 673; Toscan, *Carnaval*, pp. 1702 (*giostra* and *giostrare*), 1709 (*lancia*) and passim; Villon, *Poems*, p. 59; Jones, *Secret middle ages*, pp. 257–58. In one tale, Bandello is especially prolific with sexual metaphors about the amorous joust: Bandello, *Novelle*, vol. I, pp. 484, 487, 489.

As we have seen in Chapter 1, however, the lance was not only penetrative but also ejaculatory, when it burst or broke once it hit the "shield" or target. The sexualized lance featured in the visual eroticism of Botticelli's *Mars and Venus* panel (fig. 22), appropriated by mischievous young satyrs who have playfully manipulated the weapon so that it has already penetrated a conch-shell (understood to be a reddish body cavity).[112] So too Mars' slumber indicates that he had acted sexually; he reclines in postcoital limpness, like the fingers of his suggestively positioned right hand. Alert viewers, however, see the joke and anticipate the disruption of the idyll because at any second the tip-toeing lead satyrino, cheeks already puffed out, will blow into the shell and let forth with a blaring sound that will rudely awaken Mars as well as stir the wasps hovering nearby. Like the bolt delicately balanced at the end of Mars' left hand but about to drop dramatically, the narrative deferment will soon be impelled forward, into the very buffoonery planned by the lustful imps and wryly observed by complicit Venus. The climax of the painting's joke will be like an orgasm, loud, expulsive and unsettling, provoking in viewers (and Venus?) a similar ejection of *pneuma* when they laugh.

Violence and aggression characterized many of the Greek terms for the sexual activity of the male genitals, such as a spit piercing meat, a drill, an axe hewing, a boat-pole shoving, or the ever-present wounding swords and spears.[113] The metaphorical conceptualization extended to the medical field too. Certain Greek theories explained the mechanism that formed male or female embryos by means of a combat model, the sex determined by which parental seed prevailed.[114] Ancient Latin also supplied a rich heritage of words and metaphors, most of which represented sex as violent, the active male partner as wielding weaponry like spears, javelins, stakes and swords, and the act as striking, beating, cutting, wounding, humiliating, threatening, digging, and such.[115] In a more decorous manner, Ovid's amorous discourse had famously asserted that "every lover is a soldier" and thence every sexual encounter a

[112] For the shell, see Henderson, *Maculate muse*, p. 142 no. 160; Dempsey, *Renaissance putto*, p. 142 (which is too coy about the sexual allusion of the lance, since it is a staple of Italian literature). The vulval red opening of the conch-shell is also evident in Lorenzo Lotto's *Venus and Cupid* painting in the Metropolitan Museum of Art, New York. Key aspects of the erotic humor in Botticelli's painting were noted in Paul Barolsky, *Infinite jest: wit and humor in Italian Renaissance art* (Columbia: University of Missouri Press, 1978), pp. 7, 37–44, 202. For laughter as orgasmic, see Ch. 2, n. 89 above.

[113] Henderson, *Maculate muse*, pp. 44–45, 120–24, 169–73.

[114] "On generation" (6.1–2), in *Hippocratic treatises*, p. 3; Aristotle, *Generation of animals (GA)*, 764a7, 766a18–20; Anthony Preus, "Galen's criticism of Aristotle's conception theory," *Journal of the History of Biology* 10 (1977), 73; Michael Boylan, "The Galenic and Hippocratic challenges to Aristotle's conception theory," *Journal of the History of Biology* 17 (1984), 109.

[115] Adams, *Latin sexual vocabulary*, pp. 6, 14–22, 23–24, 124, 128, 133–34, 145–52, 198–201 (for words about play and pleasure, see 161–3, 196–98).

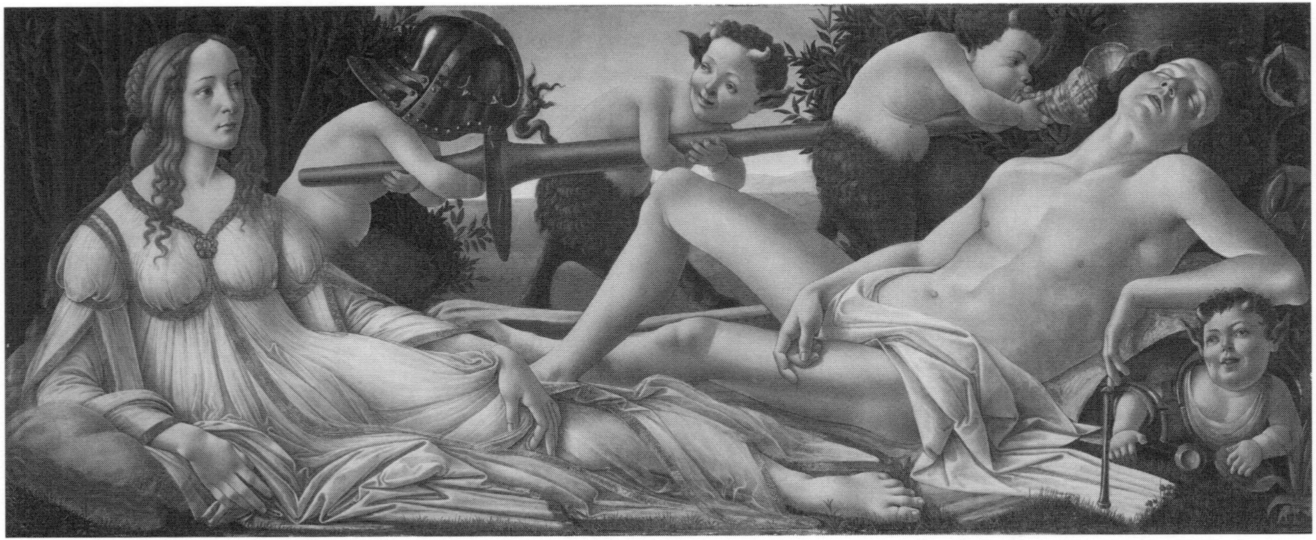

Figure 22 Sandro Botticelli, *Mars and Venus*, *c*. 1485, tempera on wood, 69.2 × 173.4 cm, London, National Gallery

nocturnal battle.[116] The trope of erotic warfare, still ensconced in the related phrase "the battle of the sexes," was familiar enough for a man to scratch Ovid's line into the exterior wall of a house in Pompeii, and the notion lived on, translated in a medieval French version of Ovid as "love is a type of chivalry."[117] Well into the Renaissance, chivalric spectacles for aristocratic display and civic pageantry adapted the metaphorical staging of eroticized violence to the technology of tournaments.

Sanctioned, manly violence informed both literary conceits and the language used to frame one's own sexual persona. Aretino claimed that, when writing sonnets to accompany the *Modi* engravings, his pen had been like the implement of a portraitist, naturalistically representing "the postures of the jousters."[118] He had reveled in writing an orgiastic "joust" in his *Ragionamento* (1534), though the lance was also figured there as "the lance with two bullets."[119] Bruni, humanist and recent holder of the Chancellorship of Florence, resorted to the imagery of erotic warfare when boasting of sexual feats with his bride in 1412.[120] The recipient of that letter, Poggio Bracciolini, later employed the erotic topos in the comic mode, making fun of the phallic *Pacialis*, "peacemaker" in two tales.[121] One had an adulterous wife propose a "game" to her husband's steward, suggesting that first they pretend to be at war, and then they would make peace. His spear thrust into her "wound" (*vulnus*) marked the battle, the conclusion with the exchange of kisses signaled peace, which punned on the liturgical Kiss of Peace as well as rituals of reconciliation and peacemaking.

The weaponry of sexual warfare was usually figured in quick, sharp, impersonal terms, but less conventionally penetrative references also occur. Sexual word play was clear when a woman referred to a man's knife (*coltel*) being necessary to put in "my sheath" (*guaina*) in Cardinal Bibbiena's influential comedy *La calandria* first performed at the court of Urbino in the carnival season of 1513.[122] But such knives may have been more than simple shafts. Some actual knives were balanced on either side of the hilt with knobs that were knowingly related to testicles, referred to in fifteenth-century documents as a "ballok-knyf" or "ballok-hefted".[123] That genital formula is followed by the

116 Ovid, *Amores*, 1.9.1, 2, 45; also *Ars amatoria*, 2.233. On the theme see Nancy Huston and Samuel Kinser, *A l'amour comme à la guerre: correspondance* (Paris; Seuil, 1984).

117 Varone, *Erotica Pompeiana*, p. 55; Bruno Roy, *L'art d'amours: traduction et commentaire de l'"Ars amatoria" d'Ovide* (Leiden: Brill, 1974), p. 181.

118 Aretino, *Lettere*, vol. I, p. 426 (no. 308, 19 December 1537).

119 Aretino, *Ragionamento*, pp. 34–35.

120 For Bruni's letter of 1412 to Poggio Bracciolini, see Ch. 1 above.

121 Bracciolini, *Facetiae*, nos. 172, 209.

122 Bibbiena, *La calandria*, ed. Paolo Fossati (Turin: Einaudi, 1967), p. 76.

123 David Mickenberg (organizer), *Songs of glory: medieval art from 900–1500* (Oklahoma City, Oklahoma Museum of Art, 1985), pp. 380–81 (a dagger from the second half of the fifteenth century, possibly from Burgundy); van Beuningen and Koldeweij (eds.), *Heilig en Profaan*,

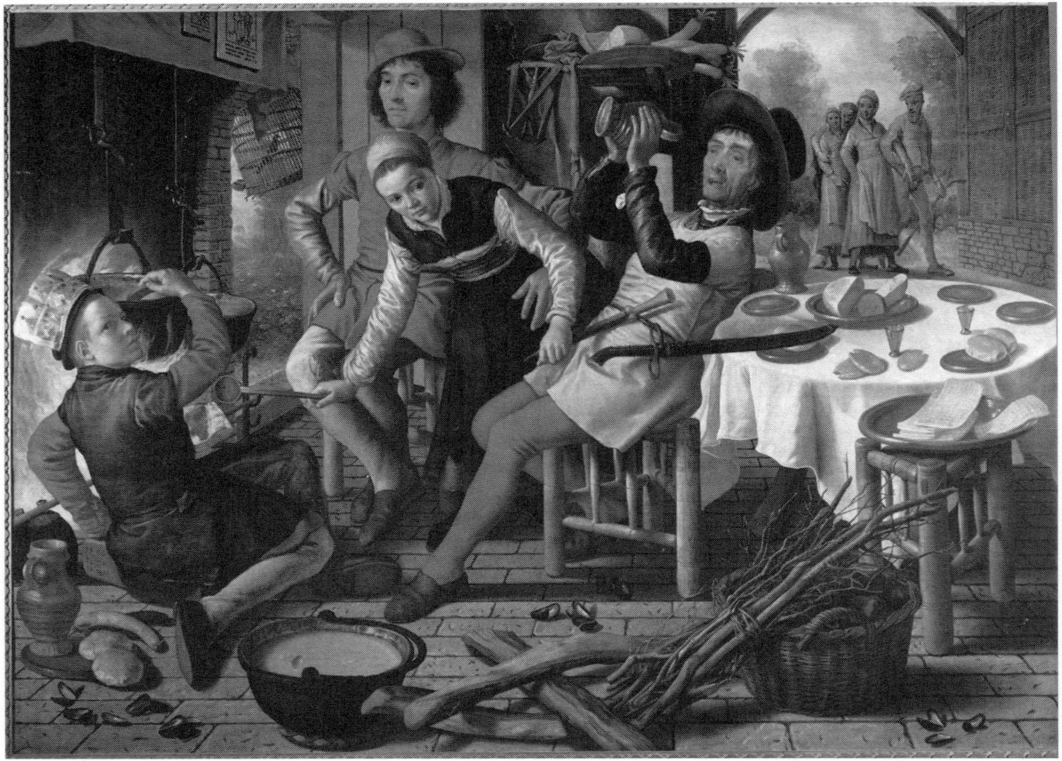

Figure 23 Pieter Aertsen, *Farmer's feast*, 1566, oil on oak wood, 142 × 198 cm, Antwerp, Museum Mayer van den Bergh

knives of two attendants in the foreground at the Duc de Berry's table in the January scene of the illuminated *Très riches heures* (*c.* 1412–16).[124] Such a knife suggestively penetrates the bag located at a fool's backside in a mid-fifteenth-century German engraving of *Dame folly*, an insertion also visible on badges. A prominent, well-dressed youth sports such a knife in Brueghel's *Netherlandish proverbs* painted in 1559, and a kitchen maid suggestively handles the bollock knife of a carousing drunkard in Pieter Aertsen's kitchen scene of 1566 (fig. 23).[125]

The well-known sexualized pole of the pilgrim's staff did not stand alone, for it was frequently represented with the pilgrim's testicular bags, influentially rendered by the poets of the medieval *Roman de la rose* and many of its illustrators thereafter, such as one illumination showing a sac bulging with two hammers, which alludes to two testicles inside the scrota (fig. 24).[126] Similarly, a suspended sword in its sheath accentuates the phallic action in the foreground of a man's hand in Beham's engraving (fig. 5) but the genital reference is underscored by the pendulous, bulbous flask attached to the weapon. Francesco Salviati's huge, disembodied set of genitals spread across over 1.6 meters of paper and being grandly processed towards a vagina not only has the clearly distinguished features of glans, coronal ridge, open orifice, vein, manly pubic hair and testicles but is also accompanied by coins that allude to semen, and the various phalli on banners or brandished dildoes all include testicles (fig. 25).[127]

According to the physician Joubert, writing in 1578, the candle was used in examinations by midwives and by women as dildoes; its tubular shape as well as medical use made it an obvious penile emblem.[128] Even so, more could be involved, as it was in Bruno's comedy *Candelaio*, where the candle was a telling device that was always carried in a man's pocket, lit after the rubbing of the

p. 286; Jones, *Secret middle ages*, p. 258, Pl. 6 (Bruegel); Olaf Goubitz, *Purses in pieces: archaeological finds of late medieval and 16th-century leather purses, pouches, bags and cases in the Netherlands* (Zwolle: Stichting Promotie Archeologie, 2007), pp. 34–35. A *c.* 1450 engraving attributed to the Master of the Playing Cards is reproduced in H. W. Janson, *Apes and ape lore in the middle ages and the Renaissance* (London: Warburg Institute, 1952), Pl. XXXVI.

124 Michael Camille, "'For our devotion and pleasure': the sexual objects of Jean, Duc de Berry," *Art History* 24 (2001), 177, 179.

125 Larry Silver, *Peasant scenes and landscapes: the rise of pictorial genres in the Antwerp art market* (Philadelphia: University of Pennsylvania Press, 2006), pp. 105–06.

126 Camille, *Medieval art of love*, fig. 139 (*c.* 1480). For the phallic pilgrim's staff, see Jones, *Secret middle ages*, pp. 256–57.

127 On Salviati's drawing of the 1540s and the later print see James Grantham Turner, "Salviati's phallic triumph," *Print Quarterly* 24 (2007), 284–86; Linda Wolk-Simon's entry in Andrea Bayer (ed.), *Art and love in Renaissance Italy* (New York: Metropolitan Museum of Art, 2008), pp. 209–10.

128 Laurent Joubert, *Popular errors*, trans. Gregory David de Rocher (Tuscaloosa: University of Alabama Press, 1989), pp. 215–21; see also Augustine, *City of God*, p. 28 for a midwife's candle breaking a hymen.

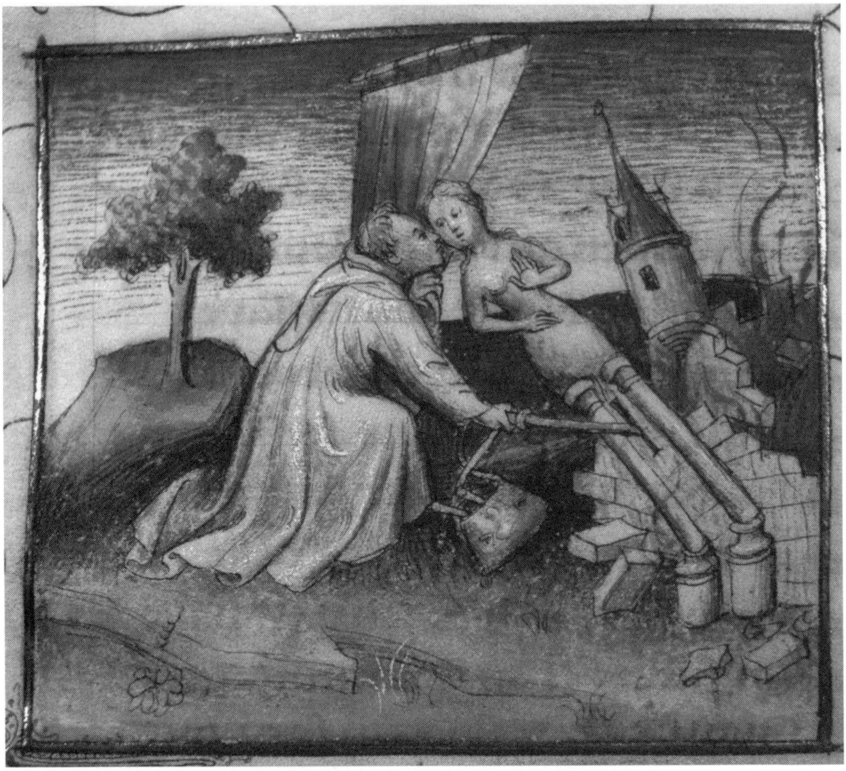

Figure 24 Parisian illuminator, *The lover reaches and penetrates the sanctuary*, from *Le roman de la rose*, *c*. 1410, Valencia, University Library, MS 387, fol. 147v-1

tinder, emitted light and heat when aroused and offered at female altars.[129] The metaphor was explicitly shifted from fire to fluid when a man retorted to a woman that "you should fear flood (*deluvio d'acqua*) more than fire" issuing from it (2.6). The same fluid output from candles would fill the little flasks (*cistelle*) of women according to a carnival song.[130] Some ancient Roman phalli served as oil lamps, the wick at the glans accentuating the output of fluid as well as heat and light.[131]

The arrow was penetrative, but quivers were also vital to the well-equipped archer. The sheer size and bulbous tip of Cupid's quiver visually suggests the phallic nature of his missiles, as though they are housed in an uncircumcised

[129] Bruno, "Candelaio," pp. 320, 358; Bruno, *Candlebearer*, pp. 102–03, 133.

[130] Prizer, "*Facciamo*," p. 198.

[131] Michael Grant, *Eros in Pompeii* (New York: William Morrow, 1975), pp. 131–33; John Clarke, *Roman sex 100 BC–AD 250* (New York: Harry N. Abrams, 2003), figs. 7, 105.

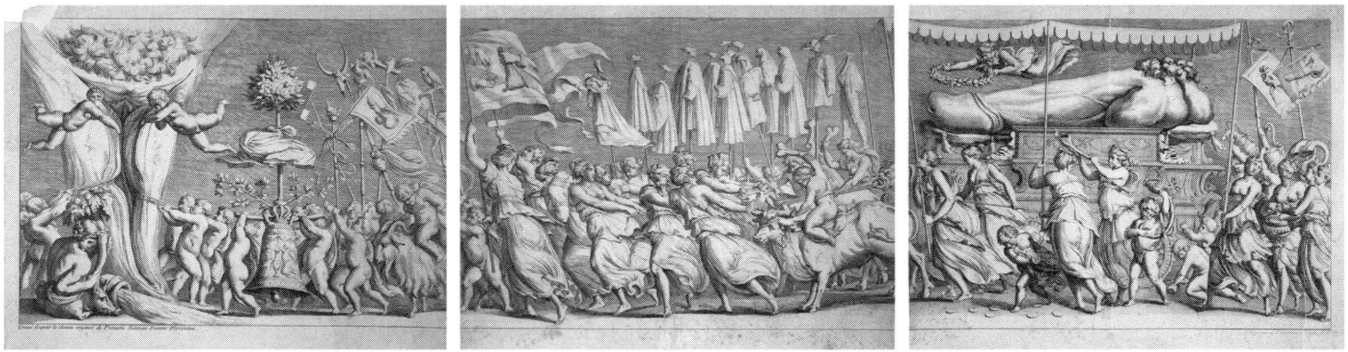

Figure 25 Anonymous seventeenth- or eighteenth-century etcher (after Francesco Salviati), *The triumph of the phallus*, engraving and etching, 38.3 × 161 cm, London, British Museum

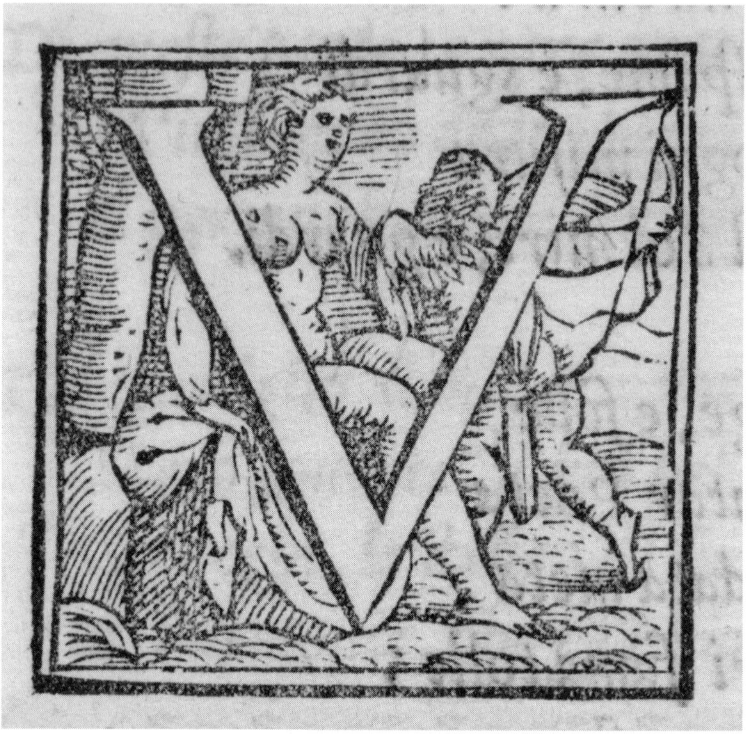

Figure 26 *Rime di madonna Gaspara Stampa* (Venice: Plinio Pietrasanta, 1554), A recto, with historiated capital V showing Venus and Cupid

penis. The anonymous carver of woodcut initials used by the Venetian print shop of Francesco Marcolini took the loaded quiver for a genital sign (fig. 26).[132] Opening the first sonnet of Gaspara Stampa's *Rime* published posthumously in October 1554, the V of *Voi* contains Venus with Cupid. The boy is described later in her volume as "painted already by the ancients, and again by the moderns, as quivered, nude and blind" (263.9–11). *Faretrato* indeed he is, with an ostensible concealment of his nudity humorously enabling the depiction of a long, laden quiver dangling between his legs. Latin word play implied that a quiver was akin to a scrotal sac, for *scrotum* was like another container, *scrautum*, a type of leather quiver.[133] In Shakespeare's *Much ado about nothing* (*c.* 1598–99), a character wonders: "if Cupid have not spent all his quiver in Venice" (1.1.271–72), spending being a common term for ejaculation. Masculine quivers hold profuse, penetrating objects that

[132] Dennis Rhodes, *Silent printers: anonymous printing at Venice in the sixteenth century* (London: British Library, 1995), p. 250.

[133] Adams, *Latin sexual vocabulary*, pp. 74–75.

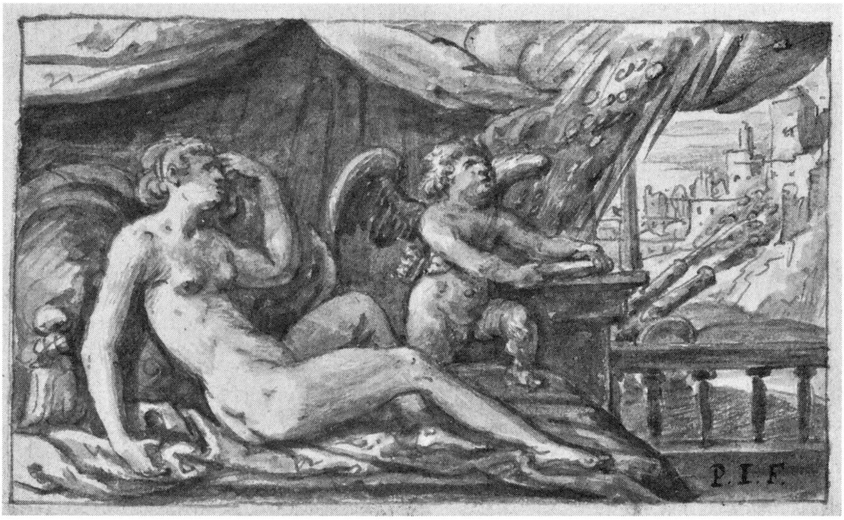

Figure 27 Pieter Isaacz, *Danaë*, *c*. 1608, drawing, pen and brown ink with blue wash, from the *Album amicorum* of Ernest Brinck van Harderwijk, fol. 246r, The Hague, Koninklijke Bibliothek

fluidly arc through the air, delivered by a bow that was more like the penis in function.

The technology of war, of firearms like pistols and handguns, or cannons, gradually engendered double entendres too, especially verbs such as "discharge" and "shoot."[134] At great force and with the aid of heated air (*pneuma*), the weaponry expelled balls like bullets or pellets that could be likened to male "seed." The conflation of cannon balls with semen is especially clear in Pieter Isaacz's amusing drawing of *Danaë* dated *c*. 1608 (fig. 27).[135] At near parallel angles, cannon raised high discharge large round objects in the background while similarly shaped coins fall between Danaë's legs and into Cupid's shallow bowl in the foreground. Jupiter's lust for Danaë was infamously expressed in a shower of

[134] For English, see Samuel Pepys, *Samuel Pepys' penny merriments*, ed. Roger Thompson (London: Constable, 1976), pp. 234–35; and for words like ball, bullets, cock (a pistol), go off, discharge and shoot see Partridge, *Shakespeare's bawdy*, pp. 73, 80, 94, 115, 161, 182; Williams, *Glossary*, pp. 35, 58–59, 73, 99, 143, 237, 276–77; Williams, *Dictionary*, pp. 17–18, 391–92, 258, 631–33, 667, 1238–39. Italian seems to have been slower to incorporate firepower, but some words were applicable, like *drizzare* (to erect, to raise up, to cock a gun), *scaricare* (discharge) and *tirare* (to shoot, to fence, to deliver a blow, and so on): Toscan, *Carnaval*, pp. 1050, 1059, 1690, 1745, 1759, and passim; Boggione and Casalegno, *Dizionario*, pp. 242–43, 341–2, 346, 349–50, 370.

[135] Eric Jan Sluijter, *Rembrandt and the female nude* (Amsterdam University Press, 2006) p. 231, which regards the cannon as a contrast to how easily gold surmounts her walls, whereas I see a humorous analogy. For "coin," see Ch. 5 below.

gold, a glistening rain often rendered as a stream of coins eagerly gathered by Cupid, venal Danaë or her servant (fig. 34). Thus, the drawing wittily presents not only the common metaphor of coin for semen, but also that of a weapon's discharge. Cannon bombardment will breach the walls of a city just as Jupiter was able to penetrate Danaë's secluded prison atop a tower.

Actions and symbols that have instituted and reinstated power have centered on more than just a penetrative, violent penis, incorporating in particular the testicles and semenotic energy as further markers and celebratory signs of masculine potency and authority. Men represented on their backs might be expected to signal disempowerment, yet workshop drawings of such a pose by artists like Michelangelo and the Carracci brothers sketch the legs lifted and apart, genital package on display, in bold acts of macho exhibition.[136] Bonding and boasting have strategically overcome moments of unease. Humor works somewhat similarly in the case of cassone and other domestic paintings such as Domenico Veneziano's tondo of the Magi (now in Berlin), addressing female as well as male audiences and often related to the establishment of a new conjugal household, which depict stallions from the rear, their large testicles clearly visible. The conspicuous genitals stress masculine might and foster amused moments of connection between viewers, including husband and young wife, or parent and child.

The word "phallus" has been a useful analytical tool when applied in modern times as a metacategory of interpretation, but it must be carefully distinguished from historical presence and preoccupations. In many ways, the noun works best not as a value but as a descriptor (phallus = male genitals, often but not always exaggerated, represented in the context of power and domination), while the adjective is especially pertinent as a metaphor applied to genital symbols or social structures and processes of power. Theoretically, it is transferable and we have seen it used, for instance, by subgroups like jousting sons and disruptive wearers of badges. Wordsmiths, artists, jokesters, medical theorists and others, including some women, tended to play in numerous directions with genital signifiers. What for Plato encapsulated irrationality or for Augustine epitomized the loss of prelapsarian innocence would for psychoanalysis signify the melancholic impossibility of fulfillment. On the other hand, nostalgia conjures up a powerful dream of authentic, coherent selfhood, and numerous words, deeds and images seek to give embodiment to that fantasy, from badge wearers declaring carnivalesque defiance or jousters performing orgasmic masculinity to rulers adopting mythological guise in order to show themselves as virile as Jupiter.

[136] Paul Joannides, *The drawings of Michelangelo and his followers in the Ashmolean Museum* (Cambridge University Press, 2007), pp. 168, 173; Clare Robertson and Catherine Whistler, *Drawings by the Carracci from British collections* (Oxford: Ashmolean Museum, 1996), p. 82.

Part II

Projecting male sex: models and metaphors

4 Physiology and anatomy

Angry at Adonis' disinterest in her, Shakespeare's Venus retaliated by telling the youth: "thou art no man, though of a man's complexion."[1] His ruddy skin indicated that his body was properly masculine in that it evinced the core qualities of heat and dryness, yet Adonis was not acting in the manner she expected, ignoring the goddess of sexual desire in favor of hunting pursuits. His psychic and physical processes were not in balance. The punning accusation assumed that readers understood standard medical theory: when a body's *complexio* or "temperament" was in order, typical men were hot and dry, typical women were cold and wet, though the exact equilibrium within those parameters varied according to factors like age, climate, diet, the seasons or astrological configurations.[2] In particular, the quality of heat was believed to mark male bodies, along with the presence of testicles that produced a particular strength of semen. According to both anatomical and physiological criteria, there was much that distinguished male from female bodies, and the penis or its lack was a minor factor.

Humoral medicine

The Pythagoreans and later Hippocrates and his followers in the fifth and fourth centuries BCE formulated the basics of complexional or humoral theory, which was particularly elaborated by the Greek-writing physician Galen in second-century CE Rome. Effective as a comprehensive system of organization, explanation and therapy, it was expanded in later centuries and propagated by way of texts such as the *c.* 1025 synoptic *Canon* of the physician Avicenna, translated from Arabic into Latin after 1170. For centuries, the *Canon* was a

1 William Shakespeare, *The poems*, ed. John Roe (Cambridge University Press, 1992), *Venus and Adonis*, line 215. For overviews on humoral medicine, see Ambroise Paré, *Œuvres complètes*, ed. J.-F. Malgaigne, 3 vols. (1840–41), rpt. (Geneva: Slatkine Reprints, 1970), vol. I, pp. 31–79; Noga Arikha, *Passions and tempers: a history of the humours* (New York: HarperCollins, 2007).

2 The four humors were blood (which was hot and wet), yellow bile (hot–dry), black bile (cold–dry) and phlegm (cold–wet), a preponderance of which caused, respectively, the sanguine, choleric, melancholic and phlegmatic temperaments.

basic textbook in medical schools that had developed from the later twelfth century in major universities at Bologna, Paris, Padua and elsewhere. Other translations into Latin of key Arabic texts, or of Greek works that had survived in Arabic versions, re-energized the humoral system of medical knowledge in Europe, where it was discussed and disseminated by way of learned men, some cloistered, others employed at courts and universities, and by a growing number of men practicing in the burgeoning cities. Renaissance philological and Hellenic scholarship spurred the printing of Greek editions and improved translations, including publication of Galen's work in various editions beginning with the Latin *Opera* in 1490 and the issue of the Hippocratic corpus in Latin in 1525.

Oral transmission and local, even incidental practice by women as well as men continued apace, and medical knowledge was acquired in the shops of barber-surgeons and apothecaries, at bathhouses and the battle front, from herbalists and neighbors, local midwives and itinerant gelders. Complexional balance was crucial to popular and learned medicine alike, though the former placed more emphasis on evacuation and purgation for therapeutic purposes, the latter on dietary regulation. Distinctions between Latin and vernacular medical theory are less important in my study than the widespread concepts and metaphors that imbued the daily lives of lay and professional alike.

Considerable agency was granted to individuals to maintain their own health, chiefly by managing the six so-called non-naturals, "air, exercise and rest, sleep and waking, food and drink, repletion and excretion, and the 'accidents of the soul,' or passions and emotions."[3] Sexual activity was a medicalized topic, for coitus was added to the non-naturals in the early twelfth century due to its potentially harmful or beneficial effects and thereafter "l'exercice Vénérien" remained an important factor in one's health.[4] People often diagnosed and treated their own ailments, changing their diet and amount of warm clothing, ingesting various potions, purging their bodies violently, and analyzing their urine even after uroscopy had begun to go out of fashion. The non-natural factors of temperature, diet and timing were crucial in the advice midwives and local women gave Samuel Pepys in 1664 when he inquired about begetting children, along with the favoring of mutual desire and a bed raised higher at its foot.[5]

[3] Nancy Siraisi, *Medieval and early Renaissance medicine: an introduction to knowledge and practice* (University of Chicago Press, 1990), p. 101; Paré, *Œuvres*, vol. I, pp. 62–79.

[4] Danielle Jacquart, "Medical explanations of sexual behavior in the middle ages," in Helen Rodnite Lemay (ed.), *Homo carnalis: the carnal aspect of medieval human life* (Binghamton: Center for Medieval and Early Renaissance Studies, State University of New York at Binghamton, 1987), pp. 4, 18 n. 8; Giovanni Marinelli, *Thresor des remedes secrets pour les maladies des femmes* [trans. Jean Liébault] (Paris: Jacques Du Puys, 1585), p. 57 (first published in Italian in 1563); Cadden, *Sex difference*, pp. 272–75.

[5] Pepys, *Diary*, vol. V, p. 222 (26 July 1664).

Since equilibrium was the ideal state of health, levels of intake and excretion were carefully monitored, at least by men, especially at times of illness. Thus, men's diaries often record what they ate (by the painter Pontormo, for instance, or the scientist Robert Hooke), and those of Hooke and the Scotsman William Drummond, as well as Pepys on occasion, noted the expenditure of semen.[6] Like Pepys after him, the Elizabethan alchemist and natural philosopher John Dee kept notes on his wife's menstrual pattern and their sex life. Montaigne's record of visits to various Italian baths in 1580–81 to treat his stones included detailed measurements of his urine output and records of his meals. Self-management of one's health engendered quantification and the concomitant awareness of the expenditure of bodily resources, like semen, or of the complexional basis of sex characteristics.

Adonis' actions did not accord with his complexion. Women were understood to be pale-skinned because of their moisture and coolness, men darker due to their drier and hotter nature, a naturalized difference reinforced by gender roles that situated ideal women indoors while men were active in the public sphere and thus more exposed to sunlight and wind.[7] Having a plethora of aqueous elements that were inherently unstable, women were softer, more impressionable, irrational and changeable, like wax to be imprinted and impregnated. Paintings of Adonis refusing Venus' entreaty executed by Titian and his workshop in the 1550s and 1560s accentuate the disparity between irrational longing and its tragic denial by heightening pale feminine flesh against the youth's firm, ruddy body.[8]

Depictions of the "first parents" Adam and Eve also reinforced humoral notions of sex difference. Albrecht Dürer's magisterial engraving of *The Fall* (1504) contrasts Adam's hard, dry, muscular flesh with Eve's softer body (fig. 28). Despite their idyllic, outdoor circumstances in the garden of Paradise, Eve is pale whereas more shading conveys Adam's darker coloration. Hairs on his chest and more extensive pubic hair also indicate the man's naturally more heated state, which caused the "excreting" of hair. Although Eve reaches out to accept the

[6] Jacopo da Pontormo, *Diario*, ed. Emilio Cecchi (Florence: Le Monnier, 1956); Robert Hooke, *The diary of Robert Hooke M.A., M.D., F.R.S. 1672–1680*, ed. Henry Robinson and Walter Adams (London: Taylor & Francis, 1935); Montaigne, *Complete works*, pp. 867–1039 passim; Deborah Harkness, "Managing an experimental household: the Dees of Mortlake and the practice of natural philosophy," *Isis* 88 (1997), 256. For Drummond, see Ch. 5 below. Between 3 September 1672 and 30 March 1679, Hooke recorded sixty-one ejaculations and several dreams about sex.

[7] On the visualization of humoral theory, see esp. Raymond Klibansky, Erwin Panofsky and Fritz Saxl, *Saturn and melancholy: studies in the history of natural philosophy, religion and art* (London: Nelson, 1964); Zirka Filipczak, *Hot dry men, cold wet women: the theory of humors in western European art 1575–1700* (New York: American Federation of Arts, 1997).

[8] Harold Wethey, *The paintings of Titian: complete edition*, vol. III: *the mythological and historical paintings* (London: Phaidon, 1975), pp. 188–94, 241–42; Peter Humfrey, *Titian: the complete paintings* (Ghent: Ludion, 2007), pp. 249, 257, 297, 338–39.

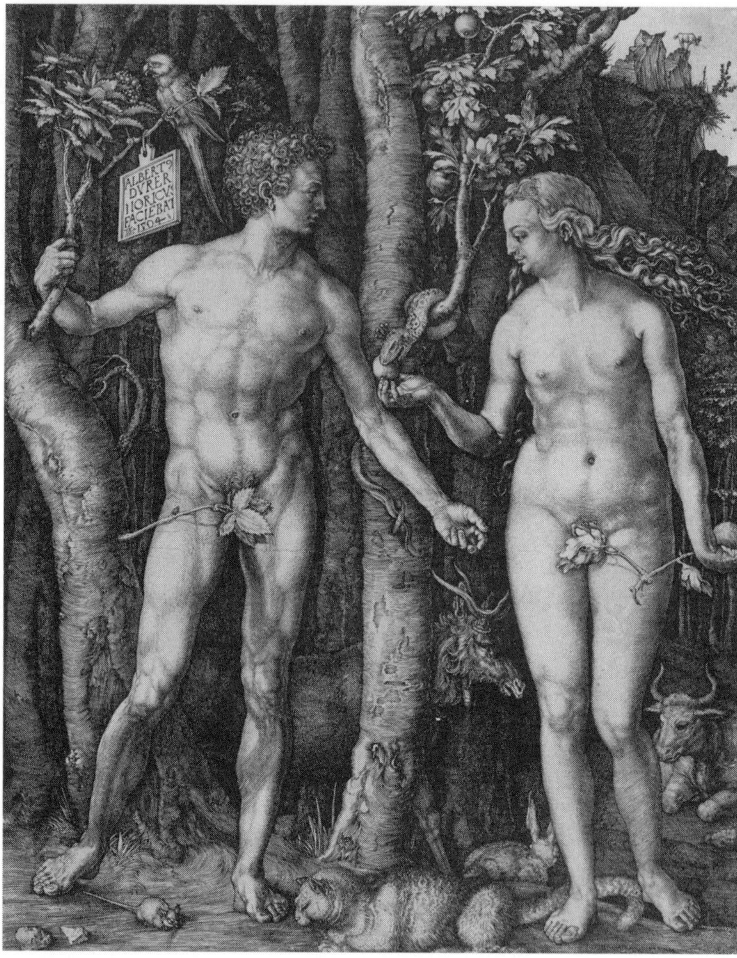

Figure 28 Albrecht Dürer, *The Fall*, 1504, signed and dated, engraving, 249 × 191 mm, London, British Museum

tempting fruit from the serpent, the upper arm remains close and her body is more contained than Adam's. The basic physiological principle of greater masculine heat is reinforced by his wider gestures and more open and assertive stance, with legs farther apart, commanding more space and being more innately active. Like Adam and Eve, the bodies of men and women were related by simultaneous contrast and complementarity in the early modern system.

Heat and masculinity

When Hooke "caught cold in my pole" in 1678 it was implicitly a dire condition that struck at the core of his male being.[9] Premodern medical epistemology assumed what Stephen Greenblatt has called the "caloric model of sexuality," that is, it was based on heat or thermal energy.[10] This physiological basis of determining sex could be taken further, since it was fundamental to the overall ideology that masculinity was about initiative, radiation and projection.

Aristotle and Galen each placed a high priority on the centrality of the masculine perfection of heat in the process of reproduction. But the natural philosopher of the fourth century BCE allotted to women a "passive" or receptive, less important role whereas the later physician Galen, while following much of the Aristotelian scheme, gave more credence to the earlier Hippocratics and thus assigned value to a mother's contribution to conception. Partly because of different paces and routes of translation and transmission, Aristotelian ideas predominated during the medieval period, but by the early sixteenth century Galenic notions had made serious inroads. However, as Joan Cadden has astutely shown for the medieval period, most medical opinions tended to deal in compromise and even confusion, taking from each system, often by way of intermediary commentaries, and attempting reconciliation.

Aristotle defined a woman as "an infertile male; the female, in fact, is female on account of inability of a sort, viz., it lacks the power to concoct semen out of the final state of the nourishment . . . because of the coldness of its nature."[11] Heat gave the male body the ability "to concoct, to cause to take shape, and to discharge, semen possessing the 'principle' of the 'form'" (*GA* 765b10). Aristotle's model of gendered biology established a basic difference between an active generative principle (Form) that was male and passive Matter that was female. His impact was notable from the thirteenth century, when all of Aristotle's works were translated into Latin. The influence was reinforced in university curricula by Avicenna's *Canon*, which sought to reconcile the two systems, though it tended to be more critical of Galen. Thence the Dominican natural philosopher Albertus Magnus (d. 1280) and his pupil the theologian Thomas Aquinas (d. 1274) instilled Aristotelian thinking in philosophy and theology. Dante's vernacular *Divine comedy* followed suit in the early decades of the fourteenth century, stating that in sexual intercourse "there the two mingle, one to passive ways / Adapted, but the other formed to act."[12]

9 Hooke, *Diary*, p. 344 (14 February 1678).

10 Stephen Greenblatt, *Shakespearean negotiations* (Berkeley: University of California Press, 1989), p. 85.

11 Aristotle, *GA*, 728a17–21; see also 729a10, 25, 730a25ff, 766b15–28.

12 Dante, *Purgatorio*, 25.46–48. I have used the translation by Dorothy Sayers.

"Female," defined Aristotle, "is that which receives the semen, but is unable to cause semen to take shape or to discharge it," and from this inability to form or ejaculate semen followed "of necessity that male animals are hotter than female ones" (*GA* 765b15). The more heated bodies of men converted (concocted) the residue from nourishment and blood into sweat, body hair and semen, but women contributed no formative semen to generation, only nurturing matter (menses) in the womb, and they expelled the excess of less pure, inactive menses (*GA* 729a20–32). As the sixteenth-century French physiologist Jean Fernel put it, male semen "possesses a divine and heavenly heat, . . . in which the whole of life has its dwelling," and thus it could spark life and instill soul in an embryo.[13] Writers well into the Renaissance repeated what had become standard lore, Aristotle's opinion that "the female is as it were a deformed male; and the menstrual discharge is semen, though in an impure condition; i.e., it lacks . . . the principle of Soul" (i.e., *psyche* or spirit).[14] She could not contribute the heated "air" or *pneuma*, which was the main component of semen besides water and which contained the "soul-heat" that generated new life.[15]

Galen's variation on the theory of sex difference returned to the tenet of some but not all Hippocratic texts that both men and women produced seed or *sperma*, but he applied a similar ranking to that of Aristotle when he defined *sperma* as "the active principle of the animal, the material principle being the menstrual blood."[16] According to Galen's study of the body's anatomical and physiological structure, *On the usefulness of the parts*, "the female is less perfect than the male for one, principal reason – because she is colder."[17] The

13 Fernel, *Physiologia*, p. 547 (with parallel Latin).

14 Aristotle, *GA*, 737a25–30. Her normal deformity is also mentioned at 775a16–17. Reiterations include Boccaccio, *Corbaccio*, p. 233; Baldassare Castiglione, *Il libro del cortegiano*, ed. Giulio Carnazzi (Milan: Biblioteca Universale Rizzoli, 1987), p. 215; Joubert, *Popular errors*, p. 107; Crooke, *Mikrokosmographia*, p. 60, quoting Spenser's *Faerie queene*.

15 Aristotle *GA*, 736a1, 736b33–37, 742a15, 762a20.

16 Galen, *Natural faculties*, trans. Arthur John Brock (Cambridge, MA: Harvard University Press, 1952), pp. 131, 135; Galen, *On semen*, ed. and trans. Phillip de Lacy (Berlin: Akademie Verlag, 1992), pp. 87–89, 145ff passim. Galen's *De semine*, first translated into Latin by Niccolò da Reggio in 1317 (Galen, *On the usefulness of the parts of the body*, trans. Margaret Tallmadge May (Ithaca: Cornell University Press, 1968), p. 6), should not be confused with the Pseudo-Galenic *De spermate*, which focused on heredity and is the chief source for the theory of a seven-celled uterus.

17 Galen, *Usefulness*, p. 628, also pp. 382, 630. See also Galen, *Semen*, pp. 176–77. Aristotle too believed women were cold, but more often the Hippocratic authors had regarded female bodies as "hotter": Ann Ellis Hanson (trans.), "Hippocrates: *Diseases of women* 1," *Signs* 1 (1975), 572; Helen King, *Hippocrates' women: reading the female body in ancient Greece* (London: Routledge, 1998), pp. 32–33. The entire *De usu partium* first appeared as an independent, Latin publication in 1528 and was often printed thereafter: Richard Durling, "A chronological census of Renaissance editions and translations of Galen," *Journal of the Warburg and Courtauld Institutes* 24 (1961), 233–34, 243, 255, 292.

thermal basis to sex difference remained fundamental in medieval and early modern medicine and culture, in learned tomes, midwifery manuals and beyond. One of the characters in Castiglione's influential manual on courtly behavior (1528) noted that "man is by his natural qualities more perfect than woman, who by temperament is frigid as man is warm. And warmth is far more noble and more perfect than cold, because it is active and productive" (3:17). Having lost their testicles, eunuchs were womanish due to their "deficiency of heate."[18] The assumption of masculine heat informs the many descriptions of the devil's organ as a cold, hard, unnatural and unmanly thing, or his semen as cold, present in chapbooks and women's confessions when they were accused of witchcraft.[19]

Temperature was the sole, sufficient basis of defining the difference between the sexes for the French physician and anatomist André du Laurens in 1593: "The Male is originally the hotter . . . The Female is the colder."[20] According to a passage he added to a later edition and which was slightly expanded by the English anatomist Helkiah Crooke in 1615:

> man should be hotter, because his body was made to endure labour and travell [travail], as also that his minde should bee stoute and invincible to undergoe dangers, the onely hearing whereof will drive a woman as wee say out of her little wits. The woman was ordained to receive and conceive the seede of the man, to bear and nourish the Infant, to governe and moderate the house at home, to delight and refresh her husband.[21]

As we saw in Chapter 1, sexed differences were intertwined with gendered behavior.

Physiology had anatomical consequences. Since heat caused the protrusion of male genitals, sex changes were explained as cases in which the body's heat had altered and thence brought forward the masculine parts. Because Nature always moved towards the more perfect state, nearly all transformations recognized in the literature were from female to male. In 1573 it was self-evident to Paré that the lesser heat of women meant that they lacked "the ability to push out what by the coldness of their temperament is held" within.[22] Once a body's heat grew "more robust, vehement, and active," the genitals were pushed outward and thus proved to be male. In the famous case he cited, of the shepherd Marie Germain, energetic activity chasing a flock had created enough heat for testicles to descend from what had previously been considered a female body. It was

18 Ambroise Paré, *The collected works of Ambroise Paré translated out of the Latin by Thomas Johnson from the first English edition, London, 1634* (Pound Ridge, NY: Milford House, 1968), p. 27.

19 See, for example, *Mother Shipton* (first published in 1641), in Pepys, *Pepys' penny merriments*, p. 79; Roper, *Witch craze*, pp. 83, 89, 90, 93, 94, 96, 98; Toulalan, *Imagining sex*, p. 76.

20 Du Laurens, *Opera anatomica*, p. 282, trans. in Crooke, *Mikrokosmographia*, p. 271.

21 Du Laurens, *Historica anatomica*, p. 371; Crooke, *Mikrokosmographia*, p. 274.

22 Paré, *Monsters and marvels*, pp. 32–33.

specifically the heat of a young girl's passion (being "enflamed with the violence of love") that caused such extroversion according to the French physician Jacques Ferrand when writing in 1610.[23] The overheating of the female body due to lust was unnatural, remedied by the dose of fluid cast on her fire in the Hippocratic model, taken literally by Somerset men who threw one woman in a stream and flung beer at others.

The heated, active, exterior and projective essence of masculinity was made more vivid, understandable and seemingly inevitable by means of numerous analogies and metaphors in medical discourse, including heated kitchens and warmed seals. The *Anatomia vivorum* from Salerno (*c.* 1225), for example, taught that male semen acts on menstrual blood and "causes bubbling like yeast in dough" and that the female reproductive system "bears the same relation to the male generative organ as a seal bears to its impression in wax."[24] *Matrix* (mold) was used for the womb and medieval terminology associated the supposed cells of a womb with the receptive molds or die used to mint coins, rendering the masculine element in that case as the hot molten metal being poured into containers, along with the assertive action of a stamp or seal that might mark soft metal or wax.[25] Hence in 1466 the sexually frustrated man in "The legacy" of the satirical French poet François Villon bemoaned that "I need fresh fields to plough / And another die for coining in."[26] One of the many ballad sheets Pepys purchased in the seventeenth century had a wife cleverly complain of her husband, a metal worker of pewter, that "A Man of much mettle I took him to be, ... But alas, ... he'll seldom cast into the mould that he should."[27] The female body was to be repetitively beaten and stamped with masculine impress, or warm liquids were poured within; further heat was produced by coital friction.

The metaphor of the blacksmith was particularly telling. One commentator on the anonymous *Secrets of women*, originally penned by a monk in the late

23 Jacques Ferrand, *De la maladie d'amour ou mélancholie érotique* (Paris: Denis Moreau, 1623), p. 12; Jacques Ferrand, *Erotomania, or a treatise discoursing of the essence, causes, symptomes, prognosticks, and cure of love, or erotique melancholy* (Oxford: L. Lichfield, 1640), p. 14. Other examples include du Laurens, *Opera anatomica*, p. 283; Duval, *Hermaphrodits*, pp. 417, 421, 436–37; Crooke, *Mikrokosmographia*, pp. 204, 250, 271.

24 George W. Corner, *Anatomical texts of the earlier middle ages* (Washington: Carnegie Institution of Washington, 1927), pp. 103, 105.

25 Adams, *Latin sexual vocabulary*, pp. 105–08; Corner, *Anatomical texts*, pp. 69, 70, 85; Jacquart and Thomasset, *Sexuality and medicine*, pp. 37, 204 n. 70. The "mould" (and "soyl") of an island in "a pornographic fantasy-travel book" of 1683 hence *does* refer to "sexual parts," cf. Laqueur, *Making sex*, p. 160.

26 Villon, *Poems*, p. 5; and see Williams, *Dictionary*, pp. 272–73 (coin). See Ch. 5 for the womb as a receptacle for coin.

27 Pepys, *Diary*, vol. V, p. 413, *The seven merry wives of London*, cited in Williams, *Dictionary*, p. 913, where "mould" is mistakenly taken to mean vagina. "Mettle" most often meant sexual vigor but sometimes the connection to semen is evident: pp. 882–83.

thirteenth century but frequently copied, translated and printed in the ensuing centuries with an attribution to Albertus Magnus, likened the potency of male semen to the hammering blacksmith fashioning iron with a hammer. Another image that would also have had a vivid impact from pulpit or confessional was the common carpenter, who "alone is the efficient cause, and the house is the effect . . . so the male seed alters the female menses into the form of a human being."[28] The distinction appeared in vernacular texts and informed the self-presentation of the mid-fifteenth-century architect Filarete when he compared his patron to the generative father of a palace, himself to its dependent, gestating mother.[29]

In the heated environs of a forge, the master craftsman initiated repetitive motion of the hammer impressing itself on the feminine anvil. In the second half of the twelfth century, a Latin poem by Alan of Lille influentially argued against sodomy by having Nature complain that once-manly hammers were turning away from anvils, which were producing no spark, that is, seed.[30] Much the same grievance was voiced around 1275 by the personification of Genius in the *Roman de la rose*, who commanded sodomites and celibates to use their two "hammers" (that is, testicles) so that anvils would not rust and perish. "Hammer away, use forge and bellows," they were urged, "think about multiplying yourself."[31] Renaissance poetry kept the metaphor alive.[32] The exclusively masculine nature of exertion at the hot forge is also emphasized in numerous depictions of Vulcan at work, often assisted by the hammering Cyclopes, as he is in a drawing by Francesco Primaticcio of the 1540s that shows the fire god (identifiable by his lame leg) repetitively pumping large bellows to add *pneuma* and heat to his forge.[33] In a subsequent print by Enea Vico and some other variants, the dual nature of these two large leather, scrotal sacs is especially evident.

Artisanal agency was represented as a naturally male initiative and prerogative in other medical metaphors too. Aristotle influentially pictured a generative father as a swordsmith, carpenter, painter or modeler, contributing

28 Helen Lemay, *Women's secrets: a translation of Pseudo-Albertus Magnus's "De secretis mulierum" with commentaries* (Albany: SUNY Press, 1992), p. 64.

29 Examples of the paternal builder include *The problemes of Aristotle* (Edinburgh: Robert Waldgrave, 1595), E 2v–3r (more or less a translation of the *Secrets of women*); Filarete, *Treatise on architecture*, trans. John Spencer (New Haven: Yale University Press, 1965), vol. I, pp. 15–16.

30 Alan of Lille, *The plaint of nature*, trans. James Sheridan (Toronto: Pontifical Institute of Medieval Studies, 1980); Jan Ziolkowski, *Alan of Lille's grammar of sex* (Cambridge, MA: Medieval Academy of America, 1985), pp. 29–30. One of the verbs he uses for the proper production of seed is "to coin" or to "stamp with an image."

31 De Lorris and de Meun, *Roman de la rose*, vol. III, p. 94 (lines 19766, 19771); de Lorris and de Meun, *Romance of the rose*, p. 326.

32 See Ch. 8 for examples of poetry by Ariosto and Michelangelo.

33 *Primatice: Maître de Fontainebleau* (Paris: Musée du Louvre, 2004), pp. 43–44, 268–70.

formative shape and movement to the raw, feminized material.[34] Galen developed the idea, chiefly in relation to sculpture, writing of raw material like blood being akin to the wax that was then "subjected to the artificer."[35] The artist was either the allegorical figure of female Nature or the actual, renowned sculptor Phidias. Or, it was semen, "the artificer analogous with Phidias, whilst the blood [female "seed" or menses] corresponds to the statuary's wax." The medieval theologian Aquinas embedded the craft analogy of "active male virtue" in Church doctrine, influenced by Albertus Magnus, who drew upon the sculptural image, likening menstrual blood to passive marble while male-only semen was similar in action to the sculptor with his chisel.[36]

Artistic creativity remained a masculine, generative process during the Renaissance too. In 1502 the anatomist Alessandro Benedetti described embryological development, beginning with the heart and finishing with other parts, being "finally completed as if in a painting (*pictoris imitatione*)."[37] "Nature resembleth the Painter, making the lively portraiture of a thing" when fashioning the embryo so that it resembled the parents according to Paré in 1573.[38] The ongoing resonance of such metaphors is due to more than convention, for they gelled with medical theory and everyday gender ideology, which in turn was naturalized so that it seemed to fit with corporeal experience.

Anatomy: penile function

Since the phallus has become the predominant corporeal sign of privileged access to power and public action, then it could be said that humoral heat was phallic, so fundamental was it to the body and actions of manliness. The penis, on the other hand, was not pre-eminent in anatomical discourse. Testicles were nearly always treated first, and at greater length because they were considered the true seat of virility. The secondary place of the penis is clear in the criteria used to assign maleness to bodies, as we saw in the case of Elena/o in Chapter 1. According to Paré, an hermaphrodite with distinct female characteristics ejaculated and she had a male member, so neither of those details was unique to male bodies. What made the distinction clear was that "la femme hermafrodite" did not have an erection, that the "male member" had no prepuce and did not issue seed or urine and that

34 Aristotle, *GA*, 724a20, 32, 725a25, 729b15, 730b10–30, 735a5.

35 Galen, *Natural faculties*, pp. 129–33; Galen, *Semen*, pp. 71, 81, 155, 157–59 (citing Polyclitus), 181, 187.

36 Joseph Needham, *A history of embryology*, 2nd edn. (New York: Abelard-Schuman, 1959), pp. 91, 93; also, for example, Jacquart and Thomasset, *Sexuality and medicine*, p. 59; Cadden, *Sex difference*, pp. 62, 127–28; Fernel, *Physiologia*, p. 540.

37 Benedetti, *Anatomice*, p. 172; trans. in Lind, *Studies*, p. 99.

38 Paré, *Œuvres*, vol. II, p. 638; Paré, *Collected works*, p. 888.

there was "no vestige of scrotum or testicles."[39] Maleness depended most on the ability to produce semen in testicles and emit it from a complete "member viril." With a nod to pleasure, anatomists represented the penis as an organ with a sensitive head, but it had two functions, to deliver semen and to enable urination. The very act of intercourse could be defined succinctly in terms of semen. The *Tacuinum sanitatis*, a popular thirteenth-century Latin version of an eleventh-century Arabic treatise on diet and health, said that coitus was "the union of two for the purposes of introducing the semen."[40]

Size was about projective function, not virility per se, which resided in the testicles. To Galen, the penis "has been elongated to be most suitable for coitus and the excretion of semen."[41] Too short a penis, and the semen could not make it to the womb, too long and the semen cooled off before impregnation and the spirits were harmed.[42] Avicenna thought that women would not be pleased by a small penis because it would inadequately position semen, not that it did not live up to modern penile obsessions about size.[43] The thought was echoed in popular literature. In an English chapbook of the 1680s a childless marriage was blamed on the husband's small equipment, "a Fiddle-string, that will make no musick to a Womans Instrument," for which the wife could find no remedy. "No Woman can indure so vile a wrong, / As too too short, or have it too too long."[44]

Intercourse from the male point of view was not so much represented as penile penetration through flesh into a deep interior as the outward projection of a naturally more heated body whose chief coital function was to direct a stream of precious fluid to a feminized receptacle. During the 1490s, Leonardo's cross-sectional drawing of coitus depicted many ancient and medieval but enduring ideas about the act of generation (fig. 29).[45] Each person's spine is prominent because vessels record how "soul" is conveyed from the spinal marrow to the prominent testicles where semen is produced; dissection of the penis in other sketches on the sheet show it with two channels, one for semen, one for urine; the uterus, which is receiving a flow of semen, has an uneven shape because it was thought to consist of seven cells; and from that rises a vessel leading

39 Paré, *Monsters and marvels*, p. 27.

40 Ibn Butlan, *Le Taqwim al-Sihha (Tacuini Sanitatis) d'Ibn Butlan: un traité médical du XIe siècle*, ed. and trans. Hosam Elkhadem (Louvain: Peeters, 1990), pp. 214–15.

41 Galen, *Usefulness*, pp. 632, 655.

42 For example, Aristotle, *GA*, 718a18–26; Henri de Mondeville, *Die Chirurgie des Heinrich von Mondeville: nach Berliner, Erfurter und Pariser Codices*, ed. Julius Leopold Pagel (Berlin: A. Hirschwald, 1892), p. 56 (crediting Galen and Avicenna); Jacopo Berengario da Carpi, *Isagogae breves*, 2nd edn. (Bologna: Benedict Hector, 1523), fol. 20v; Giovanni Marinello, *Le medicine partenenti alle infermità delle donne* (Venice: Giovanni Valgrifio, 1574), fols. 53v, 63v; Crooke, *Mikrokosmographia*, pp. 210–11, 212; Sharp, *Midwives book*, p. 24.

43 Cf. Laqueur, *Making sex*, pp. 50, 101. The length issue is instead understood at p. 31.

44 Pepys, *Pepys' penny merriments*, pp. 262–63.

45 Charles O'Malley and J. B. de C. M. Saunders, *Leonardo da Vinci on the human body* (New York: Henry Schuman, 1952), p. 460; Keele, *Leonardo*, pp. 243–46, 350.

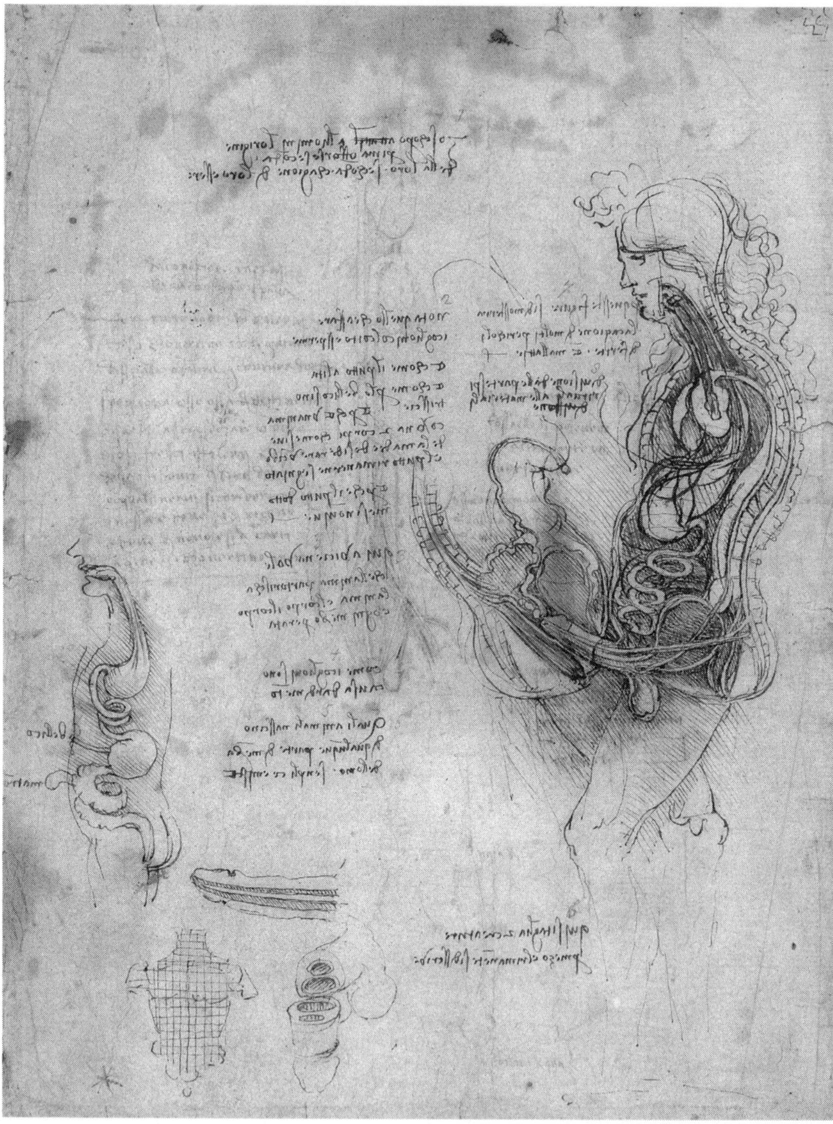

Figure 29 Leonardo da Vinci, *Coition of hemisected man and woman*, *c*. 1492–94, pen and ink, 273 × 202 mm, Windsor, Royal Library

directly to the breast, where menses was supposedly converted into milk. Other than as a close surround for the erect penis, the vagina is not described in detail by the ink pen, whereas the cervical area has opened out and extends down in order to suction up the ejaculated sperm, which is represented as separate globules, indicating consecutive spasms. Other drawings by Leonardo, and his notes, also show an interest in size and "fit" between penis and vagina.[46] Male bodies were paradigms of extromission and generative force, female bodies of reception and containment.

The basic model of coitus did not change in the sixteenth century. To the English surgeon John Banister, who published a manual in 1578 that largely summarized information from the researches of Vesalius (1543) and especially Realdo Colombo (1559), a "fit" between the "peculiar instrumentes" of male and female reproduction required a man "to reach out" and a woman "aptly to conceive ... Unto man, for the apt acte of generation, the omnipotent maker hath given a member ... most fit for the effusion of seede into the wombe."[47] To note the two functions was traditional and unremarkable, and the dual use fostered visual and verbal play about multiple fluids exiting from the penis.[48] Vesling's respected textbook of 1641 repeated the standard assessment of penile use: to "cast seed into the bottom of the Womb."[49] One a vernacular text for British surgeons, the other a short Latin summary of up-to-date information for university students that was reissued several times and soon translated into English and German, each book repeated standard anatomical doctrine.

Anatomical illustrations, which became more common due to the opportunities of print technology and the influence of the many woodcuts in Vesalius' *Fabrica* (1543), visually tell the story of the penis as a body part that stands outside the body due to innately powerful male heat and "reaches out" in order to fulfill its function of projecting seed and urine (fig. 30). Vesalius' plate of the disembodied male organs of generation illustrates the testes at several stages of dissection and has a front and rear view of the penis, seminary vessels, bladder and kidneys. The penile shaft mimics erection in that it has been stretched out and shown elongated according to Galen's observation. The splayed cleavage of flesh at either side in the area closest to the body in the frontal view is suggestive of forward motion, an impression reinforced by the triangular tip or tapered cone of the glans. As with most of Vesalius' images, the plate was often copied for other texts and became the standard view of male genital anatomy for over a century. By the time the penis was visually dissected in Vesling's first illustrated edition of his anatomical

[46] Keele, *Leonardo*, pp. 350–54.

[47] John Banister, *The historie of man, sucked from the sappe of the most approved anathomistes* (London: John Day, 1578), fols. 85r, 87v. The statement about the penis as a delivery system was ubiquitous, appearing for example in Crooke, *Mikrokosmographia*, pp. 210–11 (from Bauhin, *Theatrum anatomicum*, p. 202).

[48] Simons, "Bodily fluids."

[49] Vesling, *Syntagma*, p. 64; Vesling, *Anatomy*, p. 25.

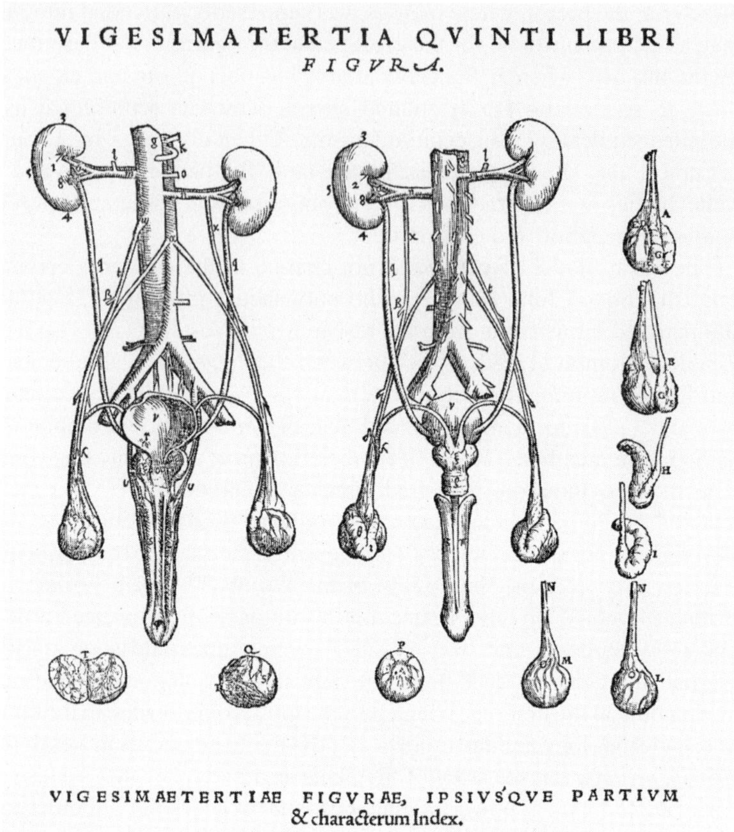

Figure 30 Andreas Vesalius, male organs of generation, *Fabrica* (Basel: Johannes Oporinus, 1555), Book V, Figure 23, p. 374

text in 1647 (fig. 31), it had become a streamlined, aerodynamic missile like the head of an arrow, spear or dart, in which sliced and parted flesh resembles wings or fletched feathers to aid in swift and sure delivery.

Anatomy: testicles, libido and virility

Testicles often counted amongst the body's select, principal members due to their role in libido and reproduction, and their causal relationship to virility was commonly remarked. Since Aristotle, they were associated with *pneuma* (*spiritus* in Latin), what Aristotle envisaged as a kind of breath, spirit or vital

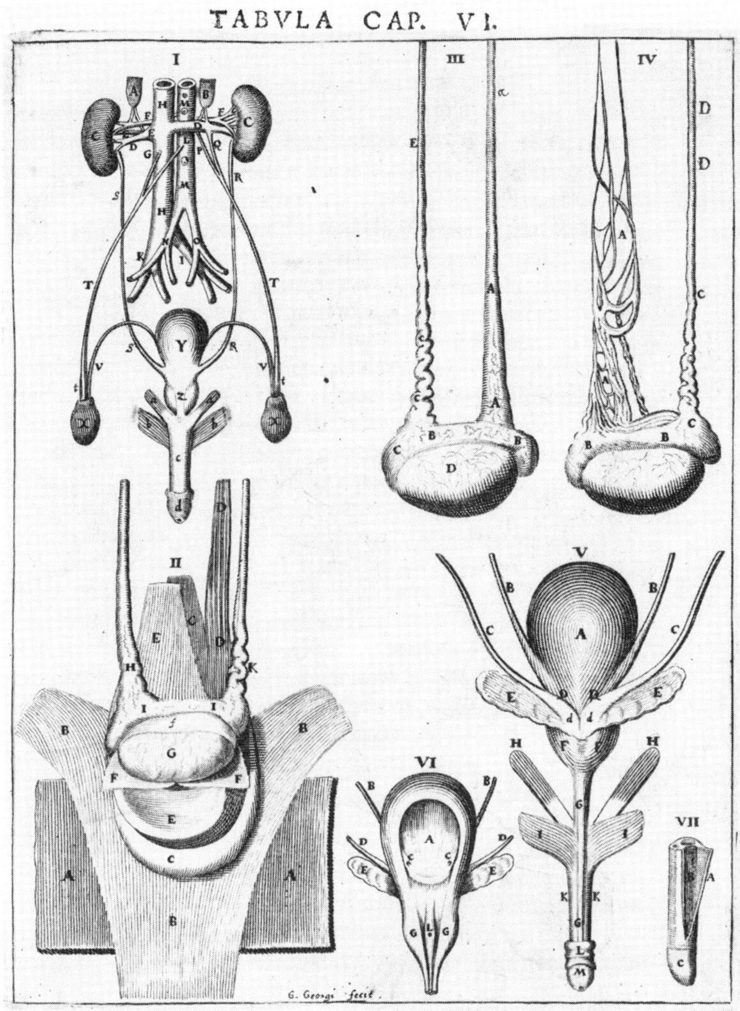

Figure 31 Johann Vesling, male reproductive system, in *Syntagma anatomica*, 2nd edn. (Padua: Pauli Frambotti, 1647), Table 6

force.[50] With variations, Aristotle and Galen understood that men's heated spirit was converted into the whitened "foam" of semen, though the former located the process in blood vessels while the latter prioritized the testicles and this idea

[50] For theories about *pneuma*, see Preus, "Galen's criticism," 73–74; Boylan, "Galenic and Hippocratic challenges," 96. Galen also associated "vital *pneuma*" with sperm: Galen, *Semen*,

was more influential.[51] Furthermore, sexual pleasure was due to expulsion, "to the fact that not only semen but also *pneuma* is emitted" (*GA* 728a10), and before that libido was aroused by the build up of seed.

According to Galen's treatise *On semen* (first printed as an independent text in 1533 but available for several decades already in his *Opera*), women and men each experienced desire only because they had testicles (what are now called ovaries in the female case) and produced semen.[52] If testicles were excised, men lost "their virility and, as one might say, their masculinity," and removal from a female would mean that then "it never feels sexual desire, . . . and it loses, as one might say, its femininity."[53] Men changed more if they were castrated, becoming chilled "as though deprived of a second source of innate heat, and all their strength collapses as if they had grown old." They lose their beards and other bodily hair, have no sexual desire and "have small veins . . . like women." Chiefly on the basis of observing sterilized sows, Galen said that "the female animal . . . becomes similar to the castrated male," implicitly entering an older, undesiring state, one even colder than that of the normative female. The effect of castration on *complexio* as well as on the body was often cited. While working in Greek-speaking areas of the Mediterranean in the 1490s, for example, the anatomist and professor Alessandro Benedetti learned that when testicles were excised "the masculine form and behavior . . . becomes feminine, for men lose their strength, boldness, habits, voices, and beard."[54]

As we have seen in the previous chapter, medical epistemology was combined with the etymological history of "testicle," for the word referred to the authority and potency of being a witness in legal proceedings, which was granted only to men. Testicular manhood informed Galen's second-century contemporary and interpreter of dreams, Artemidorus, who observed about the entire ensemble of male genitals (*aidoion*) that it "is a symbol of strength and physical vigor, because it is itself the cause of these qualities. That is why some people call the *aidoion* 'one's manhood' (*andreia*)" (1.45). That idea still underpinned the slang and euphemisms at play in early modern culture, such as the line from a song in an English chapbook of the 1680s in which a woman teaches a "bashful Young-

pp. 83, 91, 141, 214n; Galen, *Usefulness*, p. 623 and passim; Rudolph Siegel, *Galen's system of physiology and medicine* (Basel: S. Karger, 1968), pp. 183–92; Jacquart and Thomasset, *Sexuality and medicine*, pp. 48–50.

51 Galen, *Semen*, pp. 109–11, 135. Aristotle believed the testicles were merely counterweights, like those used on looms: *GA*, 717a35, 787b25. For a representative sample of later opinions on the "use" of the testicles, including the citation of Aristotle's analogy, see Crooke, *Mikrokosmographia*, pp. 243–45, a translation from du Laurens, *Historica anatomica*, pp. 346–47, first published in du Laurens, *Opera anatomica*, pp. 236–41.

52 On the printing and translation history of *De semine* see Durling, "Chronological census," 258, 259, 279–80, 291; Phillip de Lacy's "Introduction," to Galen, *Semen*, pp. 13–42.

53 Galen, *Semen*, pp. 121–25, hereafter quoted again, and from p. 137. See also Siegel, *Galen's system*, pp. 228–29.

54 Benedetti, *Anatomice*, p. 160; Lind, *Studies*, p. 97.

man" so that "his Courage began for to move."[55] As manly fluid and "spirit" inflated his penis so did his confidence and virility grow.

From courage to voice, the testicles were endowed with extensive influence. For all his attention to dissection, Leonardo's observations of the late fifteenth and early sixteenth centuries were filtered by what were then the canonical texts on anatomy, particularly in the earlier years. One of the questions he set himself to investigate was: "How are the testicles the cause of ardor?" (fig. 29). Even when musing later on the male generative organs around 1506–13, he echoed standard opinion: "Testicles witnesses of coitus. These contain in themselves ardor, that is, they are augmenters of the animosity and ferocity of animals. Experience shows this clearly in castrated animals" like bulls, boars, rams and cocks which "are left very cowardly."[56]

Vesalius' *Fabrica* of 1543 echoed Galen in many ways, including the belief that the testicles were where blood and spirit was turned into perfect semen, and that this testicular faculty "exists in males for the sake of strength and virility and in females for the sake of femininity."[57] The phrasing often occurred in subsequent texts, such as Paré's vernacular manual on anatomy for French barber-surgeons (1575), which also noted that testicles "by a certaine manly irradiation . . . breed or encrease a true masculine courage."[58] It was a medical commonplace that key characteristics of virility were what would today be considered behavioral features, like ardor, courage and mental and physical toughness, all traceable to testicular presence.

The "one-sex model," the "unequal two-seed theory" and semenotics

Laqueur famously argued in *Making sex* (1990) that from classical antiquity until the eighteenth century a "one-sex/one-flesh model" dominated, "where the boundaries between male and female are of degree and not of kind."[59] The late eighteenth century witnessed "a new model of radical dimorphism, of biological divergence." His evidence was primarily anatomical, mainly drawn from Galen, and relatively little attention was paid to humoral theory or physiology. Deeply influential for more than a decade, the argument played a leading role in the Foucauldian orientation of late twentieth-century cultural studies toward the discursive construction of sex. Physical sex and social gender were shown to

[55] Pepys, *Pepys' penny merriments*, p. 278. [56] Keele, *Leonardo*, p. 350.

[57] Andreas Vesalius, *De humani corporis de fabrica libri septem* (Basel: Joannis Orporini, 1543), p. 525; Andreas Vesalius, *On the fabric of the human body: a translation of "De humani corporis fabrica libri septem," Book V: the organs of nutrition and generation*, trans. William Frank Richardson and John Burd Carman (Norato, CA: Norman Publishing, 2007), p. 157.

[58] Paré, *Collected Works*, p. 120. [59] Laqueur, *Making sex*, p. 25, hereafter quoted from p. 6.

be intertwined, because "sex, as much as gender, is made."[60] Claims based on the assumption of scientific fact about the body were understood to be situational, to be meshed with their context and making. Yet the supposed similarity and overlap of bodies, their seeming lability and equivalence that was then made much of in scholarship of the late twentieth and early twenty-first century, fostered the neglect of corporeal materiality and the effect of power upon the conceptualization of bodies.

Here I hope to re-engage with the materiality and differences of human flesh and the ways in which these mattered in medical, cultural and everyday terms. Of far greater weight and perseverance than the one-sex model was what I call the "unequal two-seed theory," a scale of hierarchical value between male and female bodies based on the core elements of semen, testicles and heat.[61] I focus on just three problematic aspects of the "one-sex" analogy: the degree to which it was outweighed by those semenotic differences, its relatively minimal and sporadic occurrence and finally its genre and context.[62]

When agreeing with Aristotle that women were less perfect than men, Galen's *On the usefulness of the parts* gave two reasons, the first regarding innate differences in complexional heat. Then he turned to anatomical dissection: "All the parts, then, that men have, women have too, the difference between them lying in only one thing, . . . namely, that in women the [genital] parts are within [the body], whereas in men they are outside."[63] Ever the rhetorician and teacher, Galen suggested a thought experiment: "turn outward the woman's [reproductive parts], turn inward, so to speak, and fold double the man's, and you will find them the same in both in every respect." Turn the man's system inward, and scrotum would be in the place of the uterus, testicles (ovaries) outside, and the penis would occupy the space of the vagina, its

[60] Ibid., p. ix.

[61] Cadden's nuanced study occasionally refers to the "two-seed model" or "two-seed system" (*Sex difference*, pp. 18, 53), but does not draw attention to differences between female seed and male semen.

[62] Other critiques of the one-sex model include Katharine Park and Robert Nye, "Destiny is anatomy," *The New Republic* 204 (18 February 1991), 53–57; Cadden, *Sex difference*, pp. 177–83; Gail Kern Paster, *The body embarrassed: drama and the disciplines of shame in early modern England* (Ithaca: Cornell University Press, 1993), pp. 16–17, 79–83; Janet Adelman, "Making defect perfection: Shakespeare and the one-sex model," in Viviana Comensoli and Anne Russell (eds.), *Enacting gender on the English Renaissance stage* (Urbana: University of Illinois Press, 1999), pp. 23–52; Monica H. Green, "Bodies, gender, health, disease: recent work on medieval women's medicine," *Studies in Medieval and Renaissance History* 3rd ser., 2 (2005), 6–12; Helen King, "The mathematics of sex: one to two, or two to one?," *Studies in Medieval and Renaissance History* 3rd ser., 2 (2005), 47–58; Katharine Park, *Secrets of women: gender, generation, and the origins of human dissection* (New York: Zone Books, 2006), pp. 186–87. I am grateful to Katy Park for sharing with me her incisive analysis of the one-sex idea in her forthcoming article "Itineraries of the 'one-sex body': a history of an idea." Her comments on an early draft of this chapter were invaluable.

[63] Galen, *Usefulness*, pp. 628–29.

glans now being a woman's external genitals. Notably, the anatomy of male and female bodies was largely the same except for this contrast in their reproductive systems, one "turned in," the other "outward and projecting." Galen's *On semen* made the same fundamental point about internal and external position, when discussing the stages of fetal formation.[64]

Crucially, within a page or so *On the usefulness of the parts* returned to the matter of heat, noting that the semen or seed produced by male and female bodies was also different. "Of course, the female must have smaller, less perfect testes, and the semen generated in them must be scantier, colder, and wetter," because she is a less perfect, cooler, moister creature.[65] Her semen has far less generative capacity but has other uses, chiefly "inciting the female to the sexual act and in opening wide the neck of the uteri during coitus" in order to receive male semen, and to moisten passageways. Laqueur has claimed that Galen "might actually have meant that it [that is, female seed] worked like a penis."[66] But this reading confuses physiology with anatomy, female fluid with male solid. It assumes that a penis will *necessarily* "incite" women and it misunderstands the premodern function of the penis, which was rather to deliver semen to the end of a channel that had, in the Galenic system, opened because the *woman's* body had released seed and eagerly desired male *semen*, not the penis per se. Each notion, one-sex and unequal two-seed, focused on physical differences, in that the woman's genitals were interior and her semen inferior, because she was colder. No contradiction was discerned in texts that quickly described the anatomical analogy and then went on to cede women the production of seed that was distinctively lesser.

Michael Stolberg has recently argued that the one-sex idea had begun to falter by the late sixteenth century, more than a century earlier than Lacqueur discerned. Stolberg found that several somatic differences were observed at that time, beginning with the fact that female testicles were said to differ "very much in size and substance from those of the male."[67] However, several important

[64] Galen, *Semen*, pp. 189–93.

[65] Galen, *Usefulness*, p. 631; also pp. 642–45, 647, 654 passim, from which the following is drawn. For heat, see also Galen, *Semen*, pp. 176–77, and there too female semen was thinner and colder, "more suitable than all else for nourishment" of the male seed and the embryo, around which it formed a membrane: pp. 87–89, 99, 153, 175–77, 216.

[66] Laqueur, *Making sex*, p. 45.

[67] Michael Stolberg, "A woman down to her bones: the anatomy of sexual difference in the sixteenth and early seventeenth centuries," *Isis* 94 (2003), 286 (the earliest citation is Lodovicus Vassaeus of 1553). See also the responses: Thomas Laqueur, "Sex in the flesh," *Isis* 94 (2003), 300–6; Londa Schiebinger, "Skelettestreit," *Isis* 94 (2003), 307–13. Winfried Schleiner, "Early modern controversies about the one-sex model," *Renaissance Quarterly* 53 (2000), 180–91, had already pointed to the anatomical objections of du Laurens in the late sixteenth century, and debates were also indicated by Ian Maclean, *The Renaissance notion of woman: a study in the fortunes of scholasticism and medical science in European intellectual life* (Cambridge University Press, 1980), pp. 28–46.

factors are overlooked by Stolberg. First, Galen had already emphasized testicular difference, as we have seen.[68] Secondly, *pace* Stolberg, the "watery or, at times, yellowish fluid" within the ovaries or female "stones" (testicles) had also been noted by the Hippocratics, Galen, Avicenna and many others.[69] If female seed was thought to exist, as it sometimes was by medieval authors well before the revival of Hippo-Galenic theories in humanist medicine, it was always said to be inferior, less distilled, weaker, thinner, less effective in the process of fetal formation (except when, in some theories about sex determination, a particular father's semen must have been weaker because the child was female).[70]

The one-sex homology only appeared in several medieval texts, abetted by translations from Arabic rather than from any direct influence from Galen's works. The translation into Latin (after 1170) of Avicenna's Arabic *Canon* and the writing of the *Anatomia vivorum* (*c.* 1225), which was chiefly informed by Avicenna's influential textbook, re-introduced the one-sex rubric to European anatomy.[71] Avicenna went on to distinguish between male and female testicles on the basis of size, shape and location. Thereafter, the homology was a similarly brief introductory statement in the section on the female reproductive system, appearing in one medical genre, anatomies and the related manuals for surgeons, whose labor required a basic comprehension of anatomy. The quick mention of the homology in the works of surgeons Lanfranco of Milan (completed in 1296) and Henri de Mondeville (*c.* 1306–20), which were translated

[68] Other examples include the *Second Salernitan demonstration*, in Corner, *Anatomical texts*, p. 65; Thomas Raynald, *The byrth of mankynde* (London: Thomas Raynold, 1545), fol. 14v; Ambroise Paré, *De la génération de l'homme* (1573), in *Œuvres*, vol. II, pp. 636–67; Scipione Mercurio, *La commare* (Venice: Giovanni Battista Ciotti, 1601 edn., first published 1596), in Maria Luisa Altieri Biagi, Clemente Mazzota, Angela Chiantera and Paola Altieri (eds.), *Medicina per le donne nel cinquecento: testi di Giovanni Marinello e di Girolamo Mercurio* (Turin: UTET, 1992), p. 74.

[69] The quotation is from Stolberg, "A woman down to her bones." Examples include "On the nature of the child," 31.3, in *Hippocratic treatises*, pp. 21, 128; Avicenna, *Liber canonis*, 351r (Bk. III, fen. 20, tr. 1, ch. 3); Monica Green, "The *De genecia* attributed to Constantine the African," *Speculum* 62 (1987), 314–15; Berengario, *Isagogae breves*, fol. 22r; Raynald, *Byrth of mankynde*, fol. 14v; Thomas Vicary, *A profitable treatise of the anatomie of mans body* (London: Henry Bamforde, 1577), M iii verso; Crooke, *Mikrokosmographia*, pp. 218–19; Sharp, *Midwives book*, p. 34.

[70] On various attempts to explain parental influence in the determination of foetal sex, see Preus, "Galen's criticism," 65–85; Boylan, "Galenic and Hippocratic challenges," 83–112; Jacquart and Thomasset, *Sexuality and medicine*, pp. 34–35, 61, 64, 65, 139–43. Lucretius, *De rerum natura*, 4:1209–32, reiterates an old theory primarily held by the Greeks Pythagoras, Democritus and Epicurus that believed both parental seed exerted some sway, a scheme that did not necessitate absolute equality between the two seeds. More common explanations for sex determination, amongst those who believed female seed played any part, resorted to a left–right model (concerning the testicles or what was believed to be several uterine chambers) or environmental/humoral theories about such factors as temperatures, winds or the quantity and strength of male sperm.

[71] Avicenna, *Liber canonis*, 360r (Bk. III, fen. 21, tr. 1, ch. 1); Corner, *Anatomical texts*, pp. 88, 103, 104; see also Cadden, *Sex difference*, pp. 64, 119. The *Anatomia vivorum*, not cited by Laqueur or Stolberg, circulated in manuscript and was included amongst some of the printed editions of the collected works of Galen, an association that guaranteed its ongoing influence. For the sources, date and transmission see Corner, *Anatomical texts*, pp. 35–41.

into several vernaculars, did not cite Galen's *On the use of parts* (only translated into Latin in 1317).[72] Guy de Chauliac's encyclopaedic *Great surgery* (completed in 1363) was the exception, for it quoted Galen's passage, but otherwise, as Katharine Park has shown, the homology did not feature in new medical texts until the turn of the sixteenth century.[73]

Before Vesalius' groundbreaking *Fabrica* (1543) and at a time when anatomical publications proliferated, five or so sixteenth-century authors made mention of the homology. No doubt some were influenced by printed editions of Galen, though the Latin translation of *The usefulness of the parts* was first printed in 1528, so they may have taken account of works like Lanfranco's (first printed in 1490). Galen's *On semen* had been known for longer, circulating in manuscript then appearing in the Latin complete works of 1490, but the one-sex model there also does not seem to have been immediately influential. The earliest sixteenth-century appearance of the idea occurred in Alessandro Benedetti's *Anatomice*, penned in the 1490s but first printed in Venice in 1502, by a surgeon and lecturer who had worked in Greek-speaking areas of the Mediterranean. If he knew Galen's Greek texts, however, they made little impact for he used only a single analogy, between the cervix and the glans, and that was not where Galen drew a parallel, whereas it does appear in Peter of Abano's *Conciliator* (1303).[74] In the same year and city Gabriele Zerbi mentioned the idea in his *Anathomia*, whereas it appeared with more detail in two books by the Bolognese surgeon Jacopo Berengario da Carpi published in 1521–22.[75] Interestingly, both authors cite Avicenna as well as Galen, yet raise the matter of anatomical similarity in relation to whether women could become men. Instead, Niccolò Massa's anatomical book issued in 1536 as an "introduction for young men" to dissection repeats the

72 For Lanfranc's *Chirurgia Magna*, see Lanfranco of Milan, *Lanfrank's "Science of Cirurgie"* ed. Robert von Fleischhacker (New York: Scribner, 1894), p. 175, expanded in Lanfranco of Milan, *A most excellent and learned woorke of chirurgerie, called Chirurgia parua Lanfranci* (London: Thomas Marshe, 1565), p. 75. On Mondeville, see his *Chirurgie*, p. 53, hence also in a fourteenth-century Provençal version, Max Gorosch, *La notomia de Anric de Mondavilla* (Avignon: Centre d'Études Occitanes, 1975), p. 60, and Vicary, *A profitable treatise of the anatomie*, M ii recto, virtually repeated in Thomas Geminus, *Compendiosa totius anatomie delineatio: a facsimile of the first English edition of 1553 in the version of Nicholas Udall* (London: Dawson's of Pall Mall, 1959), A iiii recto. A putative edition of Vicary from 1548 does not survive.

73 [Guy de Chauliac] Guigonis de Caulhiaco, *Inventarium sive Chirurgia Magna*, ed. Michael R. McVaugh, vol. I: *Text* (Leiden: Brill, 1997), pp. 52–53; Park, *Secrets of women*, pp. 186–88; Park, "Itineraries of the 'one-sex body': a history of an idea." Neither Lacquer nor Stolberg cites Lanfranc, Mondeville or Chauliac.

74 Benedetti, *Anatomice*, p. 174. For Peter see Ch. 6 n. 85 below.

75 For Zerbi and Berengario see Park, *Secrets of women*, pp. 186–88; Park, "Itineraries" (which also discusses Charles Estienne's delayed publication of 1545). Berengario and Estienne are discussed in Laqueur, *Making sex*, pp. 79–81, 90, 130–33. The homology appeared at the head of the discussion of the uterus in Berengario's *Isagogae brevis* (1522), fols. 18v, 22v, which follows the division of the *Anatomia vivorum* between an early comparison of seminal vessels and fluids, and the later description of the uterus.

inversion several times, once more when comparing the female reproductive system to the normative male.[76]

In all these cases, the inside-out analogy was quickly made in a sentence or so, and was usually noticeable for its isolation. It was not integrated with subsequent information and was muted by descriptions of differing seed and seminal systems, which presented the male body as more perfect. The history of this matter is as much about the rarity of actual observation at dissections, and about manuscript transmission then the impact of printing, as it is a principle that can be traced back to causative changes in erotic or social history. Medical discourse was slow to alter learned opinion, and the homology of male and female reproductive systems was a cursory, introductory and conventional remark.

The text most critical of received opinion at its time was Vesalius' *Fabrica* (1543), which nevertheless continued to contrast the female uterus, semen and testicles to superior versions in the male reproductive system. Male and female bodies were implicitly parallel in many ways, each with testes, seminal passages and semen, but the standard contrasts whereby the female instances were always lesser also applied, particularly because the female body was colder.[77] Vesalius did not explicitly state the standard rubric about one sex, nor suggest the thought experiment of inversion. This, the single most influential anatomical text of the Renaissance, noted similarities in substance and function between particular parts of the male and female reproductive systems but so too did Vesalius observe differences, and no theoretical conclusion was drawn.

The exact causes for the irregular reiteration of the one-sex notion are unclear, though the new wave of medical humanism does not explain either Chauliac's attention to Galen so early nor Benedetti's near disregard, given his Hellenic interests, and Vesalius was rather resistant. Perhaps the sixteenth-century efflorescence was one way in which authors interested primarily in morphology could frame a professional opinion on the status of female bodies. Tales of sex change, including those reported by Pliny and others more easily disseminated through print, were one factor suggesting that female bodies were not always and necessarily the polarized opposite of normative male structures (and notably they were always thought to alter into the more perfect male state). The wider impact of Galen's corpus was leading to even fuller acceptance of the idea that women's contribution to generation was more substantial than had been supposed under a primarily Aristotelian theory (but not equal to male semen). Far from indicating that the choice was already decided between polarization of the sexes or their existence on a complexional or anatomical continuum, the one-sex idea perhaps enjoyed a brief heyday precisely because the choice remained debatable.

[76] Lind, *Studies*, pp. 203–08 (not cited by Laqueur or Stolberg).
[77] Vesalius, *Fabrica*, pp. 535–37 passim.

If chronology, context and genre cast the one-sex notion in a new light, so too does a consideration of function. Qualifying terms that accompany many descriptions, such as "quasi," "as it were" or "resembles to a certain degree" ("quodammodo instar," in the case of one of Vesalius' captions), indicate that the notion is more what Janet Adelman called "a loose analogy," and what I suggest is akin to an introductory teaching device.[78] Galen drew the analogy for pedagogical purposes of demonstration and his discussion of the reproductive systems in *On the usefulness of the parts* had quickly returned to men's more perfect, heated state. "Everything in the male is the opposite" of what is in the female, he said, using the example of the penis elongated in order to "excrete semen," so the overall scheme was about complementary opposites.[79] And the idea did not inform any of his later discussion. Notably, many anatomies and all surgical manuals were practical, teaching books, uninterested in the philosophical aspects of medical theory. The predominance of the one-sex opposition in that genre indicates that it was, like Galen's own statement, more an aid to visualization and memorization than the summation of a complex theory of sexual oneness.

Changes in the sixteenth century

Much of the unequal two-seed theory continued through the sixteenth and into the seventeenth centuries, though there were several shifts in medical discourse and imagery that further underscored women's lesser, different nature. The "discovery" of the clitoris by anatomists led to debates which partly assessed it according to criteria based on the male model of semen and projection. The rise of gynecology as a professional, male pursuit was driven by the notion that female bodies were different, and resulted in the expansion of the quantity and focus of medical texts, already increasing due to greater use of the printing press. And printed images contributed to the standardization of anatomical knowledge. One of Vesalius' illustrations of the uterine system has been used as proof of the one-sex analogy, but we will see that there is another way of looking at it, which accords with the basic principle that femininity was about being colder, recessive and receptive.

The one-sex idea increasingly made little sense, especially after anatomists announced the "discovery" of the clitoris in publications of 1560 and 1561. The later publication, by the anatomist at the University of Padua Gabriele Falloppio, was as much philological as anatomical, mentioning the ancient Greek term *kleitoris* and finding a comparison with this "kind of penis (*istius penis*)" in Latin translations of two Arabic sources (Avicenna and Albucasis).

[78] Ibid., p. 381 (*sic*, 481); Avicenna, *Liber canonis*, Bk. III, fen. 21, tr. 1, ch. 1 (the womb was "quasi conversum instrumentum virorum"); Adelman, "Making defect perfection," p. 26.

[79] Galen, *Usefulness*, pp. 628–32.

He also reiterated the position of Aristotelian, one-seed theorists by noting that "the *testes* in women do not seem to be made for the production of seed" while observing, with important equivocation, that the uterus had a shape "almost similar to the inverted member of the male."[80]

The death-knell of the two-seed and one-sex ideas was already beginning to be tolled as early as the mid- to late sixteenth century, joining the momentum of growing criticism of Galen's writings in the face of new knowledge gained from dissections.[81] In particular, Winfried Schleiner and Stolberg have drawn attention to du Laurens' dismissal of the commonality between male and female reproductive systems, which the French anatomist linked with the issue of sex change. The professor and royal physician first published his reasons for believing the supposed inversion "absurd" in 1593, and elaborated them in 1600. He observed that "no similarity comes in between the vagina and the male penis; none between the uterus and the scrotum; neither in the structure, form and size of the testicles the same, nor in the distribution and insertion of the spermatic vessels."[82]

To the claim that the clitoris was a species of penis, du Laurens countered that it was much smaller and had no duct for semen.[83] His criteria were about size and fluids, and those standards were used to evaluate the differences between the vessels and semen, bolstered by the thermal scale of the complexional system. More extensively than earlier writers, du Laurens demonstrated dimorphism, but he too emphasized different perspectives at different moments. He had, for instance, adapted an image from Vesalius and altered the captions so that a vessel between the female testicles and the womb was ejaculatory (fig. 32: in fig. II, ss were labeled "Principium vasis eiaculatorii"). However, this similarity in terminology and function demonstrated not equivalence but the degree to which the male and semen-centric standard was considered applicable to the female body. Furthermore, the function was allocated to neither female testicles nor vagina, and hence du Laurens broke from the Galenic inversion. A small image of the entire uterus with the testicles was placed near the margin in the middle right of du Laurens' illustration (fig. V), taken from the final page in Vesalius' drastically short *Epitome* first published in 1543. The accompanying text in both cases drew no parallel or contrast

80 Schleiner, "Controversies," 183, translating from the *Opera omnia* edition of 1600. On the clitoris, see Realdo Colombo, *De re anatomica* (Venice: Nicolai Bevilacquae, 1559), p. 243; Gabriele Falloppia, *Observationes anatomicae*, ed. Gabriella Righi Riva and Pericle Di Pietro (Modena: S.T.E.M. Mucchi, 1964), vol. I, fols. 192v–193v (facsimile of the 1561 first edition); Park, "Rediscovery of the clitoris," pp. 170–93.

81 For the slow decline of Galenism, see Owsei Temkin, *Galenism: rise and decline of a medical philosophy* (Ithaca: Cornell University Press, 1973), pp. 134–92.

82 André du Laurens, *Historica anatomica* (Frankfurt: Rhodius, 1602), p. 552, translated in Stolberg, "Woman down to her bones," 287. This is the same as du Laurens, *Historica anatomica* (1600), pp. 358–60, which is an enlarged version of du Laurens, *Opera anatomica* (1593), pp. 263–64, and was translated into English in Crooke, *Mikrokosmographia*, pp. 249–50.

83 Reiterated in Duval, *Hermaphrodits*, pp. 65–66.

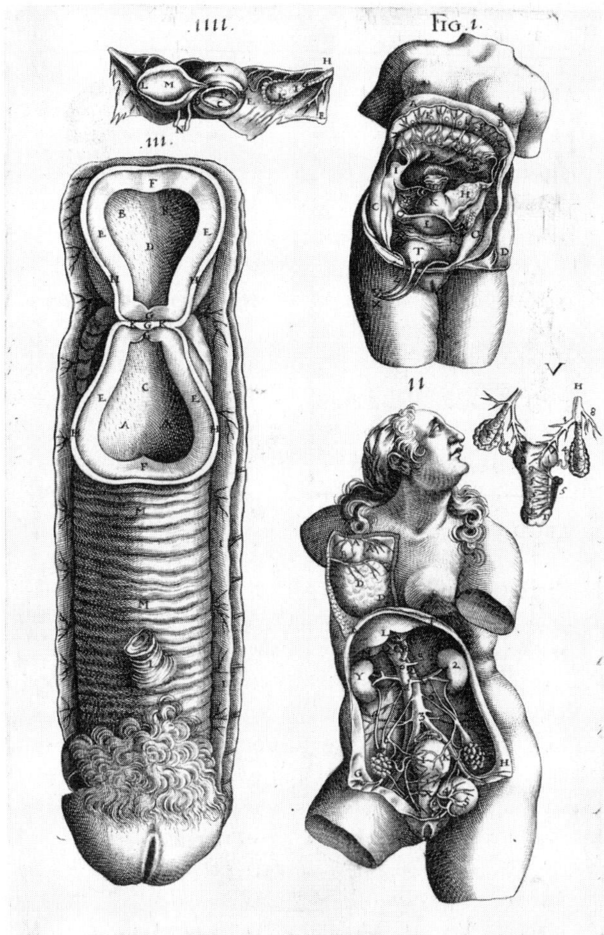

Figure 32 André du Laurens, female uterine system, in *Historica anatomica humani corporis* (Paris: A. Mettayer et Ourry, 1600), p. 257

with male genitals. Rather, when discussing his reuse of the image in 1615 Crooke likened the form in fig. V to a pear, and other metaphors like "sheath" or "embrace" speak to what was envisaged in uterine–penile conjunction.[84]

To a substantial degree, proponents of the one-sex model rely for their core evidence on the source of du Laurens' figure III on the left, Vesalius' much-copied

[84] Crooke, *Mikrokosmographia*, pp. 226–27, directing the reader to Table IX, fig. iii, on p. 224, and p. 250 for "a sheath to receive the virile member." See, for instance, Duval, *Hermaphrodits*, pp. 60, 61, 70–78 ("conduit ou gaine du membre viril"). "Vagina" was used for the scrotal "sheath": for example, Bauhin, *Theatrum anatomicum*, pp. 182–83; Crooke, *Mikrokosmographia*, p. 206.

Plate 27. It depicts what was considered the entire uterine system, including external genitalia and "neck of the womb" or vagina. Yet, taken out of context, it has been read in modern terms solely in relation to the penis. To Londa Schiebinger, "one need only refer to Vesalius' remarkable image of the female genitalia portrayed as a male penis" for the case to stand.[85] However, none of the early modern texts I have consulted points to Vesalius' popular illustration as a demonstration of the one-sex analogy. It is not closely modeled on Galen's thought experiment because it is not turned inside out and, crucially, female testicles are not attached. The one-sex assertion works only if the claimed homology applies exclusively to the penis, which is an anachronistic, Freudian assumption. Sixteenth-century viewers may not have been quite so struck by similarity with just one part of the male genitals. Unlike illustrations of the projecting penis (figs. 30–31), the female uterine system is a relatively blunt, static body part weighed down by the bulbous chamber of the womb.

The image primarily depicts a tube and receptacle to *receive* the penis, just as Aristotelian philosophy and Galenic anatomy described, to hold it close in order to draw in or "embrace" and direct semen to the uterus.[86] The image agrees with Vesalius' text, in which the standard complementarity of male emission and female reception began the chapter on the penis.[87] The Vesalian uterus bisected and literally opened out through dissection begins to make of the presumptively male reader a sexual partner emitting seed that is awaited eagerly by the receptive organ. Vesalius' sixteenth-century image of a close-fitting tube leading to the uterine cavity, reprinted and plagiarized countless times in later anatomical texts, shows the receptive response envisaged by both medical authors and Leonardo (fig. 29).

Depicting a complementary vessel, the woodcut accords with the Biblical one-sex model as it were, in which two shall become one, a phrase first occurring after Eve is made from Adam's rib in Genesis but repeated by Jesus and Paul in the New Testament.[88] More generally, God's creation of two sexes forms the preface in medieval gynecological texts like the *Trotula*, which is evidenced in a woman's "opposing frigidity and humidity," her consequent weakness and a man's rulership. His task is to pour seed into the woman "just as seed is sown in its designated field" and she must "receive the seed poured fourth in the lap of Nature."[89] Hence, the sexual innuendo was

85 Schiebinger, "Skelettestreit," 310; also Laqueur, *Making sex*, pp. 82–85 and passim; Laqueur, "Sex in the flesh," 300–6.

86 For example, Raynald, *Byrth of mankynde*, fd. 10r. 87 Vesalius, *Fabrica*, p. 527.

88 Genesis 2.24; Matthew 19.5–6; Mark 10.6–7; 1 Corinthians 6.16; Ephesians 5.31.

89 *The "Trotula": a medieval compendium of women's medicine*, ed. and trans. Monica H. Green (Philadelphia: University of Pennsylvania Press, 2001), p. 71; Monica H. Green, *Making women's medicine masculine: the rise of male authority in pre-modern gynaecology* (Oxford University Press, 2008), p. 50.

clear in a late seventeenth-century English chapbook in which a man suggested to his sweetheart that "first let's try if all things will agree together when they meet."[90]

Du Laurens' argument against the one-sex model was soon debated and most professional authors agreed with the marginal comment in Caspar Bartholin's *Anatomicae* of 1611: "The similarity (*similitudo*) of the Yard and of the Womb, ridiculous (*inepta*)."[91] All parties critiquing the one-sex homology were contributing to debates about such issues as sex changes, hermaphrodites, tribades and the acceptability or implausibility of the Aristotelian notion that women were necessarily imperfect, a topic that featured in the rising literature written and published on gynecology by men.

Monica Green and Helen King have identified and analyzed the rise of gynecology amongst male practitioners from the fifteenth century on. That very specialization indicates how much female bodies were perceived to be different, a disparity given new articulation and authority with the publication of Hippocratic texts from 1525 which stated as a basic principle that "the healing of the diseases of women differs greatly from the healing of men's diseases."[92] In particular, that difference was physiological and uterine, for it involved not only the thermal scale and a different degree of moisture but also the elemental Hippo-Galenic precept that management of menstruation (her excess "seed") was crucial to a woman's health (most saliently but not exclusively because it was thought crucial for pregnancy). Indeed, another Hippocratic passage was specific: "the womb is the origin of all diseases of women."[93] A great deal of the gynecological literature therefore concentrated on female "seed."

Traditionally heading sections on the womb in anatomical discourse, the one-sex homology took up a few sentences in the growing genre of gynecology, when books in that chiefly vernacular genre prefaced the main substance with an overview of reproductive anatomy. From the field of philosophy, gynecological literature increasingly proposed that the female body was sufficient in itself, designed to carry out the task of childbearing to perfection. Whereas du Laurens' first discussion of the one-sex model occurred as one of the "questions"

90 Pepys, *Pepys' penny merriments*, p. 102.

91 Bartholin, *Anatomicae*, pp. 98, 113–14; [Bartholin], *Bartholinus anatomy*, pp. 53, 61–62. See also, for example, Bauhin, *Theatrum anatomicum*, pp. 210–11, translated in Crooke, *Mikrokosmographia*, pp. 216–17; cf. 249–50, 270–77 from du Laurens.

92 Hanson (trans), "Hippocrates: *Diseases of women* 1," 582. On sixteenth-century publications and influence see King, "Mathematics of sex," 47–58; Helen King, *Midwifery, obstetrics and the rise of gynaecology: the uses of a sixteenth-century compendium* (Aldershot: Ashgate, 2007), pp. 11, 18, 29; Green, *Making women's medicine*, pp. 26, 248, 267, 275–77, 346 nos. 12–13, 349 no. 30, 352 no. 52, 354 no. 66.

93 King, "Mathematics of sex," 51; King, *Midwifery*, p. 11. See also Green, "Bodies, gender, health, disease," 8–10. Cf. Laqueur, "Sex in the flesh," 305.

to be argued in the book on procreation (Book 7), in the first chapter of the following book, which was on the embryo, du Laurens refuted Aristotelian claims about imperfection because Nature's work was never mistaken. When the focus shifted to the female body's role as a pregnant being then, in du Laurens' words, "the two sexes of male and female do not differ on the level of essence, as to form and perfection, but only as to accidentals, namely temperature, and structure and position of the genitals."[94] The father had performed his task to perfection and now the mother would do hers.

Male and female bodies were considered equal in certain respects but also different, judged by the determining criteria of anatomical teleology. As long as the unequal two-seed idea held, then each type of producer of seed had been made perfect by Nature for that task. The belief was solidly established by the mid-seventeenth century, infiltrating books for the vernacular market.[95] But the idea was not dramatically new. For instance, the first gynecological book of the sixteenth century, one that went on to be reissued and printed in many languages, had stated the case. Eucharius Rösslin's *Rosegarten* (1513), as translated into English in 1545 by Thomas Raynald, first made it clear that the seeds were different ("nothing so firme, perfect, absolut, and myghty in woman as in man"), and then denied the Aristotelian claim of female "imperfection or lacke," because Nature was perfect: "For the woman in her kynd, and for thoffice and pourpose wherfor she was made is even as absolute and perfect as man in his kynd."[96] Each was of a different kind, yet suited to its task, impregnation and incubation respectively; the woman's body notably remained utero-centric, with crucial attention also paid to her "seed," and the male one continued its semen-centered primacy.

Difference

My refutation of the one-sex model in favor of a semenotic understanding of premodern sexed bodies has been enabled by several decades of interdisciplinary research linking medical and cultural history in fruitful dialogue. Here, however, the usual findings of ambiguity, relativity and elision regarding gender and sex, which were so prominent in modern studies influenced by Laqueur, are

94 Du Laurens, *Opera anatomica* (1593), p. 280; du Laurens, *Historica anatomica* (1600), p. 367, translated from the edition of 1595 in Schleiner, "Controversies," 187.

95 For example, see R. B. [Richard Bunworth], *The doctresse* (London: JF, 1656), pp. 1–2. For the debate in Latinate medical culture, though tending to ignore early evidence, see Maclean, *Renaissance notion of woman*, pp. 28–46. Du Laurens' argument for perfection is considered a skirmish on the "metaphysical periphery" in Laqueur, "Sex in the flesh," 303, 305, whereas metaphysics was central to ancient and Renaissance writers: Park and Nye, "Destiny is anatomy," 54–55.

96 Raynald, *Byrth of mankynde*, fol. 24r. Much of Rösslin's book was based on Michele Savonarola's fifteenth-century *Practica maior*: Green, *Making women's medicine*, p. 270.

less evident. This results when power differentials are central, and when materials from more than one country and from a broader chronology are brought to bear on the issue of gendered and sexed bodies. At a different, early twenty-first-century moment, lability is less striking than the confident iteration, regulation, institutionalization and expansion of medical knowledge, which defined norms and limits. The cases discussed in Chapter 1, for example, of assigning only one sex to Elena/o and to Marie/Marin, were about complex bodies that any medico-legal system would find challenging. As in modern science, the varied responses were formulated within epistemological parameters that had proved adequate and were not overturned by a few exceptions and did not give rise to anxiety or relativism. Notably, when Galen and others discussed the effect of the excision of testicles, the factors of sex, gender and libido were not carefully distinguished, and this was not because those areas were thought unstable but because they were regarded as inextricably interconnected.

It is misleading to talk of "the physiology of the one-sex model" as though it was homogeneous, and careful calibration is needed when thinking about pre-eighteenth-century medical understanding of "the body as constituted of more or less fungible fluids."[97] While it is true that humors had some potential to alter within the body, especially during various concoctions, and that their pathways overlapped, it is also the case that the humors were distinct yet complex fluids that combined in a particular blend in each case of individual temperament or *complexio*, and in relation to the management of the non-naturals. Complexity is not the same as instability. According to strict Aristotelians, semen was not produced by women, and for those holding to the unequal two-seed theory seed was still not interchangeable or equivalent between the sexes. If it was, women ought to be able to impregnate themselves because their own masculinized semen would mate with their feminized seed, and that was a theoretical line some commentators since Aristotle had been aware of but thought absurd to cross.[98]

Blood was established as the most fundamental bodily humor and hence it was the basis for leakages and fungibility: blood was converted into milk for the

[97] Laqueur, "Sex in the flesh," 305, which is thinking primarily of blood, and of cases of bleeding men (chiefly from hemorrhoids), on which see Gianna Pomata, "Menstruating men: similarity and difference of the sexes in early modern medicine," in Finucci and Brownlee (eds.), *Generation and degeneration*, pp. 109–52; Green, "Bodies, gender, health, disease," 7–8; Monica Green, "Flowers, poisons and men: menstruation in medieval western Europe," in Andrew Shail and Gillian Howie (eds.), *Menstruation: a cultural history* (New York: Palgrave Macmillan, 2005), pp. 60–1; Michael Stolberg, "Menstruation and sexual difference in early modern medicine," in *ibid.*, pp. 90–101. An alternative way to think about change in the complexional system is suggested in Timothy Hampton, "Strange alteration: physiology and psychology from Galen to Rabelais," in Gail Kern Paster, Mary Floyd-Wilson and Katherine Rowe (eds.), *Reading the early modern passions: essays in the cultural history of emotion* (Philadelphia: University of Pennsylvania Press, 2004), pp. 272–93.

[98] For example, it is repudiated by Aristotle, *GA*, 1.18.722b14–15; Giles of Rome (Jacquart and Thomasset, *Sexuality and medicine*, p. 65); Paré, *Collected works*, p. 925; Fernel, *Physiologia*,

newborn and it was concocted into seed within both male and female bodies. Due to the complexity of the humors, the hierarchy was not incontrovertible and men occasionally lactated, or bled on a monthly basis, and in these events the norm was female, but such occurrences were still explained by a humoral system that had individual bodies necessarily expelling superfluous matter. The medical standard was clear: menstruation happened "alwayes to Womoankinde, after xiiii or xv yeares of age passed (beinge in their parfeit helth)."[99] Deviations occurred in unhealthy male and female bodies and were treatable, or the unusual occurrences were acceptable enough because thereby the body was self-regulating back into balance. Antonio Benivieni's notes on *abnormal* cases in fifteenth-century Florence reported one instance of a man with a monthly issue of blood, for which a new diet was prescribed, along with bloodletting to drain off the excess.[100] Applying standard humoral reasoning, Joubert deduced in 1578 that virgins' breasts could yield milk due to excess blood, and exceptional cases of breastfeeding men were cited, supported by the citation of Aristotle and anecdote.[101] Notably, reports about these sorts of cases declined in concert with the slow shift away from humoral thinking that took place during the eighteenth and nineteenth centuries.

Learned medicine proceeded within sophisticated and interactive parameters, but that trope of postmodern discourse, an "endless play with signifiers," was biosocially delimited. While it is today a commonplace that gender is culturally determined and therefore can change, it is not a logical conclusion from that insight that gender was necessarily and always "unstable" and "slippery." The "anxiety" so often identified in this schema, and which is endowed with causal effects, is only discerned for the masculine gender. Exceptions do not prove a rule, and it is best to remind ourselves humbly of our own culture's inability to define gender or sex in scientifically certain terms.

Anecdotes about sex change often came to accompany the one-sex rubric, as they notably had not for Galen, but such transformations were grounded in the humoral theory of thermal difference and almost invariably they were unidirectional into male bodies because Nature's divine plan operated according to the telos of perfection. Occasional statements about effeminacy most often focused on the result of surgical castration, and this was always considered a lesser, degenerative state. Old men became colder, old women dryer with age so that in each case their characteristics shifted a little toward the other sex, but age was

pp. 556–58. The discussion usually took place in the context of "false pregnancy" or *mola uteri* (see Crooke, *Mikrokosmographia*, pp. 297–99, and further references in Maclean, *Renaissance notion of woman*, pp. 36, 105–06 n. 65).

99 Raynald, *Byrth of mankynde*, fols. 33v–34r.

100 Antonio Benivieni, *De abditis nonnullis ac mirandis morborum et sanationum causis*, trans. Charles Singer (Springfield: Charles C. Thomas, 1954), pp. 26–29.

101 Aristotle, *History of animals*, 3.2012–20; Joubert, *Popular errors*, pp. 204–07.

not a destabilizing factor because it was one of the variable non-naturals taken into account by the complexional system, along with such matters as region and occupation.[102] Illness might well result in the notable case of one bodily fluid unexpectedly becoming another, and exiting from an inappropriate orifice (like menstruating through the nose, as Paré reported of his wife), but that was precisely a sign of imbalance and obstruction rather than of normative process.

The "one-sex model" was a summary statement about anatomical morphology, but it only applied to physiology to the extent that the humoral scheme regarded all bodies as complex, semi-porous containers comprised of a number of fluids which were converted to other particular fluids due to explicable patterns regarding overall concoction and equilibrium. Female bodies were distinctively marked by a plethora of blood, which was regularly expelled, and was considered weaker because it was not concocted as well as it was in perfect, heated male bodies. That women were sometimes threatened with castration or called "ballsy" in literary tales, or that a Spanish ecclesiastical court once thought a woman was castrated because she had been treated by a hernia master when seven months old, does not show "the instability of gender boundaries in early modern Europe."[103] Rather, such exceptions demonstrate the ways in which the exclusive application of the model of adult male perfection could engender local confusion, ambiguous terminology and inventive, usually misogynist humor in order to reassert the normative order. Daily corporeal experience did not entail an anxious sense of blood's likelihood to change into other effusions, say, or for a body to alter drastically one's sex, let alone again and again.

The early modern body was not comprised of a labile, virtual economy of limitless possibilities. Laqueur's daring project suited the times, providing a history of anatomy that reinforced the drive in cultural and feminist studies during the 1990s to concentrate on the instability of gender. Indeed, the book's enduring legacy is its contribution to the understanding that sex and gender are not neatly separate ontologies. But Adelman, Katharine Park and others have noted that there was a cost, "of doing away with women's bodies: there is only one sex, and that sex is male."[104] My study redresses the balance by returning to two bodies, but rethinking earlier attempts to characterize the male body, which chiefly occurred when modern scholars were focused on the female, reproductive body. When fundamental medical theory bolstered patriarchal structure, a man's body was a biologically superior being and its social power was grounded in projective, heated, active, semenotically potent and virile traits that were all

[102] On the issue of age and male bodies in medical discourse see Shepard, *Meanings of manhood*, chs. 1 and 2.

[103] Behrend-Martínez, *Unfit for marriage*, p. 79.

[104] Adelman, "Making defect perfection," p. 40; Park and Nye, "Destiny is anatomy," 56.

considered natural. Power differences were played out in medical discourse, as in practice, and the analysis of semenotics offered here is an attempt to reconsider and reconceptualize the evidence so that both men and women are embodied and embedded within their political and social context.

Coda: changes in the later seventeenth century

From the mid-seventeenth century, scientific arguments began to change considerably the conceptualization of the early modern body. The very focus of gynecological management on female seed contributed to its replacement by the *ova*. William Harvey, having already described the systemic circulation of blood (1628), announced in 1651 the primacy of the egg in mammalian generation, and he found no evidence for female semen or ejaculation.[105] In 1672, the Dutch physician Regnier de Graaf also concluded that females only produced an egg and contributed nothing further (hence he devised the name *ovaria*). Like du Laurens, but on the basis of new anatomical study, he announced that "the testes of women, in position, form, size, substance, integuments, and function differ greatly from those of the male," and the "one-sex" idea was again dismissed as "ridiculous."[106]

A few months before his untimely death in 1673, de Graaf recommended to the Royal Society in London another man from Delft, Antoni van Leeuwenhoek, for his skill in microscopy. In November 1677, the Society learned of the "animalcules" (*diertjes* in Dutch), that is, spermatozoa, he had observed in semen, and this new, visual level of scientific inquiry opened up a world in which there was no female contribution to the embryo except nutriment and incubation.[107] The age of sperm had begun, that of semen to wane. Plato's genital animal from antiquity had transmogrified into Leeuwenhoek's microscopic, swimming animalcule with a long, thin, transparent tail.[108]

105 For this and what follows, see Laqueur, *Making sex*, pp. 142–48, 158–59, 171, 182; Clara Pinto-Correia, *The ovary of Eve: egg and sperm and preformation* (University of Chicago Press, 1997), pp. 65–72, 109–11, and passim.

106 Regnier de Graaf, *De mulierum organis generationi inservientibus* (Leiden: Officina Hackiana, 1672), pp. 77, 171; translated in H. D. Jocelyn and B. P. Setchell, "Regnier de Graaf on the human reproductive organs," *Journal of Reproduction and Fertility*, Supplement 17 (1972), 106.

107 Antoni van Leeuwenhoek, *Alle de brieven*, vol. II (Amsterdam: Swets & Zeitlinger, 1941), pp. 279–99 (November 1677, printed in Latin by the Society in 1679), 334, 336, 348 (18 March 1678), Pls. XVI–XIX; Carlo Castellani, "Spermatozoan biology from Leeuwenhoek to Spallanzani," *Journal of the History of Biology* 6 (1973), 37–68; Edward Ruestow, "Images and ideas: Leeuwenhoek's perception of the spermatozoa," *Journal of the History of Biology* 16 (1983), 185–224.

108 For Plato, see Ch. 3 above, and Ch. 7 below. Leeuwenhoek's findings supported preformatism, the notion that the fetus was already formed, because he mistakenly espied vessels encapsulated in the sperm.

The modern moment is short, merely a couple of centuries or so, whereas for millennia medical models focused on semen-centric and complexional difference, and opinions varied regarding the significance of what was construed in part as opposition, in part as complementarity between male and female bodies. During the Renaissance, gynecology was established as a learned field for male practitioners and the metaphysical perfection of the female reproductive system countered the Aristotelian model of female flaw. The male body continued to be the paradigm *par excellence*, more heated, active and projective, concocting the more perfect semen within testicles that were the seat of virility and putting the penis to use as a device that delivered that precious resource to an eager womb. Coitus was a matter of friction and fluids; to inhabit a male body was to have both genital and physiological markers of distinction, centered on the anatomical axis of testicles, the complexional spectrum of higher heat value, and the physiological feature of semen. During the second half of the seventeenth century, the focus shifted from the semen of Aristotle, Galen, Avicenna and Paré to Hooke's "pole" and on to Freud's recent but not immutable phallus.

5 Value and expenditure

Understanding the value once accorded to the distinctly masculine resources of semen, testicles and higher heat provides a way in which to reconsider the interconnection of political and economic power with biological theory. The elaborate process of production and the precious elements that went into the making of semen caused it to be a pleasurable, valuable resource. Everyday assets and endeavors like coins and purses, spending and hoarding, informed a social iconography of metaphor and imagery that was integrated with a fundamental understanding of the worth of male seminal elements. Testicles were so potent that, even severed from the body, they could give rise to the goddess Aphrodite.

Semen and male parthenogenesis

According to Aristotle, semen was "a compound of *pneuma* [*spiritus* in Latin] and water . . . The cause of the whiteness of semen is that it is foam (*aphros*)."[1] Hence, he pointed out, Aphrodite, goddess of desire, was born from the combination of foam and *pneuma* generated in the ocean from the testicles of Ouranus, which were discarded when that sky god was castrated by his son Kronos. Foam-crested waves are thus conspicuously profuse in Botticelli's *Birth of Venus* of *c.* 1482–85 (fig. 33), representing the fructive semen. Forming triangular points that emphasize movement, the scudding foam sometimes lightly blends with the water but often its materiality is indicated by thicker trails of whitish paint raised above the canvas surface of the green-blue sea. Pressure where shell and shore meet results in smears and swirls of foamy paint nearby and against this force the glistening scallop rises up, optically pushing forward the gleaming white, golden-haired goddess.

A proficient Greek scholar in Florence like Poliziano may have informed the painter about the centrality of white spume, the "bianca schiuma" that appeared

[1] Aristotle, *GA*, 735b10, 736a1–22 passim, cited in Galen, *Semen*, p. 83 and often thereafter, for instance, in Fernel, *Physiologia*, p. 547.

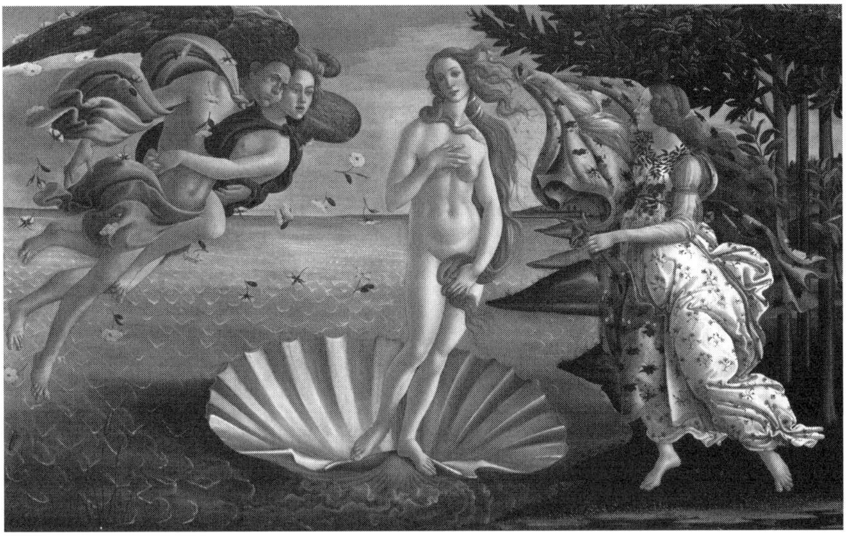

Figure 33 Sandro Botticelli, *The birth of Venus*, *c.* 1482–85, tempera on canvas, 172.4 × 278.5 cm, Florence, Galleria degli Uffizi

in his poetry written a decade or less earlier.[2] Another scholar adept in Greek and also a member of the inner literati, the Neoplatonist philosopher Ficino was the son of a surgeon so his interest in medical matters might inflect the painting too. Other fifteenth-century writers were aware of Venus' origin from the "foam of the sea (*spuma marina*)," as the possible patron's cousin Lorenzo di Piero de' Medici put it.[3] The emphasis placed on the foam in Botticelli's painting suggests he was aware of the full import of that *aphros* from the perspective of natural philosophy and medical theory.

The breath issuing from the mouths of the coupled wind gods is more than the cause of Aphrodite's propulsion shoreward. *Pneuma* has stirred up the waters, uniting it with the testicular seed, magnifying it and generating *aphros*, resulting in the male parthenogenesis of the goddess who epitomizes sexuality. Just such a picture occurred in Constantinus Africanus' eleventh-century Latin translation and adaptation of an Arabic text on coitus: "Galen also says . . . : semen is a spirit and a foamy humor. This foaminess is caused by motion, as we see in a

[2] Angelo Poliziano, *The Stanze*, trans. David Quint (Amherst: University of Massachusetts Press, 1979), pp. 50–51 (written 1475–78).

[3] Lorenzo de' Medici, "Furtum Veneris et Martis," in *Tutte le opere*, ed. Paolo Orvieto, 2 vols. (Rome: Salerno, 1992), vol. II, p. 852. Botticelli's patron was probably Lorenzo's cousin Lorenzo di Pierefrancesco de' Medici.

storm at sea."[4] Aphrodite's arrival on shore also recalls Isidore of Seville's seventh-century definition of semen: "the froth of blood shaken up like water on the rocks of the seashore, which makes the spume white, or as dark wine shaken in the cup turns white."[5] Viewers could easily grasp the notion of semen-driven creation because, even without knowledge of Greek, writers alluded to semen by way of words like "froth" or "spirit."[6] Religious imagery was another source of understanding, for the *pneuma* blown from the mouths of the winged gods is akin to the breath or spoken word from the archangel Gabriel which brings the message of motherless impregnation at the Annunciation.[7]

In cosmographic terms, the scientific scheme of creation mapped out by the ancient Greeks holds sway in Botticelli's painting, for the four fundamental elements of creation and of the human body are evident. The combined elements of water and air are about to be united with that of earth, when desire will arrive on shore to join the company of nymphs and spark fiery passion, thereby generating the fourth element. Fire is already intimated by the bright sunlight but especially by the color, motion and flame-like tresses of the goddess's hair, and it would have been brought to life when countless gold highlights shimmered under candle and lamplight. Conventionally read for some time as a Neoplatonic statement and more recently regarded as decoration emphasizing the advent of love or spring, Botticelli's canvas is also, I suggest, exploring the coupling of male intellectual creativity with desire. The solitary, male painter gives birth to an alluring creature that ensures his art's seductive resonance. The myth about parthenogenesis doubles as a tale about cosmography and art making, revolving around genital and sexual signs.

The source of "the foam of our best blood"

Aphrodite's birth was a story about the potency of semen; Greek science offered three theories to explain its source and in each case the force and value of semen derived from core bodily processes and resources. One was pangenesis, the belief that all parts of the body were involved in its production, a notion that still had adherents during the Renaissance.[8] The second and oldest theory of

4 Paul Delany, "Constantinus Africanus' *De coitu*: a translation," *Chaucer Review* 4 (1969), 57.

5 *Isidore of Seville*, 30.

6 For Italian *anima* and *spirito*, see Toscan, *Carnaval*, pp. 334, 384, 424, 498, 500, 520, 1116–17, 1129, 1410, 1499–500 (which interprets them narrowly as penile); Boggione and Casalegno, *Dizionario*, pp. 340–1, 351.

7 On breath and the logos entering the Virgin's ear, see Leo Steinberg, "'How shall this be?' Reflections on Filippo Lippi's *Annunciation* in London. Part I," *Artibus et Historiae* 8 no. 16 (1987), 25–44.

8 For example, Fernel, *Physiologia*, p. 543. For ancient and medieval theories about the origin of semen, see Preus, "Galen's criticism," 65–85; Foucault, *History of sexuality*, vol. II, pp. 130–33; Jacquart and Thomasset, *Sexuality and medicine*, pp. 52–60.

generation focused on the brain and spine, a scheme that was also outlined by Plato.[9] Arguing specifically against pangenesis, Aristotle posited a third theory, that semen was "a residue from that nourishment which is in the form of blood and which, as being the final form of nourishment, is distributed to the various parts of the body. This, of course, is the reason why semen has great potency (*dynamis*)."[10] Only the warmer heart of men converted or concocted the superfluity of food into blood then semen that was stored in the testicles. Galen also taught that the mix of blood and *pneuma* resulted in semen, but located the refinement process in liver, brain and testicles. Partly due to the impact of Latin versions of Arabic texts, this third concept, haematogenesis, predominated in European thinking from the twelfth century on, propagated in university curricula for centuries via Avicenna's *Canon*.[11]

Dante adopted the notion, thinking that semen was "blood perfect (*sangue perfetto*)" that "takes in the heart informing virtue" and moves through the veins until, "redistilled (*digesto*), it sinks where names are rude / And silence seemlier, till at length it sprays, / In nature's vessel, on another's blood" (i.e., onto uterine menses) and in the womb "it moulds as matter for its artifact" (*Purgatorio*, 25.37–51). "The most best and purest drops of blood," observed the English surgeon Thomas Vicary, were gathered "and by the labour and chafing of the testikles or stones [during coitus] this blood is turned into another kinde, and is made sparme."[12]

In 1580, as a case study in how authorities rarely agreed, the French essayist Michel de Montaigne published a catalogue of medical opinions about the origin of sperm. His list suffices as an overview of Renaissance knowledge and variety about the matter:

> Pythagoras says that our seed is the foam of our best blood. Plato, the flow from the marrow of the backbone, which he argues from the fact that this spot first feels the fatigue of the business. Alcmaeon, a part of the substance of the brain; and a sign that this is so, he says, is that the eyes grow dim in those who work immoderately at this exercise. Democritus, a substance extracted from the whole mass of the body; Epicurus, extracted from the soul and the body. Aristotle, an excrement derived from the nourishment of the blood, the last that spreads through our members. Others, blood cooked and digested by the heat of the genitals, which they judge from the fact that in extreme efforts men give out drops of pure blood; wherein there seems to be more profitability, if any profitability can be derived from such infinite confusion.[13]

9 Plato, *Timaeus*, 73b–e, 86c, 91a–b; Lonie, in *Hippocratic treatises*, pp. 101–02, 115 n. 101, tracing the model back to Alcmaeon of Croton. Marrow was thus a common metaphor for innermost sexual being and for ejaculate (for example, Vignali, *Cazzaria*, p. 51).

10 Aristotle, *GA*, 724b25–726a29, here quoted from 726b10–13. See also Galen, *Usefulness*, pp. 641–42.

11 Avicenna, *Canon*, Bk. III, fen. 20, tr. 1, ch. 3; Jacquart and Thomasset, *Sexuality and medicine*, pp. 34, 53–56; Williams, *Dictionary*, pp. 113–16.

12 Vicary, *Anatomie*, M iii verso.

13 Montaigne, *Complete works*, pp. 417–18.

He went on to point out that contradictions also abounded between Aristotelian and Galenic opinions regarding whether or not women produced spermatic seed.

While medical authors produced texts conveying the sort of certitude that Montaigne scoffed at, he shared with them a belief that such learning had to be grounded in the ancients, and in books. Multiple opinions were held and, as with debates about female seed, most texts offered a blend or compromise, relying nearly always on previous textual authority rather than experimentation. Even Vesalius' *Fabrica* of 1543 arrived at no novelty in the matter of semen's source. For the time after Vesalius, one can turn to Crooke's *Mikrokosmographia* of 1615, a thorough and reprinted English compendium of current European anatomical knowledge. There are Aristotelian traces, for blood and "vitall spirits" arrive at the testicles, along with the residue from alimentation.[14] Drawing from the reinvigorated discourse of anatomy, yet repeating a Galenic idea, the text supplied details of concoction, of the processing of blood into semen, beginning in the "spermaticke or seede vessels," where "by a kind of irradiation the matter of the seede ... receive vertue from the Testicles."[15] "Virtue" relies on the Latin word for man, *vir*, and refers to manly rather than moral value. Pondering the composition of semen at greater length, the book echoed Montaigne's summation, citing Hippocrates, Pythagoras, Plato, Alcmaeon and others, ending with Aristotle's refinement of nutrition into blood. From the amalgam, Crooke proudly provided the "perfect definition of seede": "Seede is a moyst spumous or frothy and white body, made of the permistion of the surplusage of the last Aliment and of the influent or errant spirits boyled and labored onely by the vertue of the Testicles, and that for the perfect Generation of a Creature."[16]

The most common habit was to credit the mix of "blood and spirit" perfected into semen. That was the very phrase in Vesalius, akin to Crooke's "vitall spirites and much arteriall bloud," also evident in, say, Constantinus' eleventh-century tract on coitus ("humor and spirit"), or Benedetti's adoption of Aristotle's idea that the blood-derived semen was ejaculated by pulses of *spiritus*.[17] In this matter, as in many others, Vesalius' project of observation, description, naming and clarification did not overturn the Galenic tradition. From Galen had come the sense that blood incorporated all the other humors, and hence "humor" sometimes referred to either blood or its most distilled, purified form as semen. While authorities continued to disagree about the

[14] Crooke, *Mikrokosmographia*, p. 202. [15] Ibid., p. 202. [16] Ibid., p. 277.

[17] Vesalius, *Fabrica*, pp. 525–26; Crooke, *Mikrokosmographia*, pp. 201–02; Enrique Montero Cartelle, *Constantini "Liber de coitu": el tratado de andrología de Constantino el Africano* (Santiago de Compostela: Secretariado de Publicaciones de la Universidad de Santiago, 1983), p. 144; Benedetti, *Anatomice*, p. 156; Aristotle, *GA*, 728a10; Aristotle, *History of animals*, 586a15.

precise origins of semen, the preciousness of its components was always recognized.

The management of expenditure

The history of semen is partly about varying attitudes towards how much the precious resource should be conserved or spent. Far from incidental, the production and discharge of semen was the very source of sexual satisfaction yet, in the words of the Hippocratic *Generation*, "we are weakened by its loss," an exhaustion Mars experiences in Botticelli's painting (fig. 22).[18] Galen worried about male debilitation when the *pneuma* or vital force was expended too much, for then blood overheated and a man's body dried out.[19] That overall framework was given a moral edge by Christian theologians and medical authorities, who reiterated the need to control expenditure and even abstain. On the other hand, Hippocratic and Galenic teaching and subsequent medical discourse suggested that the retention of too much semen could be harmful because humoral balance had to be maintained.

While women had to menstruate regularly to expel superfluous, noxious humors, men were the opposite. They had to conserve their vital life force and manage their resources carefully in order to be virile, a belief still evident in exhortations from sports coaches that team members abstain from sex before games. Physicians like the first-century CE Aretaeus of Cappadocia believed that the self-controlled retaining of semen made a man "bold, daring, and strong as wild beasts."[20] Worries about the debilitating expenditure of semen went beyond a purely Christian suspicion of bodily pleasure. In the twelfth century, the Jewish medical authority Moses Maimonides also explained that "semen constitutes the strength of the body, its life, and the light of the eyes. Its emission to excess causes physical decay, debility, and diminished vitality."[21] At times, authors betrayed their unease about voracious women, who could be characterized as "bloodsuckers," as Bettina Bildhauer put it recently.[22] On the other

[18] "On Generation," 1.1, in *Hippocratic treatises*, p. 1; also Aristotle, *GA*, 725b5, 726b10–14; Pseudo-Aristotle, *Problems*, 4.21; Galen, *Semen*, pp. 139–41.

[19] Galen, "De Venereis," in *Opera omnia*, ed. C.G. Kühn (Leipzig: Cnoblochii, 1823), vol. V, pp. 912–13.

[20] Foucault, *History of sexuality*, vol. III, p. 121.

[21] Elliot Dorff, "The Jewish tradition," in Darrel Amundsen and Ronald Numbers (eds.), *Caring and curing: health and medicine in the western religious traditions* (New York: Macmillan, 1986), p. 27.

[22] Bettina Bildhauer, "Bloodsuckers: the construction of female sexuality in medieval science and fiction," in Liz Herbert McAvoy and Teresa Walters (eds.), *Consuming narratives: gender and monstrous appetites in the middle ages and the Renaissance* (Cardiff: Wales University Press, 2002), pp. 104–15; Bettina Bildhauer, "The *Secrets of women* (c. 1300): a medieval perspective on menstruation," in Andrew Shail and Gillian Howie (eds.), *Menstruation: a cultural history* (New York: Palgrave Macmillan, 2005), p. 72.

hand, the mistrust was also about sex and the loss of male semen in general, not just about female repositories.

Managing the expenditure of semen was central to men's regimen of self-control and health maintenance. Ideas about sexual temperance proposed by medieval theologians and priests directly informed the opinion of the royal surgeon Paré in the sixteenth century that sexually over-active men were less fertile because their seed was too often expelled and thus under-cooked, as it were, in the hot testicles.[23] Courtiers in Paré's Paris and throughout Europe already knew from sources like Castiglione's manual of comportment that "men dry out more than women in the act of procreation" (3:18). As in most Renaissance theories, whether of medicine, conduct, politics or social management, the ideal was moderation in order to keep personal and social systems in balance. Semen had to be preserved, but not to "excess," however that was defined. It had to be expended carefully for the sake of a man's health and continuing vigor, and in order for him to beget heirs. The wasted, thin frame of a man still toiling in a barren field (fig. 48) visualizes the consequences of frivolous expenditure.

The second-century Church Father Clement of Alexandria adapted the parable of the sower to warn that the seed "ought not to be wasted nor scattered thoughtlessly nor sown in a way it cannot grow."[24] The negative aspect of the traditional agricultural scenario is also evident in the Biblical tale of sinful Onan disobeying God's command to impregnate his slain brother's wife and instead having deliberately "spilled the semen on the ground" (Genesis 38.8–10). Commentaries varied as to the precise nature of this figure of wastage, though it was eventually not only masturbatory or a case of coitus interruptus but sodomitical because it placed that valued fluid in an "improper" or "preposterous" vessel, that is, anywhere but deeply implanted in uterine safety.[25] Premodern medical texts either simply assumed reproductive use of male semen or largely observed silence about matters like masturbation or sodomy. Following Peter Damian's mid-eleventh-century definition of sodomy, many theologians considered masturbation a minor form of that sin, followed in increasing order of offense, and thus penance due, by mutual masturbation,

[23] Paré, *Collected works*, p. 931. For medieval texts, see for instance Albertus Magnus, *De animalibus*, ed. Hermann Stadler vol. XV (Münster: Aschendorffsche Verlagsbuchhandlung, 1916), pp. 1352–53; Jacquart, "Medical explanations," p. 5 (William of Conches).

[24] Clement of Alexandria, *Paidagogos*, 2.91, in *Clement of Alexandria. Christ the educator*, trans. Simon Wood (New York: Fathers of the Church, 1954), p. 170. The parable is in Matthew 13.3–23; Mark 4.2–20; Luke 8.4–15.

[25] Brantôme, *Dames galantes*, pp. 31–32; Laqueur, *Solitary sex*, pp. 111–35, 147–66. Literally meaning "before-behind," i.e., ass first, the word "preposterous" indicated anal intercourse: Patricia Parker, *Shakespeare from the margins: language, culture, context* (University of Chicago Press, 1996), pp. 26–27.

intercrural sex and anal fornication.[26] Like Mary Douglas' renowned definition of pollution, sodomy entailed matter out of place.[27]

What moralizers called lust, the Neoplatonic philosopher termed bestial or vulgar love. Echoing Socrates' judgement that "love was a kind of madness," either insanity due to illness or "divine madness" caused by spiritual release, Ficino added a medical dimension to the dangers of the earthly, irrational kind.[28] Thinking only of the male body when advising students how to protect their health and thence avoid sexual intercourse, in the 1480s Ficino reiterated the standard opinion, that "the coitus of Venus . . . suddenly exhausts the spirits. It weakens the brain and attacks the stomach and the heart, troubles which could not possibly be more adverse to thought. After all, why did Hippocrates declare that coitus was like epilepsy? Because it overthrows the brain, which is sacred, and hurts it as much."[29]

Ficino then cited the canonical physician Avicenna, for the opinion that "if someone should draw seed to flow in coitus beyond what is natural, it is more harmful than if he would bleed himself forty times."[30] Ficino doubtless heard that ratio from his father, whose surgical treatments conventionally entailed bloodletting. Although Avicenna stipulated a quantitative value for semen, the principle stemmed from Aristotle, who observed that "the loss of [semen] from the system is just as exhausting as the loss of pure healthy blood" (*GA*, 725b15, 726b10). The point was that the elaborate process of distillation and concoction led to an exquisitely refined product. Avicenna's ratio became almost magical in medical and erotic discourses, repeated as though the mantra proved value as well as danger. Over the centuries, medical authorities also attributed to the loss of semen such dire consequences as atrophy of the brain and loss of eyesight.[31]

In the mid-seventeenth century, for a few years before he married, the young Scottish gentleman William Drummond recorded in his private diary, in coded

26 Mark Jordan, *The invention of sodomy in Christian theology* (University of Chicago Press, 1997), pp. 46–47, 105–06, 128–32, 145 and passim.

27 Mary Douglas, *Purity and danger: an analysis of the concepts of pollution and taboo* (1966), rpt. (London: Ark, 1984), pp. 125–26.

28 Plato, *Phaedrus*, 265a; Marsilio Ficino, *Commentary on Plato's 'Symposium' on love*, trans. Sears Jayne (Dallas: Spring Publications, 1985), pp. 158, 168.

29 Marsilio Ficino, *The book of life*, trans. Charles Boer (Woodstock, CT: Spring Publications, 1994), p. 12.

30 Scholars sometimes cite a single reiteration of the number forty as though it is unique and ludicrous, whereas the habit was widespread. Other instances include Thomas Cogan (1584) in Laqueur, *Solitary sex*, p. 196; Giuseppe Daciano's 1576 treatise on the plague (Finucci, *Manly masquerade*, p. 33 n. 87); *Culpeper's school of physick* (London: N[athaniel] Brook, 1659), pp. 285–87.

31 For coitus causing brain shrinkage, blindness and melancholy, see Jacquart and Thomasset, *Sexuality and medicine*, pp. 56, 118; anonymous, *The mirror of coitus: a translation and edition of the fifteenth-century "Speculum al foderi"*, trans. and ed. Michael Solomon (Madison: Hispanic Seminary of Medieval Studies, 1990), pp. 3, 45, 93–94 n. 21. Much later, masturbation was instead the cause of such effects.

language (calling it the act of "fatall"), the number of times he masturbated, probably to regulate the outflow and counter the worrying possibility of excessive spending.[32] John Marten's *Onania* (*c.* 1712) and Samuel Tissot's influential treatise against masturbation, first published by the Swiss doctor in 1758, brought an obsessive focus to earlier concerns that had been understated. Echoing Avicenna but for more strident purposes, Tissot warned that "the loss of an ounce of this humor would weaken more than [the loss of] forty ounces of blood."[33]

Humoral notions were spread orally and in numerous vernacular texts, not only medical and philosophical manuals but bestsellers like Rabelais' *Gargantua and Pantagruel*, penned by a physician trained at the distinguished medical school of Montpellier (bk. 3 ch. 1). Far from parodying medical orthodoxy, or twisting it to support idleness and ignorance, Rabelais cited Hippocrates and summarized standard anatomical and physiological knowledge, like Ficino. As Rabelais' humorously immoderate book illustrates, issues of physical health were in dialogue with pleasure, and indulgence was represented licitly in the comic mode. The idea that a man needed to conserve his sperm and hence his virility is the substratum of a joke in Cardinal Bibbiena's comedy *La calandria*, first staged in 1513. The assumption indicates that the audience, consisting of courtiers in cities like Urbino and Rome during carnival season, was expected to understand the notion. A wife attacked her adultery-scheming husband by saying that now she understood why he had not approached her in bed the last few nights: "planning to discharge your load somewhere else, you want to arrive at the battle as a fresh knight."[34] Drummond's later monitoring of his expenditure before marriage reflects something of this sense that semen was almost finite, or at least took time to be properly concocted, as Paré had maintained.

More often, medical concern about depletion was allied with boasts about willful over-expenditure, as though it was boldly daring to risk harm while asserting masculine desire. Joyfully obscene literature lamented loss but blamed ever-eager women for making a man, in the words of the ancient Roman *Priapea*, "ruptured, thin, fucked out, and pale" in contrast to his formerly Priapus-like state of being "bright red and brawny," as were most painted phalli. Now only "a morbid spittle is expectorated" from the pale man.[35] Aretino, that defiant penman of obscene verse and voracious verve, boasted in December

[32] David Stevenson, "Recording the unspeakable: masturbation in the diary of William Drummond, 1657–1659," *Journal of the History of Sexuality* 9 (2000), 223–39, esp. 227, 235.

[33] Elizabeth Abbott, *A history of celibacy* (New York: Scribner, 2000), p. 200; Laqueur, *Solitary sex*, pp. 195–96.

[34] Bibbiena, *Calandria*, p. 63.

[35] *Priapus poems*, 26.7–9; a prostitute drained or consumed men (34.4), adulterous women "squeezed dry in lascivious rout" their lovers (47.4).

1547 about his vigor and "revenge upon time" when he was in his mid-fifties.[36] He ostentatiously describes himself as bearded (as he is in numerous portraits), with some hair turning white, and this father of a newborn daughter looks back on "youthful escapades" without admitting for a second that he has become like other "eunuchs of time."

He is presented as a man surrounded by buxom maidservants and children's nurses who inspire his "*vivezza* and strenuous *complessione*":

> By our faith, when I but see one of these strumpets, all milk and grain, my senses, my spirits, my very vitals revive, and reviving, they live again, and living again they stand erect (*dirizzano*), and standing erect they leap into flame just like a log of wood does, which has not entirely burned out, when it is fanned by the air of the *instrumento* that begins to blow up a stormy wind. Whence, having risen lustily, I resemble a tree trunk that, when others have cut it down for heating themselves at their fire, bursts into leaves and sprigs. I do not deny that there are Platonic blockheads who in their decrepitude scarce can luxuriate in one small strike (*colpetto*) a year. But I, for myself, if I did not draw a bow (*accoccarla*) at this handmaiden or that at least forty times a month, I would hold myself to be all washed out.

Aretino brings himself alive, and swells larger than life, as images tumble over each other in a vivid conglomeration drawn from emblems (the revivified tree stump), religion (the Resurrection, and the flowering rods of Aaron and Joseph), the pastoral (amenable maidens), the rustic (blazing fire), the medical ("wind" and forty times). His productivity is about flourishing, standing, bursting and stretching the *nervus* or sinews of his "bow." Aretino brags about the release of semen tellingly said to take place *quaranta volte il mese*, a striking echo of the medical warning against being bled, or drained of vital bodily fluid more than forty times.

Similar hyperbole had been employed in obscene macaronic verse written in 1498 by the respected physician Gian Giacomo Bartolotti, a man later portrayed by Giorgione and by Titian, and probably known to Aretino. In that case, the groom had "done it" forty times on the wedding night.[37] Not cowed by the medical threat of being "washed out," Aretino appropriates the lore to invert it, by claiming he would instead "go to seed" if he did *not* emit semen. In the same month, he wrote to Sperone Speroni on the man's Neoplatonic treatise about love: "to anyone who says that by following our appetites we accelerate death, I respond that a man just so much prolongs his life as he fulfills his desires. And so say I and not Plato."[38]

36 Aretino, *Lettere*, vol. IV, pp. 188–90 (December 1547, to Gioanbattista Fossa); trans. adapted from Thomas Caldecot Chubb, *The letters of Pietro Aretino* (Hamden: Archon Books, 1967), pp. 239–42.

37 William Schupbach, "Doctor Parma's medicinal macaronic: poem by Bartolotti, pictures by Giorgione and Titian," *Journal of the Warburg and Courtauld Institutes* 41 (1978), 175 lines 228–29 ("quaranta intendas in pota, bocha, thomao," that is, cunt, mouth and ass).

38 Aretino, *Lettere*, vol. IV, p. 194.

But for the majority of men, opined Aristotle, "the sequel to sexual intercourse is exhaustion and weakness rather than relief" because semen "has some *dynamis* within itself."[39] In Greek science, *dynamis* connoted potency and masculine quality, translated into the virile *virtus* of Latin. It appeared also in Hippocratic texts, and to Aristotle it was "the first of the elements," indestructible and divine, associated with the aether of the heavens. The Pseudo-Aristotelian *Problems* (4.1) noted a similarity between sexual intercourse and death, for eyes were cast upwards in each event as though following the direction of the expiring heat. To the Christian apologist Tertullian, when writing on the soul during the early third century CE, orgasm (envisaged as a male phenomenon) brought fundamental loss: "the whole human frame is shaken and foams with semen, as the damp humor of the body is joined to the hot substance of the spirit. And then . . . in that last breaking wave of delight, do we not feel something of our very soul go out from us?"[40] More than a millennium later Aquinas attributed semen's power to a threefold heat, derived from the seed itself, the man's soul and the "heavenly bodies and notably . . . the sun."[41]

No wonder then that a long-lived figure for orgasmic release and postcoital languor was "death" or *la petite mort*, suffered after libidinous battles in which one was "killed," "finished off," spent and as though dead.[42] The humor of satirical verse written by the fifteenth-century Florentine humanist Cristoforo Landino, "Epitaph for Paolo who died while having sex," lay in its cohesion of literal with figurative death, for the defunct Paul "laid down his life just as his penis spurted."[43] Sex and its "little death" could sap not only his body but a man's very soul. "Love and death," wrote Pierre de Ronsard, "are but the same thing."[44]

I suggest that the metaphorical embrace of ideas about violence and death could countermand the medical and moral representation of sex as hazardous for men. In the face of obstacles and dangers, the understanding propounded by men

[39] Aristotle, *GA*, 725b5, 15, 736b35–737a1. For the word see I. M. Lonie's note in *Hippocratic writings*, ed. G. E. R. Lloyd (Harmondsworth: Penguin, 1978), p. 353, and his comment in *Hippocratic treatises*, p. 100.

[40] Tertullian, *De anima*, 27.5, from Peter Brown, *The body and society: men, women and sexual renunciation in early Christianity* (London: Faber and Faber, 1989), p. 17.

[41] Jacquart and Thomasset, *Sexuality and medicine*, p. 57.

[42] To cite just a few examples over a range of time and location: Adams, *Latin sexual vocabulary*, p. 159; Camille, *Medieval art of love*, pp. 131–32; Lorenzo de' Medici, "Giaccopo," in *Tutte le opere*, vol. II, pp. 824–25; Aretino, *I modi*, 1.6, 1.14, 3.5, 7.17, 13.14, 16.17; Ariosto, *Orlando furioso*, 28.17.3–4; Veronica Franco, *Poems and selected letters*, ed. and trans. Ann Rosalind Jones and Margaret F. Rosenthal (University of Chicago Press, 1998), p. 137 (13.85); Pepys, *Pepys' penny merriments*, pp. 278–79 (a chapbook of the 1680s); Chandler Beall, "A quaint conceit from Guarini to Dryden," *Modern Language Notes* 64 (1949), 461–68.

[43] Cristoforo Landino, *Poems*, trans. Mary Chatfield (Cambridge, MA: Harvard University Press, 2008), pp. 118–19.

[44] Pierre de Ronsard, *Sonnets pour Hélène*, quoted in Keith Cameron, *Louise Labé: Renaissance poet and feminist* (Oxford: Berg, 1990), pp. 74–75.

like Aretino that quintessential masculinity was heroic and valiant moderated anxiety about sexual encounters. One bravely "died" on a regular basis. Challenges were voraciously confronted; the species, the family, the dynasty, the nation, lived on. In telling words, a fissure that can stand for bodily aperture or cleft in a city's wall will be penetrated after Shakespeare's king Henry V rallied the troops in 1599 by urging them: "Once more unto the breach, dear friends, once more, / . . . when the blast of war blows in our ears, / . . . / Stiffen the sinews, summon up the blood / . . . / Dishonor not your mothers; now attest / That those whom you call'd fathers did beget you. / . . . The game's afoot."[45] If the sexual act conquered mortality by engendering heirs, death was also momentarily vanquished by the body-wrenching delights of what was only *petite* "death."

Medical texts also offered reassurance, framing copulation and desire in terms of reproduction while also pointing to the need to release semen in moderate amounts for health reasons. Melancholy, lovesickness, obsessiveness and excessive anger were amongst the unhealthy consequences of abstention, although the regimen of evacuation varied according to one's physiological complexion and moderation was always counseled. Around 1256, for the countess Beatrice de Savoie and her four daughters who were all married to princes, Aldobrandino of Siena wrote the *Régime du corps*, an early vernacular book about the non-naturals of hygiene and diet; rules for health included the advice that moderate sex "is a principle [sic] means of maintaining one's health."[46] Despite the female patronage, however, the male body was paradigmatic in the treatise, and male readers were the chief owners of subsequent copies of the popular book. Print technology expanded the audience for such advice. *Culpeper's school of physick* (1659) listed numerous medicalized diseases under "Venery," yet advised about semen that "the timely evacuation whereof avails much for the bodies health."[47]

Moneybags

Semen was like coinage that could be hoarded in its purse or spent, wastefully, pleasurably. Testicles were precious stones; semen was a vital element in the imagery of a sexualized economy. For Artemidorus, reader of dreams in the second century, a man's genital ensemble was "a sign of wealth and possessions because it alternately expands and contracts and because it is able to produce

45 Shakespeare, *Henry V*, 3.1. For sinew in the sexual sense, see Williams, *Dictionary*, p. 1250.

46 Michael Camille, "Manuscript illumination and the art of copulation," in Lochrie, McCracken and Schultz (eds.), *Constructing medieval sexuality*, p. 63; Green, "The possibilities of literacy," in Monica H. Green, *Women's healthcare in the medieval west: texts and contexts* (Aldershot: Ashgate Variorum, 2000), essay VII, pp. 23, 26–29, 32, 51 no. 17.

47 *Culpeper's school of physick*, pp. 285–87.

and to eliminate" (1.45). Priapus' balls were *gemmae*, literally buds of an apple tree in the context of *Priapea* 61.6 and also meaning gems, and the latter connotation is still epitomized in today's colloquialism "family jewels." Testicles were not only two small rocks but also "precious stones."[48] A punch line in one of Poggio's jokes proposed that two mere stones, *duos lapides*, are more valuable than gems because they produce an income or gain: they are ostensibly millstones but actually testicles.[49] These stones were apt genital metaphors for their grinding action and frictional heat as well as for their duality. In the case of a sixteenth-century carnival song written by Alfonso de' Pazzi, men pretending to be jewelers boasted that "We have precious stones / that are as big as beans; / firm and shiny / but we keep them locked up" (literally, they are under the "key," that is, below the penis). Their stock also included "large pendants / from which their pearls issue forth," by which was meant prized droplets of semen.[50]

The valuable product was stored in a scrotal "purse"; its "spending" was an expenditure to be managed carefully or enjoyed thoroughly, and impotent men were metaphorically penniless.[51] Or, after raping Lucrezia, post-coital and criminal Tarquin was pictured as a "bankrupt beggar" in Shakespeare's *Rape of Lucrece* of 1594 (line 711). The Greek *phris* meant both leather bag and scrotum; in Latin *folliculus* (small bag or sack) or *fiscus* (moneybag) was sometimes used, with the Latinized Greek word *bursa* or purse becoming common usage from the medieval period.[52] The etymological, morphological and functional connection between leather moneybags holding coins and scrota containing semen-laden testicles gave rise to sexual jokes, visual puns and misogynist raillery against women selling themselves for sex.

Since the Roman playwright Terence, and then Augustine, Jove's spermatic "golden shower" raining down on Danaë (fig. 27) was understood to carry the

[48] For English, see Williams, *Glossary*, pp. 33–34 (bag), 35 (bankrupt beggar), 107 (ducat), 192 (load), 250 (purse), 284 (spend), 284–85 (spirit, for "expense" of), 313 (treasure); Williams, *Dictionary*, pp. 1116–19 (purse, for vagina, scrotum, condom), 1281–82 (spend), 1320–23 (stone), 1419–20 (treasure); Taylor, *Castration*, pp. 53, 106 for Heywood ("precious stones") and John Davies (rubies).

[49] Bracciolini, *Facezie*, p. 194.

[50] Aldo Castellani, *Nuovi canti carnascialeschi di Firenze: Le "canzone" e mascherate di Alfonso de' Pazzi* (Florence: Olschiki, 2006), pp. 134–36.

[51] For "spend" in Italian and English see Bandello, *Novelle*, vol. I, p. 486; Toscan, *Carnaval*, pp. 989ff, 1725, 1752, and passim (esp. *pagare*, *spendere*); Boggione and Casalegno, *Dizionario*, pp. 135–38 (commerce), 256–59 (coin and money), 375 (*borsa*); Williams, *Glossary*, p. 284; Williams, *Dictionary*, pp. 1009–10, 1281–82.

[52] Adams, *Latin sexual vocabulary*, pp. 74–76, 119. In Latin, *coleus* and *coleo* were used for balls (ibid., pp. 66–67) and *culleus* meant leather sack; ultimately from the Greek κυλεοζ (*kuleos*) for "sheath" comes the English cullion and French *couillon* for testicle or scrotum (Williams, *Glossary*, p. 87; Williams, *Dictionary*, p. 349).

valence of coins buying access to her body.[53] Augustine knew the legend signified that "a woman's purity was corrupted by gold," and he unwittingly popularized the scenario in Terence's play where a man emulated the gods by masturbating while looking at a painting of the tale. Popular renditions of the subject by Titian and his workshop from the mid-1540s through to two decades later, especially the canvas given to Philip II in Spain (fig. 34), place the falling coins against heated, golden colors and chaotic brushstrokes which capture not simply passion but specifically the complexional, red-hot desire of a supremely masculine, potent god in full eruption.[54]

Anatomists called the testicles bags, though often the womb, which was the female receptacle for semen or in the two-seed theory a producer of its own form of seed, was also a *bursa* to be opened or closed. But it is not accurate to say that a purse's "usual metaphorical association [was] with the female vulva" or

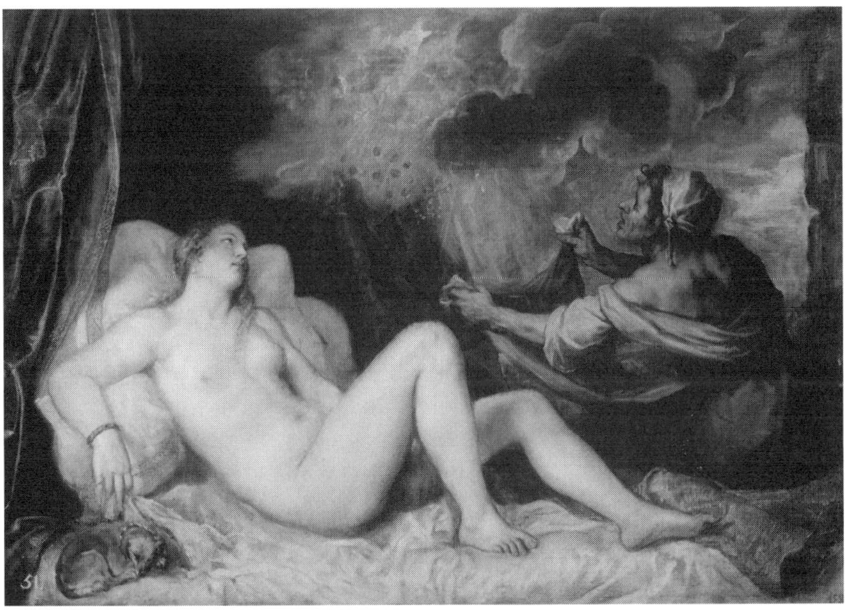

Figure 34 Titian, *Danaë*, 1550s, oil on canvas, 129 × 180 cm, Madrid, Museo Nacional del Prado

[53] Ovid, *Metamorphoses*, 4.611 ("pluvio . . . auro"); Terence, *Eunuchus*, 3.5; Augustine, *City of God*, pp. 55, 777; Gregorio Comanini, *"The Figino," or "On the purpose of painting"* (1591), trans. and ed. Ann Doyle-Anderson and Giancarlo Maiorino (University of Toronto Press, 2001), p. 70; Madlyn Kahr, "Danaë: virtuous, voluptuous, venal woman," *Art Bulletin* 60 (1978), 43–55; Salvatore Settis, "Danae verso il 1495," *I Tatti Studies* 1 (1985), 207–37.

[54] Humfrey, *Titian*, pp. 199, 250, 296.

"vaginas."[55] Like so many other ideologies and images based on the principle that the male body was the model for erotic experience, the "purse" could be either masculine or feminine. Around 1225, the *Anatomia vivorum* likened the uterus to the "scrotal pouch," and the image was adapted in the early fourteenth century by the French surgeon Henri de Mondeville as "the mouth of a purse closed by a cord," Englished in Thomas Vicary's anatomical book of 1577 as "shut togeather as a Purse mouth." But the latter also noted of the male scrotum that "this purse was ordeined for the custodie and comfort of the testikle and other spermatike vesselles."[56] Women's purses were certainly erotic objects and uterine metaphors, but to neglect the masculine aspect of purses is to apply modern fashion expectations and, more importantly, to neglect anything that does not match our standards for a "phallus." The *Roman de la rose*'s pilgrim, it will be remembered, traveled with a staff *and* an *escharpe*, a pouch or wallet inside which two "hammers" were stored (fig. 24).[57]

Crooke's English compilation of Continental sources usefully summarized standard anatomical opinion in 1615. The womb was likened to a bottle, and when gravid it resembled "a Peare or a halfe-peny purse" or on other occasions a gourd.[58] Similar logic applied to the testicles: "The *scrotum* or Cod was made as a purse or bagge," related to its similarity to "a leather sachell . . . made of tanned leather or skinnes." Jane Sharp's *Midwives book* of 1671 continued the metaphorical habit, noting that "the Cods is as it were a purse for the Stones" whereas the ovarian "Stones have not one purse to hold them both as Mens stones have, but each of them hath a covering of its own."[59] So too the cervix "will open and shut like a purse." The same metaphor thus could apply to more than one body part, and there was no neat symmetry between male and female bodies.

Such naming was reinforced by practice, for late medieval and Renaissance purses and bags, usually hanging near a man's genitals, were often designed to mimic them, somewhat akin to codpieces. Medical terminology, lay metaphor, corporeal substance and material experience closely intersected in such cases. While the bulk of men's purses and moneybags were made of perishable leather

[55] The quotations are from Camille, *Medieval art of love*, pp. 64, 65, which offers an overview of "purse" imagery in medieval culture on pp. 18, 63–65, including a lady fondling a man's purse in fig. 52. For images from the *Roman de la rose*, see his figs. 139–40.

[56] Corner, *Anatomical texts*, p. 103; Mondeville, *Chirurgie*, pp. 53, 57 (the latter for scrotum as purse); Lemay, *Women's secrets*, pp. 65–66; Vicary, *Anatomie*, M ii verso, N ii recto.

[57] Gnarled staff (*bordon noderuto*) and pendant moneybag are equally genital in the Italian version of the tale: Santa Casciani and Christopher Kleinhenz (trans.), *"The fiore" and the "Detto d'amore": a late thirteenth-century Italian translation of the "Roman de la rose" attributable to Dante* (University of Notre Dame Press, 2000), pp. 490, 494, and see pp. 376, 528 for loosening purse strings. See also Toscan, *Carnaval*, pp. 1669, 1732, 1744 and passim for *borsa*, *pietra* and *sasso*; Boggione and Casalegno, *Dizionario*, pp. 375–76, 381 (*borsa*).

[58] Crooke, *Mikrokosmographia*, pp. 222, 223 (and see p. 204 on the scrotum, partly from Bauhin, *Theatrum anatomicum*, p. 181).

[59] Sharp, *Midwives book*, pp. 17, 34 (see also 18); hereafter quoted from p. 56.

or cloth and most were not highly decorated (and hence not deemed worthy of preservation), both a few surviving exceptions and visual representations of men's bags clearly indicate their occasionally overt reference to genitals. Straps or false flaps like one on a purse from Leiden could be penile in outline, and smaller, testicular pouches for coins were often placed on the bag's external side (fig. 35).[60] A man lifting his bag's flap or pushing fingers into the pouches was brashly handling his commercial and physical equipment. What was known as a "father purse" is prominently used to signal a peasant's command in Joachim

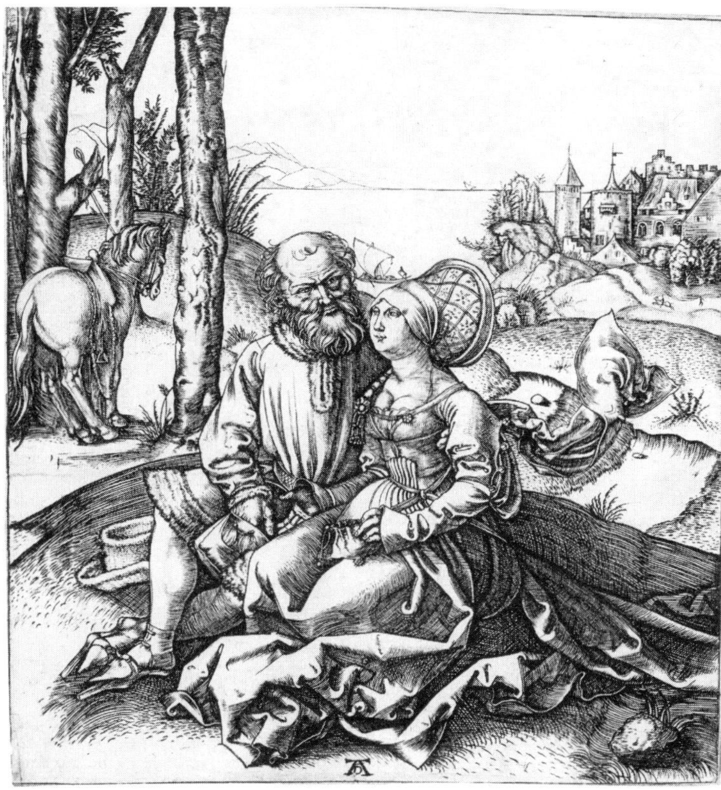

Figure 35 Marcantonio Raimondi (after Albrecht Dürer), *Old man and young woman*, *c.* 1505, engraving, 150 × 139 mm, London, British Museum

[60] Goubitz, *Purses*, pp. 16–17, 19, 28, 34–35. Surviving purses in collections such as the Victoria and Albert Museum are chiefly elaborate, delicate, decorative items for an elite that did not engage directly in commercial transactions and hence had no need for cash at hand. Such purses often contained gifts (including coins), sewing or toilette items or herbs to act as pomanders.

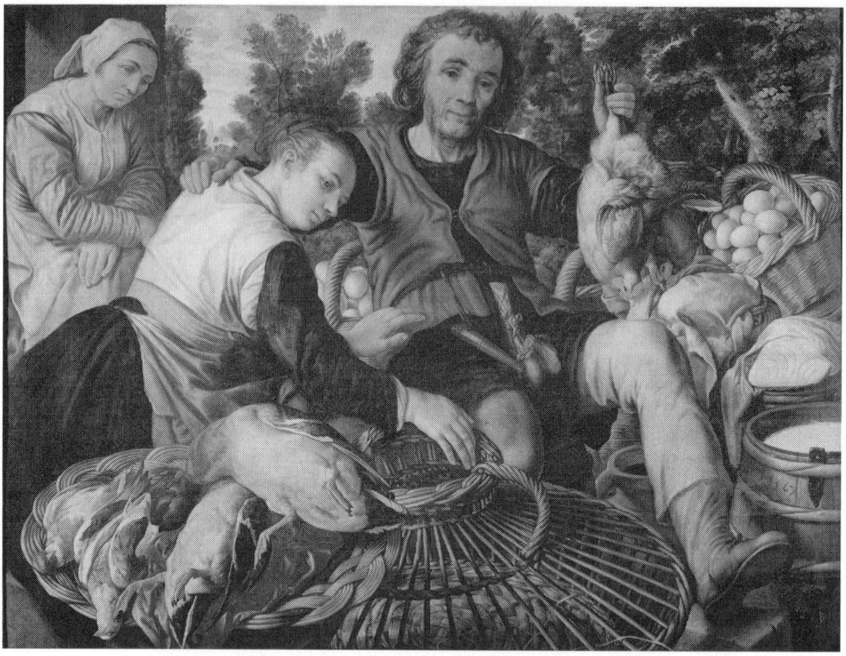

Figure 36 Joachim Beuckelaer, *Peasants at the market*, 1567, oil on oak, 109 × 140 cm, Vienna, Kunsthistorisches Museum

Beuckelaer's market scene of 1567 (fig. 36).[61] Between his legs, its penile stick rises above two scrotal sacks, although other images and surviving examples indicate that patriarchal and financial wealth was often signified by four or more pouches bulging around the central handle.

In the work of artists like Lucas van Leiden or Albrecht Dürer the fingering of a bag's interior contents, or their limp disuse, usually had amusingly sexual connotations. The large sack hanging down from Emperor Friedrick III's neck so that it dangles between Pope Paul II's legs just over his genitals, represented in various print versions of a political allegory produced by both Italian and German artists during the 1470s and 1490s, is not merely a moneybag but also an indication of the simultaneity of greed and lust (fig. 37).[62] Ostensibly, a clever way to censor the view of genitals, it acts as a visual pun on a powerful man's genital "purse" filled with coin. Its heavy load indicates venal wealth but

[61] Ibid., pp. 34, 76–78; Elizabeth Alice Honig, *Painting and the market in early modern Antwerp* (New Haven: Yale University Press, 1998), pp. 46, 57, 58.

[62] Zucker, *The illustrated Bartsch 24 Commentary part 3*, pp. 221–27; Sabine Griese's entry in Peter Parshall, Rainer Schoch et al., *Origins of European printmaking: fifteenth-century woodcuts and their public* (Washington, DC: National Gallery of Art, 2005), pp. 207–08.

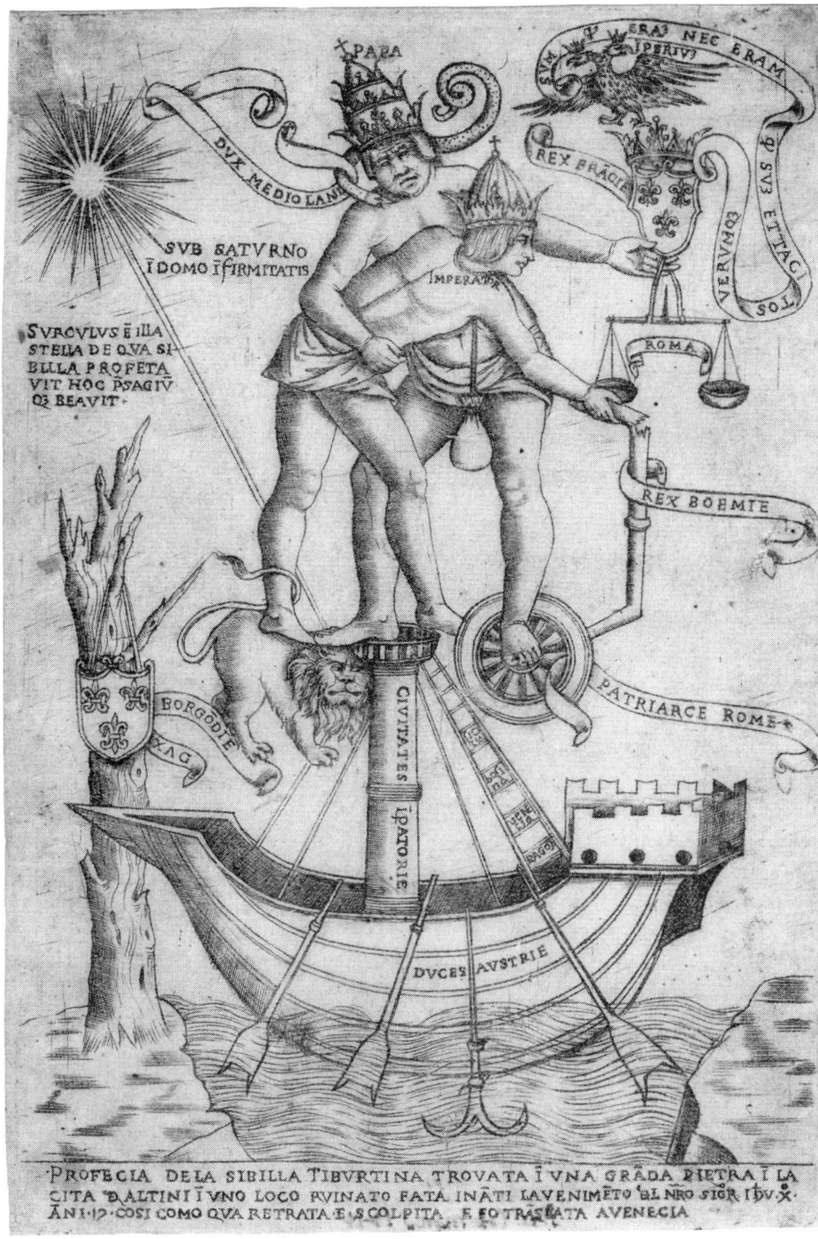

Figure 37 Anonymous (north Italian or Venetian), *Allegory of Pope Paul II and Emperor Frederick III*, *c.* 1470, engraving, 215 × 147 mm, London, British Museum

also excessive sexual drive, given the notion that it was the accumulation of semen that spurred libido.

Much visual and textual punning centered on coinage. Pompeian images of Priapus sometimes endowed him with a moneybag; in the mural at the entranceway to the House of the Vettii his heavy genitals were humorously compared to the weight of such a ponderous bag.[63] One terracotta roundel from the third century shows Danaë bombarded with phallic missiles (and she applies one to her genitals as though it is a dildo), but usually the impregnating golden semen was rendered as coins, avidly collected by Danaë, Cupid or her greedy hag of a servant, simultaneously reaping monetary and amorous reward (figs. 27, 34).[64] While the supreme god projected his seed from on high, mortal men literally flung their coin into the vaginas of bathing women in Germany, a practice observed in 1416 at Baden by the humanist Poggio Bracciolini, reported in a letter that was often published.[65] Pornographic texts from seventeenth-century England reiterated the scenario, now placing the acrobatic, exhibitionist women in brothels, but no less depending on the reader-client's understanding that the practice affirmed women's status as mere prostitutes while engaging men in the performance of the corporeal analogy between projected semen and flung coin.[66]

The theme of female prostitution recurred in the Latin comedy *Chrysis* written in 1444 by Enea Silvio Piccolomini before he became pope. A prostitute advised that "a lover's purse shouldn't be tied up tight," and because the prostitutes' "purse is empty" a man is encouraged to enter the brothel since his purse is "brand new and overflowing."[67] In a brothel, boasted a man of the 1590s who refused to take on the delicate role of a courtly wooer, "Ile freely spend my Thrise decocted bloud."[68] François Villon's mock *Testament* of the mid-fifteenth century bequeathed to his female lover, who "isn't hard up for money . . . a big silk purse / swollen with coins thick and long." He jealously cursed any other man who "slips her his *écu* or his *targe*," two words for shields,

63 Clarke, *Laughter*, p. 186.

64 For the roundel, see Settis, "Danae verso il 1495," 226, 228, fig. 52. On avaricious servants see Kahr, "Danaë," 46, 49–40. For Tintoretto's *Danaë*, see Frederick Ilchman et al., *Titian, Tintoretto, Veronese: rivals in Renaissance Venice* (Boston, Museum of Fine Art: MFA Publications, 2009), pp. 181, 183; and for two dated *c.* 1621–22, Ward Bissell, *Orazio Gentileschi* (University Park: Pennsylvania State University Press, 1981), pp. 176–78.

65 Phyllis Walter Goodhart Gordan (trans.), *Two Renaissance book hunters: the letters of Poggius Bracciolini to Nicolaus de Niccolis* (New York: Columbia University Press, 1974), p. 28. For a variant in Basel, see Pero Tafur, *Travels and Adventures 1435–1439*, ed. and trans. Malcolm Letts (London: Routledge, 1926), p. 185.

66 For the English texts but not their context see Toulalan, *Imagining sex*, pp. 186, 221.

67 Enea Silvio Piccolomini, *Chrysis*, in *Humanist comedies*, ed. and trans. Gary Grund (Cambridge, MA: Harvard University Press, 2005), pp. 287, 317. See also Prizer, "Games of Venus," 26–27, 32, 48.

68 *The poems of Sir John Davies*, ed. Robert Krueger (Oxford: Clarendon, 1975), p. 181.

but *écu* was also a gold coin (914–17). He alone wanted the privilege of "spending" money on/in her.

Two badges from around Villon's time, excavated in London and Middleburg in Holland, depict a large purse filled with just such "coins thick and long," that is, several phalli, which are represented in the usual manner with glans and testicles.[69] The joke is about the body turned inside out, the world upside down, for the *borsa* now contains more than just a pair of testicles (or the two hammers seen in fig. 24), and it promises a ridiculous plenitude because so many "coin"-producing items nestle in the "purse." Given the seminal symbolism of coins, it is likely that semen rather than a testicle was indicated in a magic ritual to cause impotence in the groom, recorded by Thomas Platter in 1598 when he was studying medicine in the south of France.[70] The sorceress threw a coin over her shoulder as well as tied a knot in a lace, thereby blocking the penis and inappropriately ejaculating seed, to be remedied only by unknotting the lace and retrieving the coin.

The emblematic image of hands offering a large moneybag signified sexual as well as fiscal gluttony in a group of vices drawn by Michelangelo in the background to *The dream* of *c.* 1533.[71] Lust is represented not only by a kissing couple but in genital details later largely erased, though these are legible in contemporary copies made on a maiolica plate (1545) and several engravings (fig. 38).[72] A disembodied hand next to the kissing pair on the left clasps a large phallus (with glans, pubic hair and testicles) and another, upright phallus is more crudely drawn nearby. The moneybag seen to the right side of the winged trumpeter's face is supported by a hand in such a way that it seems to form two large testicles, and it resembles the scrota hanging from the grasped phallus which is visible on the other side of the central figure but on the same horizontal axis. Only one of the lustful bodies to the left is clearly female with breasts; the rest are ambiguous or masculine as they engage in eating, drinking and coupling. The genital sign recurs in Salviati's rambunctious *Triumph* (fig. 25), where a similar hand and moneybag are flourished on a banner, but now

69 Jones, *Secret middle ages*, p. 267. For other jokes by Villon about purses, see his *Poems*, pp. 63, 91, and Ch. 4 above for minting.

70 Thomas Platter, *Journal of a younger brother: the life of Thomas Platter as a medical student in Montpellier at the close of the sixteenth century*, trans. Seán Jennett (London: Frederick Muller, 1963), p. 171; cf. Ladurie, "Aiguillette," p. 95.

71 Maria Ruvoldt, *The Italian Renaissance imagery of inspiration: metaphors of sex, sleep and dreams* (Cambridge University Press, 2004), pp. 152–53; Bernardine Barnes, *Michelangelo in print* (Aldershot: Ashgate, 2010), pp. 67–68, 197; Stephanie Buck (ed.), *Michelangelo's Dream* (London: Paul Holberton, 2010).

72 For the detail and eleven copies, see Ruvoldt, *Imagery of inspiration*, pp. 182, 211 n. 7, with the plate reproduced as Pl. 51, the print as Pl. 70; see also Robert Liebert, *Michelangelo: a psychoanalytic study of his life and images* (New Haven: Yale University Press, 1983), pp. 307–11; Buck, *Michelangelo's Dream*, pp. 167–70 and passim.

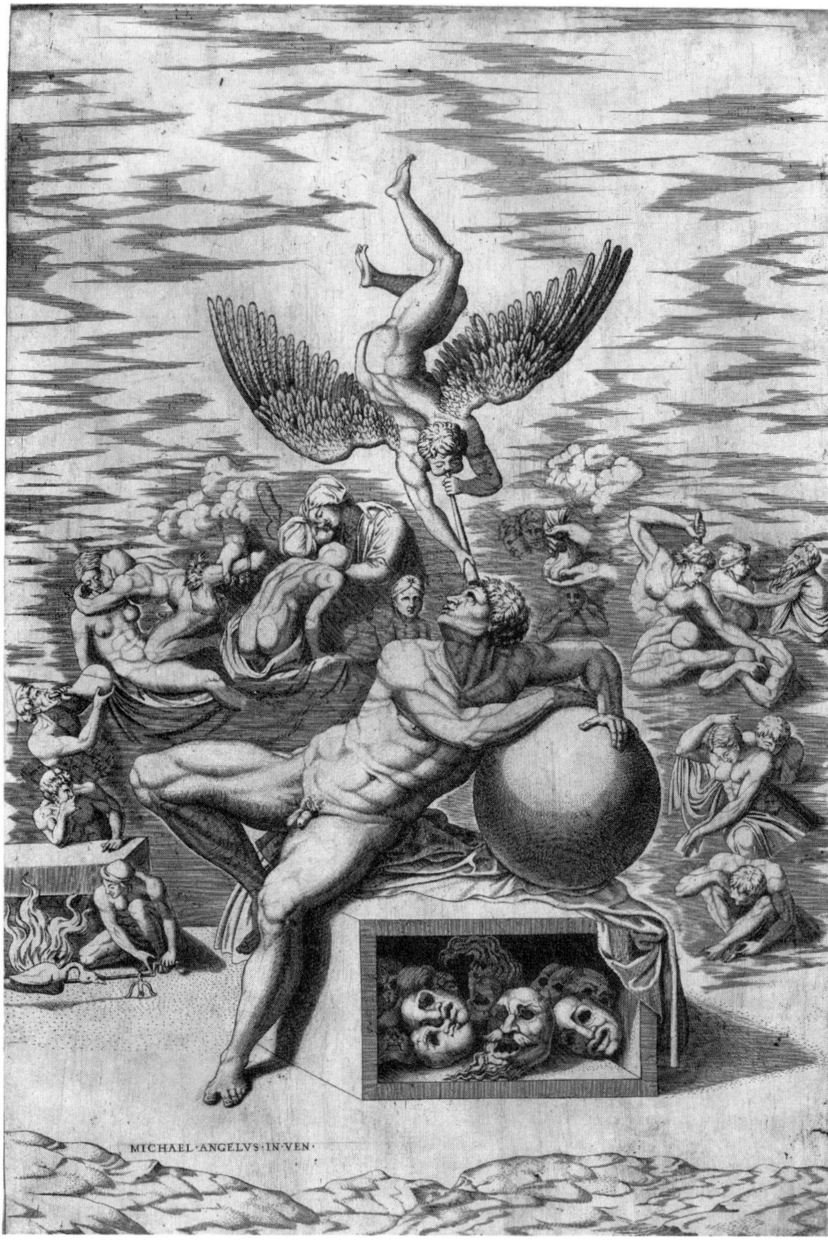

Figure 38 Unknown engraver, formerly attributed to Nicolas Beatrizet (after Michelangelo), *The dream*, *c.* 1545, engraving, 436 × 295 mm, London, British Museum

adjacent to two more hands counting coins, forming a celebratory emblem of the prostitutes' physical and monetary triumph.

Theft and deceit are central to the theme that has been dubbed by modern scholars "Unequal lovers" or "Ill-matched couples." "From Chaucer onward," Taylor reports, English literature represented "old men with shriveled testicles but full moneybags [who] acquire beautiful young wives and are duly cuckolded by young men with ripe scrotums and empty purses."[73] Especially from the late fifteenth century, the theme was also popular in images, chiefly though not exclusively in northern Europe. The earliest surviving examples are prints by the Housebook Master from the Middle Rhine area, dated to *c.* 1472–75, which were copied in reverse in the 1480s by another German artist Israhel van Meckenem.[74] Each printmaker depicted a half-length couple in two images, one showing a young woman courted by an older man with a large moneybag, the other taking up the antithesis by imagining a youth wooing an old woman for her money. Simplified and with even more caricatured figures, the two scenarios were rendered in one woodcut by an anonymous German artist during the 1510s (fig. 39).[75]

A variant on the theme placed a woman standing between two men of unequal ages, taking an old man's money to buy the attentions of a young dandy. In Urs Graf's woodcut of *c.* 1511–12 (fig. 40), a gaming board, cards, a lute, a large goblet and fruits all accentuate licentious indulgence.[76] These attributes of transience are offset by the skull and bones below, with banderoles inscribed "Consider the end – that is my counsel: when everything finishes with death." The moral point addresses all three characters, for the mercenary love of the beplumed youth and the rapacious desire of the conniving woman for lucre as well as fleshly pleasure are matched by the old man's yearning. Aged enough to use a cane and possibly impotent (suggested by the limp cloth hanging over his belt, possibly an emptied purse, as well as the "broken" handle of his cane), the man has forgotten the dignity of a patriarch; the forked nature of his beard underlines the notion that he has been cuckolded, possibly by a wife who is still wearing her bridal crown. In one now-lost example of the woodcut, an inscription in the blank banderole above the figures indicated that some discerned a homoerotic implication, in that the old man speaks of like being attracted to like,

[73] Taylor, *Castration*, p. 107. For "Literary sources from Plautus to Shakespeare," including the *Roman de la rose* and Boccaccio's *Decameron* (2.10, 7.9), see Alison Stewart, *Unequal lovers: a study of unequal couples in northern art* (New York: Abaris Books, 1977), pp. 13–34.

[74] Fritz Koreny (ed.), *Hollstein's German engravings, etchings and woodcuts 1400–1700*, vol. XXIV: *Israhel van Meckenem, Text*, ed. Tilman Falk (Blaricum: A. L. van Gendt, 1986), p. 188, and vol. XXIV A: *Plates*, Pls. 488–89; Stewart, *Unequal lovers*, pp. 41–42, 90, 120–21, 139–40. These may stem from lost engravings by Master E. S. (active *c.* 1450–67), according to Stewart, *Unequal lovers*, p. 143. On the general theme, see also W. A. Coupe, "Ungleiche Liebe: a sixteenth-century topos," *Modern Language Review* 62 (1967), 661–71.

[75] Stewart, *Unequal lovers*, pp. 61–63, 143.

[76] Ibid., pp. 32–33, 87, 93, 98, 100, 173–74; Bartrum, *German Renaissance prints*, pp. 216–17.

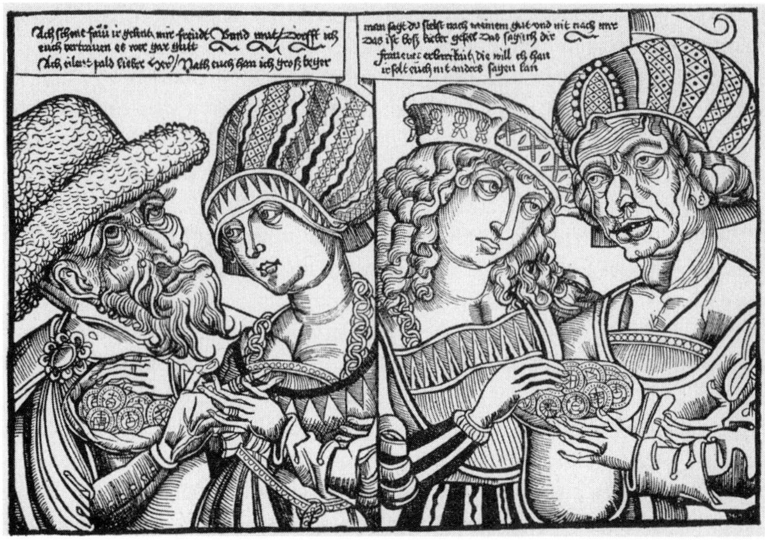

Figure 39 Anonymous (German), *Unequal lovers*, *c.* 1510s, woodcut

and he wants to get in the middle.[77] Following this logic, the woman is sodomitically transferring the older man's "seed" to an inappropriate receptacle, the youth's slightly furtive hand.

Intergenerational rivalry between older, richer men and younger lovers was joined by the related theme of older men courting younger women with the aid of monetary inducement, a satirical exaggeration of the common demographic pattern of an age disparity in marriage. This disparity is the theme of Marcantonio Raimondi's copy in reverse done around ten years after Dürer's engraving of *c.* 1495, showing a bearded man reaching into his purse to pay a young woman who holds out her hand and opens her own purse in readiness to receive the particularly pleasurable "remuneration," of both semen and coin (fig. 35).[78]

[77] "Birds of a feather flock together, I therefore want to get in the middle [i.e., between the two young lovers]": Stewart, *Unequal lovers*, pp. 100, 134 (for "love triangles" see pp. 173–79).

[78] Stewart, *Unequal lovers*, pp. 20–21, 24, 115, 120, 163, 165, and for a Leonardesque composition see pp. 10, 140–41, 145, 169–71; Bert Meijer, "'L'arte non deve schernire': sul comico e sul grottesco al Nord," in *Rabisch: il grottesco nell'arte del Cinquecento: L'Accademia della Val di Blenio, Lomazzo e l'ambiente milanese* (Milan: Skira, 1998), pp. 69–72, and his entry on a drawing attributed to Jacob Hoefnagel, pp. 141–42; Larry Silver, *The paintings of Quinten Massys* (Montclair: Allanheld & Schram, 1984), pp. 143–45, 223–24, which also discusses Massys' *Ill-matched pair* of the 1520s. Further Italian examples include one or more paintings by Jacopo de' Barbari (Stewart, *Unequal lovers*, pp. 94, 97, 108, 116, 117, 141–42), and Cariani's painting in the Hermitage (Rodolfo Pallucchini and Francesco Rossi, *Giovanni Cariani* (Milan: Credito Bergamasco, 1983), p. 122).

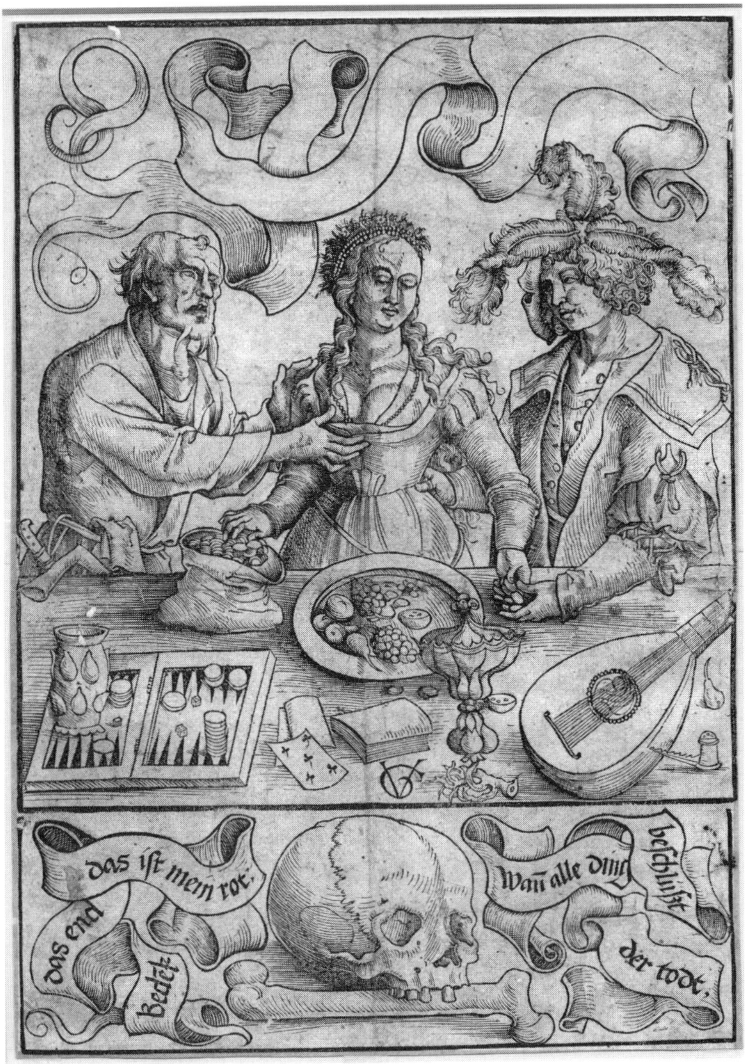
das ist mein rot.
das end
Bedeüt
Wan alle ding
beschlüst
der todt.

Figure 40 Urs Graf, *Young woman with an old man and a youth*, *c.* 1511–12, woodcut, 325 × 224 mm, London, British Museum

In dotal systems, matrimony was arranged at the elite level after the bride's family promised a sizable dowry; everywhere in Europe marriage was a key vehicle for the transfer of property between generations and families. The requirement of some guild regulations that a widow could only maintain the business if she remarried, usually to a man experienced in the trade, probably exacerbated economic and erotic tensions around differences in age. At times, the stock pattern is reversed in the images, and an aging woman avidly buys the attentions of a young swain. Coin and seed, each stored in sacks, are thus overlapping resources to be managed wisely or ill.

The satirical theme was played out in numerous prints, as well as a considerable number of paintings, especially from the Cranach circle, and it was at the heart of noisy charivari performances outside the homes of widows or widowers who remarried, particularly if the partners were much younger.[79] The stock character of the ill-married woman was a feature in such genres as Italian comedies, French songs and German prints, suffering the impotence or incompetence of an aged husband and thus exhausting his already weaker, depleted seminal resources while spending his money and her cuckolding attentions on a young male lover who is usually shown as a fop, similar to Graf's wooer (fig. 40).

The multivalence of the "purse" might suggest that an opened purse punned on the receptivity of a woman's uterine vessel, but the point of this misogynist imagery was more about her mercenary nature or sexual favor shown to a man, and his eagerness to expend, rather than his fertility as a parental agent. An Italian carnival songster asked a woman to "open your purse and take the pheasant in hand," with no intention that the dalliance would result in pregnancy, and Dürer's scenario with both purses unfastened in a secluded rural spot (fig. 35) does not suggest licit domestication either.[80] Sexual license and material indulgence are clearly the focus of each partner in the "unequal lovers" type (figs. 35, 39–40). Most often, the purse being opened is male and the hand's load is coin; the young woman is usually sly, suggesting that the old man will be sucked dry of both his financial and physical resources. Men fondling young women while their own purses were pilfered or voluntarily emptied signified not only the luring of maidens into prostitution or "ill-matched" marriage but, especially given the position of some of those purses hanging near the genitals, also visually punned on the kind of manual satisfaction the male client or husband was hoping to receive.

The full nuance of these images has not been understood because the depiction of coinage has been taken literally, as merely a configuration of fiscal payment. Agostino Carracci's *Ogni cosa vince l'oro* from the 1580s (fig. 41)

[79] For charivari and concerns about the "pool of available mates" see Platter, *Journal*, pp. 172–73; Muir, *Ritual*, pp. 98–104. For some of the more than forty paintings issued by the Cranach circle, see Max Friedländer and Jakob Rosenberg, *The paintings of Lucas Cranach* (Secaucus, NJ: Wellfleet Press, 1978), pp. 125–26, 149–50, nos. 282–92, 401; Bodo Brinkmann (ed.), *Cranach* (London: Royal Academy of Arts, 2007), pp. 308–13. For several by the Flemish painter Jan Massys in the 1560s, see Leontine Buijnsters-Smets, *Jan Massys* (Zwolle: Waanders Uitgevers, 1995), pp. 94–108, 170–71 no. 16, 218–19 nos. 53, 53a, 195–96 no. 36.

[80] Bruscagli, *Trionfi*, p. 440 line 44.

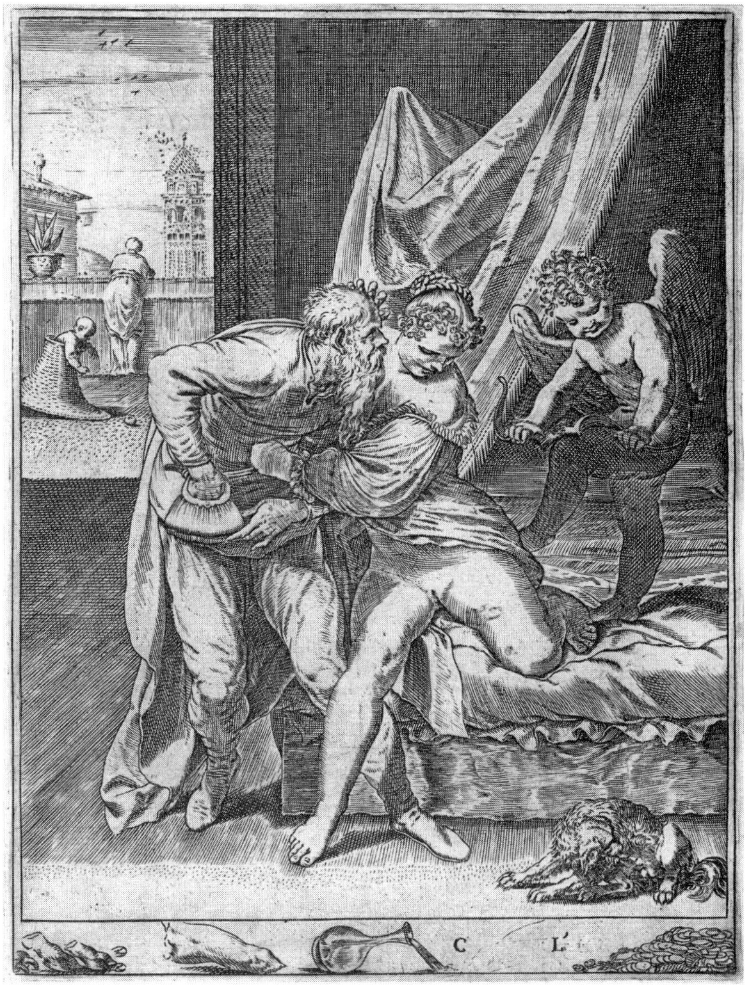

Figure 41 Agostino Carracci, *Ogni cosa vince l'oro*, *c.* 1588–90, engraving, 214 × 162 mm, London, British Museum

declares by way of a rebus that lucre conquers everything.[81] An old lecher reaches eagerly into his purse, while in the rebus wine spills and a pile of coins flow across the ground, each visual metaphors for ejaculation. Fluid effusion in the rebus is reminiscent of Samuel Pepys' experience on several occasions when his sexual enounters with women other than his wife did not include

[81] On the engraving see Simons, "Carracci's wit," 205–15.

coitus but aroused him so much that "I spent in my breeches."[82] Depictions of "unequal" lovers are moralizing lessons against the lust of both men and women, yet they also use amusing satire and hint at a degree of sexual success in the game of seduction.

In a Leonardesque composition, and other images showing a youth as the one being seduced by money (fig. 39), the extreme, "unnatural" disparity in ages is reinforced by the visual conception of partial sex reversal. The woman is mannish in her dried out humoral *complexio* and lack of voluptuous, moist flesh. The male figure is so young that he is almost feminine, still beardless, longhaired and fine of facial features. Besotted, the standard parodic character of a postmenopausal widow is willing to waste one kind of specie in order to obtain a spermatic "cure" for what ails her. A painting from the circle of Lucas van Leyden thus depicts the old woman in partly masculine attire, and dresses the strutting boy in decorative, nearly feminine fancy dress.[83] Misogynist literature not only attacked women for their lust, but these attempts to define and control masculinity often constructed the stock type of effeminate youths too. Over-dressed youths with richly embroidered caps and dazzling clothing, often with feathers or other fancy additions to their headgear, are wooers satirized as much as the women. Lucian had already imagined the scene in the second century, writing of an effeminate man courting an old woman with hopes of becoming her heir (*Rhetorum praeceptor*, 24–25).

When Isabella De Moerloose married a much older man in seventeenth-century Holland, she rationalized that in her case she was fertile but she disapproved of old, sterile women who married again, especially if the husband was young.[84] Isabella's disquiet was fed by centuries of satire and social ridicule, and she was interweaving her own autobiographical narrative with the weighty tradition of received opinion. In the previous century her compatriot Erasmus believed that "no true marriage can be made between those too old for child-bearing, or those who are irremediably sterile." He had been disgusted by the folly of skeletal women, "always in heat," who "display their withered and foul breasts" and try to seduce "some Phaon, engaged at a high fee."[85] Aretino was vitriolic about postmenopausal women too, describing a witch who resembles some of those depicted by Hans Baldung Grien (fig. 59), having

[82] For example, Pepys *Diary* vol. III, p. 191, and vol. IV, p. 317.

[83] Stewart, *Unequal lovers*, pp. 113, 181, fig. 75.

[84] Herman Roodenburg, "The autobiography of Isabella De Moerloose: sex, childrearing and popular belief in seventeenth century Holland," *Journal of Social History* 18 (1985), 527–28.

[85] The first quotation is from Desiderius Erasmus, *Institution of Christian matrimony*, trans. Michael J. Heath, in *Collected works of Erasmus*, vol. LXIX: *Spiritualia and pastoralia*, ed. John W. O'Malley and Louis A. Perraud (University of Toronto Press, 1999), p. 221 (on age differences see also pp. 325–26, 409); the second from Erasmus, *Praise of folly* (1509), trans. Hoyt Hopewell Hudson (Princeton: Princeton University Press, 1969), p. 42.

breasts that "dangled like a man's bags, but without the seeds inside."[86] Her loss of reproductive power and demeaned social status were accentuated by the negative comparison with male testicles.

The remark bears comparison with Dürer's painting of an *Old woman with a moneybag* (fig. 42), depicted as though what is not filling her sagging breast is instead stored in the bag, a sack which resembles those clutched by crones in "Unequal lover" images.[87] It holds all her wealth but, her gaze and smiling appeal seem to suggest, she will willingly part with it if an infusion of male semen can give her new life. The painting is the allegorical reverse of a portrait depicting an anonymous young man, dated 1507, and the figure perhaps

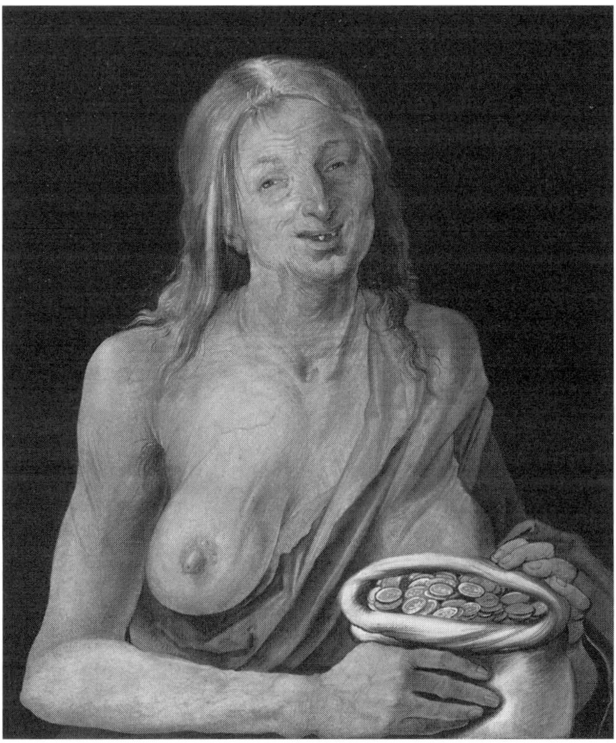

Figure 42 Albrecht Dürer, *Old woman with a moneybag*, 1507 (signed and dated on recto), oil on linden wood, 350 × 290 mm, Vienna, Kunsthistorisches Museum

[86] Aretino, *Ragionamento*, p. 54; Aretino, *Dialogues*, p. 45.

[87] Angela Ottino della Chiesa, *The complete paintings of Dürer* (Harmondsworth: Penguin, 1986), p. 106 no. 124.

represents Avarice, though the hanging breast and withheld moneybag can also characterize another vice, Envy. Further, the reference to amorous satire invokes yet a third deadly sin, Lust. The contrast of the young and the old in "Unequal lover" iconography is now divided onto two sides of a single image, and her "coins" are offered to the viewer rather than a coxcomb. Notably, the male sitter is shown with a beard and moustache developing, a masculine sign associated with testicular "force." While he is represented coming into his adult prime and displaying biological virility, she is shown as overheated (brown skinned and draped in red), infertile, empty, dried out, with hairy armpits and whiskers on her chin, bereft of the "natural" feminine *complexio* due to her age.[88] Her ludicrously large moneybag is all the more perverse for being associated with a seedless hag, whereas the portrayed man is accumulating his resources and, it is implied, ready for the marriage market.

The very conventionality of the "unequal" scenario and the effectiveness of ridicule as a mechanism of social control point to the way in which such imagery reasserted rather than subverted the authority of older men. Women of all ages and also men, including those excluded from decision making because they were too old or too young, laughed and learned lessons in restraint and preservation. One important function of the popular tales, plays, prints and paintings was to displace onto exaggerated, stock characters any anxiety about the capacity to woo a woman, perform virility or become fathers. Given the medical background, jokes about laden purses were all the more efficacious because they appeared to operate on an incontrovertibly biological basis.

Commerce

The purse was often an attribute of Mercury, god of commerce, who could be paired with Priapus in Pompeian wall paintings.[89] The fecund blessings conveyed by phallic images in patriarchal economies entailed commercial success as much as agrarian prosperity or familial fertility. Trade, commerce, trafficking and dealing were practices that commonly stood euphemistically for sex (and were sometimes literally a part of such transactions).[90] Seeking vengeance against a

[88] For previous descriptions of old women see, for example, Boccaccio, *Corbaccio*, pp. 54–55, 137 n. 250, and frontispiece; Michael Vickers, "The sources of Invidia in Mantegna's *Battle of the sea gods*," *Apollo* 106 (Oct. 1977), 270–73; Roper, *Witch craze*, pp. 160–78; Patrizia Bettella, *The ugly woman: transgressive aesthetic models in Italian poetry from the middle ages to the Baroque* (University of Toronto Press, 2005).

[89] Philippe Morel, "Priape à la Renaissance: les guirlandes de Giovanni da Udine à la Farnésine," *Revue de l'art* 69 (1985), 18–19; Clarke, *Laughter*, pp. 118, 186–89.

[90] See, for example, Aretino, *Ragionamento*, p. 106 (*traffico*); Toscan, *Carnaval*, pp. 197, 988–1005, 1022, 1031, 1038, 1718 (for words such as *danaro*, *ducato*, *mercanzia*, *mercato*, *negozi*, some of which are over-read as penile or anal only); Boggione and Casalegno, *Dizionario*, pp. 135–38, 378; Tessa Storey, *Carnal commerce in Counter-Reformation Rome* (Cambridge University Press, 2008), pp. 24, 162–64.

man who sexually used her but then refused marriage, Elizabeth Francis "willed Sahtan [sic] to waste his goodes," and the man's subsequent death featured in her statement to the Chelmsford court in 1566 when she was tried for witchcraft.[91] Usually, female prostitutes were the goods on sale but virginity was considered a commodity on the marriage market and any sexualized person could be presented as merchandise. It was "her commodity" an English clothier tried to feel when he thrust his hand under a woman's clothing, and other words like "wares" recurred in anecdotes and fiction too, in several languages.[92] Sometimes the investment had too high a price. The character Marescalco in Aretino's comedy of the same name, whose erotic interest was solely focused on boys, believed that "wives are merchandise on which you can lose one hundred per cent."[93]

Female bodies were "shops" in which valuable money would be spent. One of the jokes collected in the fifteenth-century book attributed to Poliziano has a wife seated at the household's entrance on a feast day, her legs apart, evoking the husband's response that she should close the store (*serrassi la bottega*) because it was a holiday and all the shops were shut. Rather than bring her legs together, the woman retorted that he has the key but has not come to lock up. Keys were a well-known metaphor for the penis, and hence her rejoinder suggested that he was impotent because he was not using his key.[94] The derogatory reference to female shops was familiar to doctors, aristocrats, artists like Leonardo da Vinci and scholars. When humanists in Rome around the years 1510–12 praised the wealthy banker Agostino Chigi as another Augustus, one of them devised a cleverly nasty quip for Chigi's mistress Imperia, who understood Latin well herself. The verse went: "Your (Imperia), Augustus, she is no empire, but she / With her name changed is called Emporium."[95] That is, the famed courtesan sold her sexual wares in a large store, Chigi being only one of the merchants frequenting her roomy establishment, which was enlarged due to overuse.

But shopping and trading were not confined to male–female pairs, nor to fiction and jokes. In 1590, a Camaldolese friar creatively propositioned a nearly naked novice with the lines: "I see that your shop is open . . . and that you have oysters, if you wish I will oysterize you."[96] The sense seems to be that the rear view of the

[91] *The examination and confession of certaine wytches at Chensforde* (London: William Powell, 1566), n.p.

[92] Quaife, *Wanton wenches*, p. 168. [93] Aretino, *Commedie*, p. 96.

[94] Poliziano, *Detti piacevoli*, p. 100 (p. 86 has another quip about "keys").

[95] Ingrid Rowland, "Some panegyrics to Agostino Chigi," *Journal of the Warburg and Courtauld Institutes* 47 (1984), 197, which does not understand the joke.

[96] Guido Ruggiero, "Marriage, love, sex, and Renaissance civic morality," in James Grantham Turner (ed.), *Sexuality and gender in early modern Europe: institutions, texts, images* (Cambridge University Press, 1993), p. 25. The opening of oyster shells suggested sexual access to a woman and oysters were considered aphrodisiacs and symbols of sexual appetite, but male genitals are not mentioned in Liana De Girolami Cheney, "The oyster in Dutch genre paintings: moral or erotic symbolism," *Artibus et Historiae* 8 no. 15 (1987), 135–58, except for the brief indication that

youth's open, bivalve buttocks or "shell" displayed round, testicular temptations that the friar wished to fondle. In negative terms, prohibition and invective linked usury with sodomy, conceiving of both practices as perverse and contrary to nature.[97] Sodomy was condemned as sterile, unnatural sexual activity, and literal money was unable to breed whereas usury led to its unnatural replication. However, the friar adapted language used chiefly for sexual trade between men and women, offering to spend "coin" in the youth's oyster shop.

"Money" did breed, in the metaphorical arena, as the expenditure of semen paid witness to the currency of virility. Whatever a man's financial state, his virile "wealth" was flaunted in its accumultion and spending. Sexual commerce infiltrated the practice and language of the licit institution of marriage too. Public matters cannot be divided from seemingly private affairs, and I argue that interconnectedness is evident in the cross-over between the spheres of sexual metaphor, medical language and economic activity. As Carole Pateman has demonstrated, the "sexual contract" of the patriarchal social order constitutes the pattern of domination and subjection.[98] When selecting a bride, Leon Battista Alberti advised in his *Libri della famiglia* (written during the 1430s and 1440s), the future husband should treat the marriage contract like other business deals. He "should act as do wise heads of families before they acquire some property – they like to look it over several times before they actually sign a contract."[99]

While the conjugal or marital debt (*debitum*) was not literally about payment or debts but theoretically about mutual obligation, the concept was applied unequally in practice.[100] The terminology may have influenced the way in which people construed sexual commerce, as it did to witty, assertive effect in a letter written around 1607 by Maria Thynne to her husband of thirteen or so years who was too long gone in London. She blushed upon joyfully receiving his "kind wanton letters," the first of which "threatened sound payment, and I sound repayment, so as when we meet, there will be pay, and repay, which will pass and repass, *allgiges ultes fregnan tolles*."[101] Her pig Latin seems to have

oysters were thought to increase male virility (157 n. 28). Occasionally, "oyster" in English suggested testicle or semen (as it does today with "prairie oyster"): Williams, *Dictionary*, p. 983 (which reads "she hath gutted his Oyster" as penile but I suspect it refers to the emptying of scrota).

97 See Dante, *Inferno*, 15–17; Anne Derbes and Mark Sandona, *The usurer's heart: Giotto, Enrico Scrovegni, and the Arena Chapel in Padua* (University Park: Pennsylvania State University Press, 2008), pp. 59–61, 66–67; also Toscan, *Carnaval*, pp. 1006–11; Stephens, *Demon lovers*, pp. 332, 415 n. 31; Williams, *Glossary*, pp. 1463–64.

98 Carole Pateman, *The sexual contract* (Stanford University Press, 1988).

99 Leon Battista Alberti, *The family in Renaissance Florence*, trans. Renée Neu Watkins (Columbia: University of South Carolina Press, 1969), p. 115. See also Bartolomeo Scala, "Whether a wise man should marry," in his *Essays and dialogues*, trans. Renée Neu Watkins (Cambridge, MA: Harvard University Press, 2008), p. 41.

100 For an introduction to conjugal debt, see Tentler, *Sin and confession*, pp. 170–74.

101 Alison Wall (ed.), *Two Elizabethan women: correspondence of Joan and Maria Thynne 1575–1611* (Devizes: Wiltshire Record Society, 1983), pp. 37–38.

meant "you will add together (or you will collect) frequently, you will rise up," a wonderful set of puns about mathematics and intercourse, economic and somatic increase, coded in an elite if imperfect language shared in personal correspondence. The give and take, between payment and repayment, one event and the next, alludes to the sexualized household economy and the alternating motion of sex, though the husband notably takes the lead.

It is, I think, important that in social systems organizing marriage through dowry payments the physical act of sex was officially required before a new husband could begin to collect the full amount. In the ideal circumstance of first marriage, the money often enabled the man to become independent, to mark the moment of guild matriculation, for instance, or invest in a business venture, and at that time he established his own household. The principle was neatly applied to international politics in a witticism reported in 1528 by Castiglione, as an example of what was obscene when spoken in the company of ladies. At a recent banquet, a Sienese man had taunted a Florentine by claiming that his city had married the Emperor and given Florence to the ruler as a dowry. The Florentine retorted: "'Siena will first be possessed' [*cavalcata*, ridden] ('possessed' in the French sense, but he used the Italian word), 'then in good time the dowry will be discussed.'"[102] That is, Siena must first be screwed and the marriage consummated before any dowry could change hands.

To embark on the adult phase, the groom had to demonstrate virility and potency; a bride could not immediately prove her fertility, only her prior virginity and thus her value on the marriage market as an honorable woman. Without his attestation before public officials managing the dowry fund in cities like Florence or a sufficient public sign (like bloodied sheets, on occasion), avowing that consummation had occurred, his financial stake was not necessarily forthcoming. Catholic Church law required consummation that entailed the uterine placement of semen, and even marriages of international, diplomatic importance had to be consummated before large dowry payments were completed.[103] The Florentine widow Alessandra Strozzi reported in August 1477 to

[102] Castiglione, *Cortegiano*, p. 178; Castiglione, *Courtier*, p. 122.

[103] See, for example, Sanudo, *Venice: cità excelentissima*, pp. 72, 301, 302, 385; Anthony Molho, *Marriage alliance in late medieval Florence* (Cambridge, MA: Harvard University Press, 1994), pp. 30, 31 n. 16, 32, 72, 315, 318; Ferraro, *Marriage wars*, pp. 10, 28, 72, 73, 79, 80, 81, 86, 88, 89, 92, 93, 96, 102 (for the importance of blood, and the delivery of semen); Hacke, *Women, sex and marriage*, pp. 168–69. In actuality, large dowries were often paid in instalments and sometimes the full amount was never received. In preTridentine lower class and clandestine marriages, a promise to marry led to sex, which sealed the arrangement. Julius Kirshner, "The morning after: collecting Monte dowries in Renaissance Florence," in Diogo Ramada Curto et al., eds., *From Florence to the Mediterranean and beyond: essays in honour of Anthony Molho* (Florence: Olschki, 2009), pp. 29–61, points out that in Florence dowries were paid a day or two either side of consummation, by which is meant either the moment officially declared or the time of the *ductio*, when the bride was removed from her natal to her conjugal house. It is

her son on marriage arrangements she had made for her daughter, observing that "whoever takes a wife wants ready cash."[104]

Masculine entry into the normative public and economic spheres hence was demonstrated through a man's implicit ability to inseminate a woman. More than mere penetration was essential for him to begin an economically productive as well as domestically reproductive career. Church courts regularly examined annulment cases in which semen was absent or misplaced. Venetian officials, for example, heard that "he always spilled his seed outside," "my penis cannot enter far enough so that the seed can be received in the womb," or "she withdrew when I was about to spill my seed, and she made me spill it outside of her."[105]

Beyond the marital chamber, the very language of a healthy business could be discussed in gendered terms taken from complexional theory and anatomical metaphors. Over the decade of 1484–94, for example, the troubled accounts of the wool guild in Florence were "very weak," "failing," "very arid" and "cold, cold," physiological diagnoses indicating an unbalanced, largely feminine state of financial affairs, for women were cold and weak, while men were ideally dry but not overly so.[106] Attempts to manipulate Pope Innocent VIII's relationship with the Medici bank were consistently portrayed by officials in sexual terms that made the Pope feminine, the bank aggressively masculine. The work of financial seduction was described, for example, with the verb *frugare*, meaning amongst other things to stir, to seed, to finger or pick through the contents of a purse or pocket.[107] In both the metaphorical and practical realms, male bodies created, manipulated and released valuable resources that were fundamentally linked to testicles and semen.

possible that consummation sometimes occurred in the bride's natal household, immediately before the *ductio*. In any case, the attestation of consummation by the groom and male relatives of the bride was essential.

104 Alessandra Macinghi negli Strozzi, *Lettere*, ed. Cesare Guasti (Florence: Sansoni, 1877), p. 4: "chi to' donna vuol danari."

105 Ferraro, *Marriage wars*, pp. 73, 81, 88. While a deflated penis was often mentioned, this was because it therefore failed in its task of the placement of semen.

106 For the terms, but not the link with the complexional system, see Alison Brown, "Women, children and politics in the letters of a Florentine notary, Ser Pace di Bambello," in David Peterson and Daniel Bornstein (eds.), *Florence and beyond: culture, society and politics in Renaissance Italy* (Toronto: Centre for Reformation and Renaissance Studies, 2008), p. 242.

107 Florio, *Queen Anna's new world of words*, p. 198; Melissa Meriam Bullard, "'Hammering away at the Pope': Nofri Tornabuoni, Lorenzo de' Medici's agent and collaborator in Rome," in David Peterson and Daniel Bornstein (eds.), *Florence and beyond: culture, society and politics in Renaissance Italy* (Toronto: Centre for Reformation and Renaissance Studies, 2008), p. 383.

6 Pleasure and the unequal two-seed theory

Laqueur's one-sex model, with its requirement for the equivalent emission of female and male seed, supposedly gave rise to the necessity of female pleasure, which was thus a notable early modern phenomenon. It is now a commonplace to claim that, until the eighteenth or nineteenth century, medical authors believed "that conception was possible only when intercourse resulted in orgasm for both partners."[1] However, quite what constituted orgasm is unclear, due to variation and misunderstandings in premodern evidence and to modern assumptions that orgasm is a universal, constant, instantly recognizable event.

Premodern notions of female sexual pleasure varied, but were more focused on fluids and uterine reaction than on an event considered orgasmic in modern terms. Despite variations, it is striking that the most vital component of a woman's delight was reception of male seed, so much so that semen was represented as having therapeutic as well as impregnating capabilities. Aristotle's one-seed theory surmised that the absence of female seed concurrently meant that female satisfaction was irrelevant to generation.[2] The Hippo-Galenic unequal two-seed theory also operated by way of comparison with male bodies, and its understanding of the elements of female orgasm often betrayed ignorance more than erotic sympathy. The requirement for a fertile woman to reach "orgasm" was often no more than a need for some sign that she had released secretions, which were mistaken for the lesser, female version of semen. Women were considered naturally avid for more perfect, humidifying male semen, and their bodies ejaculated weaker seed in a less intense manner.

The four separate matters of seed, secretions, sexual pleasure and orgasm tended to be confused in premodern texts, and this habit continues in many modern historical studies. In particular, a post-Betty Friedan assumption that formerly "frigid" and neglected women must now always have orgasms, and a

[1] The quotation is from Thomas Foster, "Deficient husbands: manhood, sexual incapacity, and male marital sexuality in seventeenth-century New England," *William and Mary Quarterly* 3rd ser., 56 (1999), 727. See also two texts which otherwise disagree about a great deal: Laqueur, *Making sex*, pp. 2–3, 43–52; Stolberg, "Woman down to her bones," 285.

[2] Aristotle, *GA*, 727a26–30, 727b5–10, 739a25–35.

Viagra-exacerbated assumption that so must men, further fueled by values of instant gratification in mass media and advertising, means that "orgasm" is an undifferentiated, seemingly "natural" occurrence that has little history but is instead presented in terms of homogeneity and psycho-biological urgency. Yet, female bodies can experience a range of responses, from conscious "faking it" and the pleasure possible for some (though not most) women who have undergone a degree of genital mutilation, to minimal response on the one hand and intense orgasm at any age on the other.[3] Precise physiological responses, including degree of secretion, are also variable and the mere presence of some form of fluid does not guarantee orgasm, and not always pre-orgasmic satisfaction.

We need then to be cautious about reading as obvious and unproblematic any reference to female pleasure or, in more common early modern parlance, release of female seed. Many male-authored texts were based more on previous learned tradition than personal observation. Even those authors with clear sexual experience, and the few women whose articulations about desire survive, filtered their experience through concepts and metaphors that bespeak an historically specific comprehension which is often unlike our own. The celebration of eroticism evident in many early modern texts and images neither proves nor disproves the existence of new, more sensual experiences for actual women. This chapter will show that the notion of a sex-positive early modern culture for women needs to be examined more closely, and that power differences cannot be forgotten.

The issue of pleasure can be couched in other terms. Rather than reinstate the standard notion that premodern women were ideally passive in the Aristotelian sense of contributing no effective cause to generation and were hence politically marginalized, I find an alternative utero-centric model at work in much medical and cultural theory. Even Aristotelians were able to countenance the notion of a womb actively receptive of male semen, and Plato's notion of a wandering, hysterical womb long had misogynist currency. From medieval times on, via Arabic as well as Greek texts, more medical professionals believed to varying degrees the Hippo-Galenic theory of unequal female seed. That seed added something ill-defined to generation but it was not conceptualized in purely reproductive terms, for it was also an erotic agent, responding actively to male intromission, even ejaculating into the uterus. Ideal female passivity was thus modulated by acceptable female desire and agency when reception of male semen was the goal. Lustful women hungered too much for male semen, but the

[3] On variations see, for example, Carole Vance, "Social construction theory: problems in the history of sexuality," in *Homosexuality, which homosexuality? International conference on gay and lesbian studies* (London: GMP, 1989), pp. 13–34, esp. 23–26; Roach, *Bonk*, pp. 65–84 and passim.

underlying principle was the same: that women necessarily, physically depended on what only men could provide. This alternative theory of female nature is the essential complement to the male semenotic model, demonstrating that seed/semen fundamentally determined premodern understanding of biological sex.

Male sexual pleasure

Fluid (chiefly in the form of blood) became semen when it mixed with *pneuma*, and thence erection and ejaculation were pneumatic.[4] The final heated product of "spirit," according to Constantinus Africanus' eleventh-century translation *De coitu*, "fills the hollow of the penis . . . and makes it hard and stiff," pithily put by physician Peter of Spain in the thirteenth century when he wrote simply of "elevating windiness."[5] Describing the ancient Greek idea "as plainly and briefly as possibly I can" so that her words would serve midwives and also the "young men and maids" who might read her *Midwives book* of 1671, Sharp described erections in which the penis is "raised, and swels with a windy spirit."[6] The penis, she explained, "is stretched and made to swell by reason of fullness of Seed and plenty of wind."[7]

To Galen, the moisture warmed in the testicle had to be evacuated, but "an extraordinary, excessive pleasure" resulted from ejaculation because there was "also a great deal of warm pneuma requiring to be exhaled."[8] The sense of explosive release easily led to metaphors about pistol shots or cannon fire, breaking lances and swords or unloosed arrows (figs. 3–4, 27). The Pseudo-Aristotelian *Problems* simply pointed out that the friction of sexual action, experienced throughout the body, "is pleasant, as the vaporous moisture which is unnaturally enclosed escapes" (878b5–10). The penis sounds like the spout of a steaming kettle, the liquid contained within the testicles having been heated by friction. A fifteenth-century glazed red clay vessel unearthed in Brughes has just such a phallic spout, and the stubby legs underneath indicate that it was a cooking pot placed over a fire to heat its contents.[9] The makers and users of such pottery were rendering material and performative the model of

4 Aristotle, *GA*, 736a1, 736b33–37, 742a15, 762a20; also Pseudo-Aristotle, *Problems*, 953b35.

5 Delany, "Constantinus Africanus' *De coitu*," 56; Mary Francis Wack, *Lovesickness in the middle ages: the "Viaticum" and its commentaries* (Philadelphia: University of Pennsylvania Press, 1990), pp. 234, 245. See also, for example, Avicenna, *Liber canonis*, 352r (Bk. III, fen. 20, tr. 1, ch. 2); Jacquart and Thomasset, *Sexuality and medicine*, pp. 60, 79–80, 83, 147, 150, 173 (including flatulence increasing sexual desire); Benedetti, in Lind, *Studies*, p. 98; Crooke, *Mikrokosmographia*, p. 212. Hence, many believed a man should eat "all windy meats, as Pulse, Beans" to aid erection: Sharp, *Midwives book*, p. 30. Jokes about farting were partly attractive because the action was ejaculatory.

6 Sharp, *Midwives book*, pp. 13, 23, 25. 7 Ibid., p. 30. 8 Galen, *Usefulness*, pp. 640–41.

9 Koldeweij, *Geloof & Geluk*, p. 117, fig. 7.55.

ejaculation inherited from ancient medicine. With fluids rather than steam, the joke was made in surviving Greek or Roman artifacts too, for either images of pots or actual vessels occasionally feature a phallic spout.[10] Appropriately, the two elaborate vessels carried high at the far right in Salviati's classicized procession have penile spouts (fig. 25).

The Hippocratic *Generation* describes for both men and women a process of friction, heat, pleasure and discharge, though for the latter the impelling irritation occurs in the womb.[11] The male model was thus often transferred to women, and the priority of semen, pneumatic pressure and heat explains the chief medical explanation given for male–male desire too. According to the Pseudo-Aristotelian *Problems*, offering a model that was still discussed and accepted in the seventeenth century, male homoerotic desire was caused by a build up of semen in the anus, which then necessitated friction to be released; rubbing was the chief mode envisaged in such commentaries, rather than penetration per se, for semen required the application of masculine heat to be discharged from either the penis or the anus.[12]

The teleology of sex was spermatic evacuation, but what we think of as orgasm (which is today often mistakenly conflated with ejaculation) was not an important reproductive moment to Aristotelians or the Hippocratic writers. Rather, ejaculation was the objective, so much so that Foucault characterized the pattern described by Hippocrates, Plato and others as the "ejaculatory schema."[13] What I draw attention to here is not only that the theory lived on for millennia, and into the vernacular register, but that it was quite specific regarding the non-penile components of fluid, *pneuma* and heat. Moreover, it played a central role in theories of female sexual activity and pleasure.

[10] Boardman, "Curious eye cup," 288, 289; *Museu Monográfico de Conimbriga, Catalogue* (Lisbon: Instituto Português de Museus, 2000), p. 166 no. 557. I am grateful to James Grantham Turner for bringing the Roman vessel of the fourth or fifth century to my attention.

[11] "On generation" (1.1–2), in *Hippocratic treatises*, p. 1, and commentary, p. 106; for women see pp. 2–3 (4.1–2).

[12] Pseudo-Aristotle, *Problems*, 4.26. For Avicenna on the matter, see Jordan, *Invention of sodomy*, pp. 119–23. Peter of Abano's commentary was completed in 1310 in Padua and first published in 1475: Joan Cadden, "Sciences/silences: the natures and languages of 'sodomy' in Peter of Abano's *Problemata* commentary," in Lochrie, McCracken and Schultz (eds.), *Constructing medieval sexuality*, pp. 40–57. Translated extracts of Pseudo-Aristotle, Avicenna and Pietro d'Abano are in Kenneth Borris (ed.), *Same-sex desire in the English Renaissance: a sourcebook of texts, 1470–1650* (Routledge: New York, 2004), pp. 122–24, 127–40. For commentaries published in 1498 and 1608 see Derek Neal, "Disorder of body, mind or soul: male sexual deviance in Jacques Despars' commentary on Avicenna," and Faith Wallis, "Giulio Guastavini's commentary on Pseudo-Aristotle's account of male same-sexual coitus, *Problemata* 4.26," in Kenneth Borris and George Rousseau (eds.), *The sciences of homosexuality in early modern Europe* (London: Routledge, 2008), pp. 43–56, and 57–73 respectively.

[13] Foucault, *History of sexuality*, vol. II, pp. 126–30.

Female pleasure: the Renaissance heritage

Despite being naturally moist in complexional terms, a woman regularly expelled her excessive plethora through menstruation and thence longed always for the replenishing moisture provided by male semen, as well as its pleasurably warming effects. Thus the most explicit scientific statement from antiquity about sexual pleasure enshrined an essential connection between male semen and female gratification. According to the Hippocratic author of *On generation*, during intercourse a woman "experiences pleasure throughout the whole time, until the man ejaculates."[14] The explanation for the cessation of female pleasure tellingly constructs two analogies based on the defining principle that masculinity was about fluids.

> If into boiling water you pour another quantity of water which is cold, the water stops boiling. In the same way, the man's sperm arriving in the womb extinguishes both the heat and the pleasure of the woman. Both the pleasure and the heat reach their peak simultaneously with the arrival of the sperm in the womb, and then they cease. If, for example, you pour wine on a flame, first of all the flame flares up and increases for a short period when you pour the wine on, then it dies away. In the same way the woman's heat flares up in response to the man's sperm, and then dies away.[15]

The vivid model of dousing a woman's sexual flame resonated through the centuries. Without being concerned with a woman's pleasure, only his conjugal rights, the misogynist husband of Boccaccio's fourteenth-century *Corbaccio* seethed with indignation: "although first I, then each of these [other lovers of hers] in turn, poured cooling water upon her flames, she nevertheless tied herself in closer bonds" with yet another lover.[16]

Galen's insistence on two seeds did not prioritize physical or psychic gratification. When discussing the harmful nature of the retention of seed, his sole male example was the philosopher Diogenes, who rid himself of "the inconvenience caused by the retention of sperm" by resorting to prostitutes or, when such a woman was late in arriving to service him, masturbation relieved the urge in a calm, immediate fashion.[17] Pleasure was explicitly beside the point. In the same section, a midwife's attendance on a widow led to the voiding of considerable female seed due to contractions that were "similar to that experienced during intercourse."[18] Desire had more of a place in his *On semen*, in which the loss of male or female "testicles" led to the depletion of the urge to copulate, but no theoretical point was made about pleasure in conjunction with a widow's

[14] "On generation" (4.1–2), in *Hippocratic treatises*, pp. 2–3, and commentary, pp. 119–22.
[15] Ibid., p. 2. [16] Boccaccio, *Corbaccio*, pp. 47, 130 n. 216. For Somerset, see Ch. 1 above.
[17] Galen, *On the affected parts*, trans. Rudolph E. Siegel (Basel: Karger, 1976), pp. 184–85.
[18] Ibid., pp. 184–85.

report that in the course of self-treatment to release accumulated seed her convulsive experience was "like that of sexual intercourse."[19]

Female pleasure was of greater interest to medieval authors.[20] Perhaps because much of the discourse was taking place in monasteries or in universities organized along similar lines as they developed out of cathedral schools, physiological questions were asked about largely unfamiliar, intriguing female bodies. Was there, it was wondered, an equivalent to male ejaculation? Some authors believed so, mapping a fluid injection from the female "testicles" (ovaries) into the womb and/or at the vulva.[21] Before the printed publication of the work of Galen and the Hippocratic corpus (from the late fifteenth and during the early sixteenth centuries), the notion that women produced some kind of seed was already in circulation. If pregnancy resulted from pleasure, as it usually did in the two-seed theory, then raped women who fell pregnant had to be explained. Some scholars believed that at an irrational level all women responded with pleasure to sexual contact and thus the raped woman had released seed.[22]

On the other hand, prostitutes were supposedly sterile, due to their lack of delectation and hence emission. Some medical commentators averred that a whore's womb became as "slippery" as marble through over-use and therefore it could not retain male seed, an explanation that partly stemmed from a Hippocratic aphorism but was marred by mistranslation and early reliance on pigs for dissection.[23] There was no need to account for female emission in this notion of overly sexually active women with slippery, infertile wombs, which still informed both vernacular medical books and insults about whoredom that women cast at each other in seventeenth-century England.[24]

If women did not produce seed, it was easy for theorists to understand how a woman might become pregnant without pleasure. According to an oft-repeated

19 Galen, *Semen*, pp. 121–25, 151.

20 See Jacquart and Thomasset, *Sexuality and medicine*, pp. 61–70; Joan Cadden, "Medieval scientific and medical views of sexuality: questions of propriety," *Medievalia et Humanistica*, n.s. 14 (1986), 157–71; Cadden, *Sex difference*, pp. 93–98, 134–65, and passim.

21 For instance, "On Generation," 4.2, in *Hippocratic treatises*, p. 2; Cadden, *Sex difference*, p. 157 (Albertus Magnus); below, for Benedetti and others.

22 Jacquart and Thomasset, *Sexuality and medicine*, p. 64; Cadden, *Sex difference*, pp. 95–96; Patricia Crawford, "Sexual knowledge in England, 1500–1750," in Roy Porter and Mikulás Teich (eds.), *Sexual knowledge, sexual science: the history of attitudes to sexuality* (Cambridge University Press, 1994), pp. 87–88.

23 Hippocrates, *Aphorisms*, 5.62 ("those who have the womb watery do not conceive, for the seed is drowned"). The twelfth-century opinion of William of Conches was published in the sixteenth century: Finucci, *Manly masquerade*, pp. 17–18, citing the Strasbourg edition of 1567 as though it were a new text. See also Jacquart and Thomasset, *Sexuality and medicine*, pp. 25–26, 64, 80–81; Cadden, *Sex difference*, pp. 92, 94; Lemay, *Women's secrets*, pp. 67, 73, 136, 137; Crooke, *Mikrokosmographia*, p. 295.

24 Gowing, *Common bodies*, p. 115; Toulalan, *Imagining sex*, pp. 63, 88.

passage by the twelfth-century Aristotelian physician Averroes, a woman conceived after simply bathing in water containing male seminal fluid.[25] Some doctors also reported women's claims that pregnancy resulted without their having experienced emission. The bath story is striking for Averroes' credulity as well as for the willingness of later scholars to repeat an implausible tale in part due to the weight of textual authority, in part because they were invested in downplaying female contribution to the embryo. The story moved beyond medical circles, occurring for example in an important, popular guide for confessors, first published in 1514.[26]

Women were blamed for spreading the belief in fertilizing bathwater because it was an excuse to cover illicit behavior when they became pregnant, according to such texts as the popular Italian midwifery first published by Scipione Mercurio in 1596.[27] Yet the fantasy of an inseminating bath lived on, still cited by Spanish doctors in 1687 and appearing in a *Treatise on hermaphrodites* published in London by the professional pornographer Edmund Curll in 1718.[28] The baby conceived in the bathwater is, on the one hand, another tale that could exacerbate male concerns about the insecure nature of their paternity but, on the other hand, as Joan Cadden notes, "the concept of female pleasure dissociated from the emission of seed . . . absolved men of a reproductive interest in women's sexual satisfaction."[29] Furthermore, the pornographic efficacy of male semen so potent that it could impregnate by remote control, as it were, is a case of medical theory offering assurance rather than exacerbating anxiety.

On the whole, the Arabic tradition was more at ease with medical and poetic discourse about pleasure and this had an influential impact in Europe, in addition to conveying Hippo-Galenic ideas about female seed. From the last quarter of the twelfth century, Avicenna's translated *Canon* described women's pleasure as multiple, due to the two-seed theory in which women received two kinds of seed-centric delight: "delectation from the motion of the sperm that is in them, and . . . delectation from the motion of the man's sperm in the mouth of the womb, descending to the womb."[30] Physicians were advised not to let

25 M. Anthony Hewson, *Giles of Rome and the medieval theory of conception* (London: Athlone Press, 1975), pp. 87, 88; Jacquart and Thomasset, *Sexuality and medicine*, p. 66; B. F. Musallam, *Sex and society in Islam: birth control before the nineteenth century* (Cambridge University Press, 1983), pp. 48, 64, 136 n. 35; Lemay, *Women's secrets*, pp. 66, 67. Averroes' work was translated into Latin in the 1280s.

26 Tentler, *Sin and confession*, p. 201, by the Dominican Sylvester Prierias Mazzolini.

27 Mercurio, *Commare*, pp. 51–55, 257–59; reiterated, for instance, in Crooke, *Mikrokosmographia*, p. 294, which dismisses Averroes' story as "a right old wives tale" on p. 286.

28 Behrend-Martínez, *Unfit for marriage*, pp. 76–77; Roger Thompson, *Unfit for modest ears: a study of pornographic, obscene and bawdy works written or published in England in the second half of the seventeenth century* (Totowa: Rowman and Littlefield, 1979), p. 171.

29 Cadden, *Sex difference*, p. 143; similarly, Jacquart and Thomasset, *Sexuality and medicine*, p. 67.

30 Avicenna, *Liber canonis*, 362r (Bk. III, fen. 21, tra. 1, ch. 2).

shame hinder their sexual advice to patients, because "when the woman does not emit any sperm, conception cannot take place ... [Husbands can be told that] they should watch out for the moment when the woman clings more tightly, when her eyes start to go red, her breathing becomes more rapid and she starts to stammer."[31] Especially in works influenced by Avicenna, physicians advised male patients to practice foreplay, first given that name as the Latin *preludia* in Andreas Capellanus' treatise on courtly love from the 1180s.[32] While the later sixteenth and seventeenth century in Europe has been identified as a newly sex-positive time, its roots are evident in much earlier medical and courtly literature.

Uterine reception and attraction

Aristotle's very definition of female was "that which receives the semen" rather than emits seed, and uterine reception was essential in the Galenic model too.[33] Receptivity was inscribed into the way people were meant to have sex, because the Church forbade all formations except what was considered best for impregnation, with the woman on her back while the man was above her and took the initiative. In sixteenth-century Spain, being on top of the female partner marked Elena/o's early sexual action as a man.[34] Images of copulating couples (fig. 15) reinforced the posture's legibility and seeming naturalness, whereas the brazen sexual effect of the fifteenth-century engraving plate partly consists of the composition of the coital couple, who are seated and without hierarchical differentiation (fig. 14). The engravings and verse of *I modi* produced during the 1520s were even more subversive and enticing, famously bringing into visible and verbal existence a plethora of sexual positions (*modi*).

The normative position of female passivity was reinforced in medical theory, jokes, stories and images. Boccaccio's gullible painter Calandrino believed himself pregnant because his wife always insisted on sex with her on top.[35] Instead, secular badges delighted in a sexual world upside down: the vulval

31 Avicenna, in Jacquart and Thomasset, *Sexuality and medicine*, pp. 130–31. Virtually no other writer was as detailed and clear about the convulsive peak of orgasm.

32 Baldwin, *Language of sex*, pp. 161–69; Helen Rodnite Lemay, "Anthonius Guainerius and medieval gynecology," in Julius Kirshner and Suzanne Wemple (eds.), *Women of the medieval world: essays in honor of John H. Mundy* (Oxford: Basil Blackwell, 1985), pp. 331–32 (printed posthumously in 1481 at the town of Pavia where he taught at the university); Luigi Belloni (ed.), *Il trattato ginecologico-pediatrico in volgare: Ad mulieres ferrarienses de regimine pregnantium et noviter natorum usque ad septennium di Michele Savonarola* (Milan: Società Italiana di Ostetricia e Ginecologia, 1952), p. 41 (written *c.* 1460 in the court of Ferrara); anonymous, *Mirror of coitus*, pp. 35–38, 79–82; Paré, *Generation*, in *Œuvres*, vol. II, pp. 640–42.

33 Aristotle, *GA*, 765b15; Galen, *Semen*, p. 85; Galen, *Usefulness*, pp. 631, 655.

34 See Ch. 1 for Elena/o, and also Jehanne. 35 Boccaccio, *Decameron*, p. 560.

queen is borne by penile minions (fig. 10), another phallus bows before a mighty vulva, the cat has caught the phallus bird, a female blacksmith hammers at a phallus on her anvil, a merely genital animal has been crowned king (fig. 12). The effect is to disavow yet thereby acknowledge norms, blatantly celebrating and simultaneously mocking different models of sexual delight.

Even Aristotle's theory of passive, receptive femaleness envisaged uterine action. The womb attracted semen like a vacuum: it "draws up the semen in the same way that conical vessels which have been washed out with something warm draw water up into themselves when they are turned mouth downwards."[36] Reporting what women told him, Galen referred to "grasping the semen," and dissections then showed him that indeed the womb was like Plato's influential notion of the hysterical uterus, what Galen called an "animal desirous of procreation." His analogy too was that the womb acted "to draw the semen to itself and enfold and hold it . . . like a physician's suction cup."[37]

Leonardo's drawing of coitus (fig. 29) depicts the cervix opened out and each side of the uterine wall stretched down into the vaginal channel, beginning to draw up globules of male semen. In the mid-1550s, the French physiologist Jean Fernel painted an especially eager, anthropomorphic picture of this snatching womb, which draws the semen towards itself like a cupping glass and

> sucks the male semen out of its own cervix . . . And so the womb entices semen in this fashion, provided it is strong and empty, and eager for love; and if there is to be conception, the woman has a pleasurable presentiment that her womb is impatient; and, with a marvelous longing for the semen, it is pushed out into the private parts, so that it faces the semen and receives it, or rather, seizes it, with its mouth as if with a hand. Then it holds on very greedily to what it has received, . . . grasping it . . . and . . . contracting upon it.[38]

The personified womb was like an alluring, ever-sexually voracious woman, dependent on superior male semen. Significantly, according to the papal brief of 1587 male semen only answered the female appetite if it was what was called *verum semen*, that is, it had to be properly processed in testicles and have a masculine consistency rather than be of the weaker, watery kind that characterized women's "seed."[39] Hence, marriages with eunuchs were disallowed, not

[36] Aristotle, *GA*, 739b10–15; see also Lonie, in *Hippocratic treatises*, pp. 210, 267.

[37] Galen, *Semen*, pp. 67–69, with other cases of the suction cup noted at p. 209. For the animated, eager womb see Plato, *Timaeus*, 91c–d; Galen, *Semen*, p. 75, and *Usefulness*, p. 646. Very similar language for the uterine embrace is evident in texts like Raynald, *Byrth of mankynde*, fol. 11v; Berengario, *Isagogae breves*, fol. 21v; Crooke, *Mikrokosmographia*, pp. 232, 234, 295; Sharp, *Midwives book*, pp. 31, 33, 63, 75.

[38] Fernel, *Physiologia*, pp. 567, 569.

[39] McGrath, *Controversy*, pp. 31–41 (for the information, but not the medical understanding of the difference in the semen).

due to sterility but because the concupiscent purpose of marriage would not be satisfied.

In *Natural faculties*, Galen's analogy was magnetic, ascribing to male and female seed "a faculty for attracting blood similar to that possessed by the lodestone for iron" (2.3.85). Female seed avariciously drew to itself the blood-derived male semen it desired. Popular texts like the *Secrets of women*, first written in Latin in the late thirteenth century but widely disseminated for centuries thereafter in numerous translations and variants, likened the womb to a magnet attracting sperm and sucking in the penis.[40] In the mid-seventeenth century Nicholas Culpeper's vernacular midwifery still believed in the womb's "Magnetick Vertue" which enabled it to draw semen "as the Load-stone draws Iron," echoed in 1671 by Sharp's midwifery.[41] Averse to much use of similes or analogies, Vesalius' renowned *Fabrica* (1543) simply reported uterine attraction with terms like "grasp" and "embrace," characterizing the cervix as involuntarily opening when "being desirous of male semen, it attracts this to itself by a natural movement of suction."[42] He also resorted to Plato's metaphor of the womb "like a sort of animal," and thought it beneficial that women could not consciously control the greedy beast because otherwise "women could refuse to have children unless they wanted to."[43]

Far less suspicious and more poetic is the description of a century later by the French physician Lazare Rivière, here quoted from Culpeper's translation printed in 1655:

> her Genitals ought to swell at the instant of Generation, that her womb skipping as it were for joy, may meet her Husbands Sperm, graciously and freely receive the same, and draw it into its innermost Cavity or Closet, and withal bedew and sprinkle it with her own Sperm, powred forth in that pang of Pleasure, that so by the commixture of both, Conception may arise.

The tone was particularly enthusiastic because it was situated in a chapter on sterility, under the instance of "passions of the mind ... especially hatred between Man and Wife." High rhetoric is put to use in order to encourage women to be not "averse from this kind of pleasure," which causes her to produce insufficient "quantity of Spirits."[44]

[40] Lemay, *Women's secrets*, pp. 121, 178 n. 108; Jacquart and Thomasset, *Sexuality and medicine*, p. 23; Paré, *Collected works*, p. 887.

[41] Sharp, *Midwives book*, p. 53; Culpeper, *Directory for midwives*, p. 27 (also pp. 77, 85, 90, 97, 126, 130). It is probably a misunderstanding of this analogy that explains the view that women insert iron into their vagina which then wounds the penis: Lemay, *Women's secrets*, pp. 88–89.

[42] Vesalius, *Fabric*, pp. 174, 180, 205. See also Raynald, *Byrth of mankynde*, fols. 10r, 14r.

[43] Vesalius, *Fabric*, pp. 174, 176, also 144.

[44] Lazarus Riverius, *The practice of physick* (London: Peter Cole, 1655), p. 503, from his *Praxis medica* (Paris, 1640). Hostility between the two partners was an important cause of sterility: Marinello, *Medicine*, fol. 55v.

In 1671 Sharp informed her readers of the standard opinion that the first proof of pregnancy was that the woman would "feel the womb shut close, and a shivering or trembling to run through every part of her body," with the second sign being that "the pleasure she takes at that time is extraordinary."[45] Spasms or contractions due to what was thought of as immediate closure may have been mistaken for orgasm, or vice versa. Whatever the symptomology or the reproductive outcome, the cause of female pleasure was thought to be uterine reception of seed, chiefly or wholly originating from the male body. If the female body was a void craving to be filled, the lack was semen-centric and embryonic not penile.

Metaphors made the womb an animal hungering for food and fluid that only the male body could supply. Vulval creatures on badges demonstrate the active volition envisaged in Leonardo's drawing, medical lore and numerous metaphors (figs. 10, 13). These vulval signs represent what Vesalius and other anatomists considered the entire uterine system, and the exhibition of eager uterine appetite picks up on language already evident in ancient Greek humor and medicine, creating obscene innuendo from nutrients or foods and the act of eating. The mid-fifteenth-century physician Savonarola was not unusual when he described the womb as having "a great appetite and delight" to receive semen.[46] Montaigne's additions to his *Essays* after 1588 included a passage on Plato's penile and uterine animals, showing a solid grasp of medical opinion. To him, the womb was "a gluttonous and voracious animal which, if denied its food in due season, goes mad, . . . until it has sucked in the fruit of the common thirst and therewith plentifully irrigated and fertilized the depth of the womb."[47] Although Caspar Bartholin denied the applicability of Plato's metaphor, the womb was even more a ravening beast for that early seventeenth-century anatomist, because it "gapes to receive the Yard, as a Beast gapes for its Food."[48]

Women eagerly picking "fruit" from a phallus tree, depicted in various contexts such as manuscript margins, wood caskets and the fresco of a public fountain in the Italian town of Massa Marittima, allude to taboo oral sex as well as to uterine hunger.[49] So too does the female figure obeying the inscription

45 Sharp, *Midwives book*, pp. 50, 82. 46 Finucci, *Manly masquerade*, p. 21.

47 Montaigne, *Complete works*, pp. 651, 654. Other uses of the metaphor include Rabelais, *Gargantua*, 3.32; Bandello, *Novelle*, vol. I, pp. 485, 489.

48 Bartholin, *Anatomicae*, p. 126; repeated in *Bartholinus anatomy*, p. 70; Thomas Bartholin, *Anatome*, 4th edn. (Lyon: Joan. Ant. Huguetan, & Soc., 1677), p. 274. The comment recalls Galen, *Semen*, p. 75.

49 Michael Camille, *Image on the edge: margins of medieval art* (London: Reaktion, 1991), p. 148 fig. 81; Camille, *Medieval art of love*, p. 109 fig. 95; George Ferzoco, *Il murale di Massa Marittima: the Massa Marittima mural* (Florence: Consiglio Regionale della Toscana, 2004); Adrian Hoch, "Duecento fertility imagery for females at Massa Marittima's public fountain," *Zeitschrift für Kunstgeschichte* 69 (2006), 471–88.

("Come get your good fruit, women") and helping herself to the phallic "fruits" on offer in a basket painted on an Italian maiolica plate (fig. 43). The phalli amidst their bed of leaves recall the glass "fruits" or dildoes that arrived in just such a basket at the end of a banquet at the nunnery where Aretino imagined an orgy in 1534.[50] In the language of a mid-seventeenth-century English jokebook, in which a wooer offers special "meats" because "you have two palats, and the best below," the maid depicted on the maiolica plate is employing one palate while alluding to the other.[51] If used to display or serve edibles, the maiolica plate itself saucily offers "fruits" for everyone's amusement. Merry play with female hunger was, at other times, presented in threatening terms because utero-centric agency co-existed with the femme fatale stereotype. Remembering the dangers of spermatic expenditure, an Englishman complained in 1641 that he

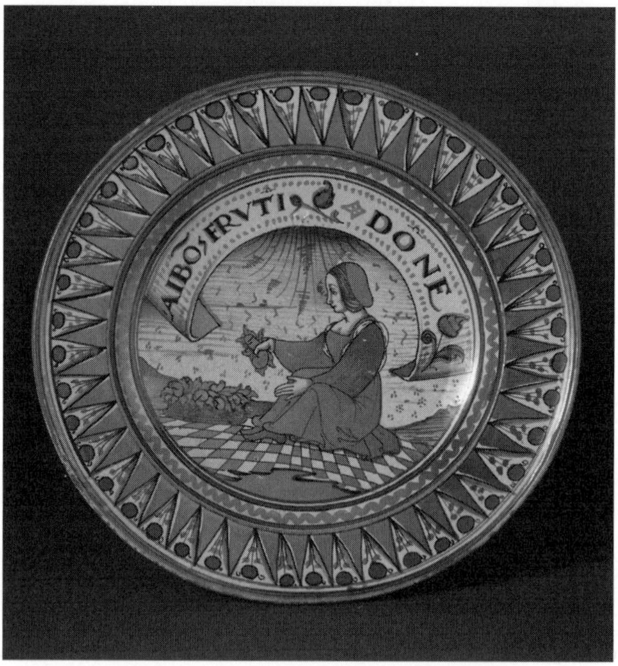

Figure 43 Deruta, *Woman with a basket of phalli, inscribed "Come get your good fruit, women,"* c. 1500–25, maiolica, 34.9 cm diameter, Paris, Musée du Louvre

[50] Aretino, *Ragionamento*, pp. 20, 31, 52; Wolk-Simon's entry on the plate, in Bayer (ed.), *Art and love*, p. 215 no. 106.

[51] John Mennes et al., *Facetiäe: Musarum Deliciae* (1656), as cited in Williams, *Dictionary*, p. 430.

had been sapped and impoverished by his mistress' "greedy desire," for she had made him "the cadaver of her love to feede her helluous gorge."[52]

The nature of women's "seed" and pleasure

Various female discharges or secretions were often misread as straightforward parallels to male ejaculate. Aristotle, however, had pointed out that women's fluid secretion during intercourse "is not seminal; . . . there is a discharge from the uterus, which though it happens in some women does not in others."[53] He confused secretion with leucorrhea ("the whites" in Renaissance English) and later authors could mistake everyday lubrication, secretions due to arousal, smegma, discharge and even blood with what was thought to be female semen.[54] The analogy with hunger led to the influential *Secrets of women* ascribing the release of woman's seed to "delectation just like saliva runs out of the mouth of a starving person."[55] Professional discourse employed the metaphor too. The famed and influential anatomist Mondino de' Luzzi, who introduced dissection to the curriculum at the University of Bologna, wrote in 1316 that women's ovaries were "not truly testicles like those of the man"; further, Aristotelian opinion was supported by the observation that women produced "a humidity similar to saliva which is the cause of female pleasure."[56]

Menses and female seed were commonly conflated, as they were in the *Secrets*, where an aroused "vagina dilates and ejects the menses."[57] The much-reprinted English version of the medieval text, the anonymous *Problems of Aristotle* (first published in 1595), claimed that a woman's "seed" had to be red because it was made of menstrual blood.[58] Women could also associate menses with female seed and thence desire. Lacking access to learned medicine, they nevertheless believed and continued to disseminate views that must have been widely held. Fertility carried great social cachet and gave

52 John Johnson, *The academy of love* (London: Humphrey Blunden, 1641), p. 8. For more English references regarding words like appetite, eat, feed, hunger, see Williams, *Dictionary*, pp. 27–28, 430, 472–74, 986–87; Williams, *Glossary*, pp. 28, 109, 122–23, 130, 166.

53 Aristotle, *GA*, 727b34–728a3. See also 728a31–35, 739a21–b3.

54 For Albertus Magnus see *Animalibus*, pp. 730, 1038–39. Other examples include Laqueur, *Making sex*, p. 106 (a German physician in 1572); John Noonan, Jr., *Contraception: a history of its treatment by the Catholic theologians and canonists*, enlarged edn. (Cambridge, MA: Harvard University Press, 1986), pp. 337–38.

55 Lemay, *Women's secrets*, p. 62.

56 Ioannem Dryandrum (ed.), *Anatomia Mundini* (Marburg: Christiani Egenolphi, 1541), fol. 24v. For the analogy to saliva see also Jacquart and Thomasset, *Sexuality and medicine*, p. 37; Cadden, *Sex difference*, p. 125 (where, also, Albertus Magnus refers instead to "sweat").

57 Lemay, *Women's secrets*, p. 76; Cadden, *Sex differences*, pp. 28, 79; Bildhauer, "*Secrets of women*," pp. 65–75.

58 Adelman, "Making defect perfection," pp. 30, 46 n. 18 (without noting the Latin source).

women a central economic and social purpose, so it was in their interest to glean knowledge from as many sources as possible.[59]

Such seems to have been the case when Beatrice de Planissoles testified before an Inquisitorial panel in 1320. This French widow was surprised that she still experienced strong desire for her lover even though she was what we would call postmenopausal. In part, she was also following the cultural habit of dismissing the sexual life of women who have passed their childbearing years, but that stereotype in turn depended on the slippage between female desire, menstruation and supposed female "seed."[60] No longer emitting "seed," Beatrice understood that she should have been experiencing only half or less of the usual yearning. Lessened desire, which often does occur in menopausal women due to hormonal changes, was framed by another, plausible explanation in premodern Europe. Beatrice wondered whether she had been cast under the spell of love magic, so much was her sexual desire unexpected.

Another case, of pleasure thwarted, is also instructive about how women understood their sexual yearnings. Isabella De Moerloose's autobiography, which was published in Amsterdam in 1695, recalled amongst other things sexual details during her two-year marriage with a provincial clergyman.[61] Wed in 1692 when she was around thirty, and he was over seventy with children from a previous marriage, Isabella regretted that he had never "given her seed," even though she had begged him on her knees "that I would rather he never touched me again than bring me so far and then leave me." He was wrong, she said, "first to awaken nature and then to fling away the seed," by which she meant not only his consistent practice of coitus interruptus but also, implicitly, the waste of her own seed. When asked how far he had taken her, she replied "to the conception," meaning that they had each produced seed that should have been mixed, or coagulated like cheese in the womb. Pleasure, then, was incomplete for Isabella, in part because she did not become pregnant, in part because her womb could not joyously receive semen; and, perhaps, in part because she witnessed male orgasm, but may not have experienced her own, or not often. Her scale of pleasure stopped at the point of releasing seed, described as "conception," yet still she reported dissatisfaction. Whether or not she orgasmed in a modern sense, the point is that her priorities and language concentrated on other

[59] Patricia Crawford, "Attitudes to menstruation in seventeenth-century England," *Past and Present* 91 (May 1981), 47–73.

[60] Jean Duvernoy, *Le registre d'Inquisition de Jacques Fournier* (Paris: Mouton, 1978), vol. I, p. 284; Patrick Geary (ed.), *Readings in medieval history*, vol. II: *The later middle ages*, 3rd edn. (Peterborough: Broadview Press, 2003), p. 216. I owe knowledge of this case to Green, "Flowers," p. 55. However, it is thought there that Beatrice "had some sense that menstruation . . . was connected to sexual pleasure," whereas I would highlight female menses/seed.

[61] The following is drawn from Roodenburg, "Autobiography of Isabella De Moerloose," 529–32 passim.

matters. Isabella was informed about the basic principles of gynecological theory: she emitted seed, it could overpower male sperm and thereby lead to the birth of a girl, and unfertilized menses would putrefy. To her, the husband's neglect of her seed was "the greatest affliction or indignity." Her valuable contribution to the marriage contract was neglected, and with it her worth as a person.

To Isabella's body, as in medical theory, a vital component of female pleasure was neither clitoral nor vaginal but uterine and fluid. Beatrice in 1320 also seemed to think of desire in relation to her womb and its now-gone menses/seed. Both women knew about the analogy with cheese making, the Frenchwoman thinking that a herb which prevented curdling might act as a contraceptive.[62] These two accounts are especially interesting because they are non-literary female-authored stories, though very conscious of their audience, in a law court in one case and, in the other, for a readership that Isabella was especially keen to reach. What is probably the description of orgasm by a Venetian weaver in 1584 is also couched in terms of common ejaculation and seed. Defending himself against the charge of impotence from his childless wife and wanting to retain the dowry, Francesco Revedin boasted that he had often emitted into her "nature" and that she had "emitted her sperm on my member while I was penetrating her."[63]

Investigating late medieval medical texts, Cadden concludes that the "lack of clarity about the female fluid or fluids involved in procreation was a persistent problem."[64] That confusion, which characterized two-seed advocates too, continued and even the weaver Revedin may be describing female lubrication rather than orgasm. The most influential vernacular gynecological manual of the sixteenth century, Eucharius Rösslin's *Rosegarten* (1513), as translated into English in 1545, was uncertain about its identification in the womb of "whyte spermy and thyn clere matter which no doubt is the woman's sede."[65] Some might dismiss this dew-like moisture, thinking it served "for no other purpose but onely to excite, move and stere the woman to pleasyr," but the author regarded pleasure as a legitimate motivation for purposes of propagation and it counterbalanced the pains of childbirth.

Anatomical descriptions were more detailed, but no less confused. By distinguishing between three female elements, menses, "genital humor" produced internally and without libido, and some other but infertile fluid that "bursts forth with such great pleasure," the humanist anatomist Benedetti tried to cope in the 1490s with the different theories of female seed. His findings included the observation that sometimes the infertile fluid "poured forth in coitus . . . with

[62] Duvernoy, *Registre*, vol. I, p. 280.
[63] Hacke, *Women, sex and marriage*, pp. 146, 151–52, 162, 164, 169.
[64] Cadden, *Sex difference*, p. 79; also Jacquart, "Medical explanations," p. 11.
[65] Raynald, *Byrth of mankynde*, fol. 27r. Parts of the text relied on Savonarola's earlier *Practica*.

so great an impetus in many that it spurts out farther like the semen of males."[66] A later professor at the University of Padua was less precise and more traditional, for Vesalius mentioned only "a thin and very scanty and watery semen" entering the womb from the ovaries, an evaluation that was fundamental to the unequal two-seed theory.[67]

Vesling's *Syntagma*, an anatomical textbook first published in 1641, stated that "such Women as are fruitful have a twofold Spermatical matter, the one watry, which moistens and refresheth the Womb, and Fruit in it, the other which is thick in the [Fallopian] *Tubae*, which is mixed with the Seed of Man to make the Conception."[68] Unlike Benedetti, however, Vesling regarded both kinds of female "sperm" as necessary for conception and gestation. The professional anatomist could not distinguish between discharge, lubrication and female seed or semen, and he did not think the production of such "juyce" had anything to do with sexual desire in most women. In 1651 William Harvey revived the Aristotelian denial of effective female seed, ironically due in part to the observation made by Galen and many since, that women's sexual fluid was too thin, of "a serous and watery consistency, like urine."[69]

Crooke emphasized the tactile quality of the "extasie" of male pleasure, focusing on the cause of "the touch of the seede upon the nervous and quicke sensed parts as it passeth by them," which implicitly requires no sexual partner.[70] Du Laurens and thence his English translator Crooke decided that much the same could be said of female pleasure, which was more fully internalized: "pleasure is not therefore conceived because the [female] seede toucheth the orifice of the wombe, but because it runneth through the spermaticall vesselles of the woman which are of exquisite sense," and her "eiaculations" were uterine.[71] The illustrated edition of du Laurens' anatomy released in 1600 had provided readers with an illustration of this ejaculating part (fig. 32).[72] The plate was a recut collection of images from Vesalius' *Fabrica*, but the captions were reduced. Figure III at the lower right used "s" for the "Principium vasis eiaculatorii," but in Vesalius that had been the "beginning of the vessel that conveys semen from the testis to the uterus." At the top left in du Laurens' figure iiii

66 Lind, *Studies*, pp. 98–99, 101.

67 Andreas Vesalius, *The epitome of Andreas Vesalius*, trans. L. R. Lind (New York: Macmillan, 1949), p. 85; his *Fabric*, p. 186 has women's semen as moister and colder.

68 Vesling, *Anatomy*, p. 27. Also, for example, Crooke, *Mikrokosmographia*, pp. 218–19.

69 William Harvey, *Disputations touching the generation of animals*, trans. Gweneth Whitteridge (Oxford: Blackwell Scientific Publications, 1981), p. 165.

70 Crooke, *Mikrokosmographia*, p. 238.

71 Du Laurens, *Historica anatomica*, p. 395; Crooke, *Mikrokosmographia*, p. 295. Other texts also characterized the woman's vessels as ejaculatory, for example: Paré, *Œuvres completes*, vol. I, pp. 154–63; Marinelli, *Thresor*, p. 43.

72 Du Laurens, *Historica anatomica*, pp. 256 for the table, 257 for the illustrations; cf. Vesalius, *Fabric*, pp. 42–43.

(fig. 32) the letter K marked the "Vasa eiaculatoria," part of what was labeled the left testicle (F), whereas Vesalius called K the "Vessel conveying semen from the testis to the uterus." Changes in terminology made the passage of seed even more comparable with male function.

Even if the term "ejaculation" was not used, aroused women were often represented as gushing with sexualized fluids. Voluptuous delight led women to pour forth (*effundo*) their seed, albeit "less and weaker" than male semen and infertile according to Fernel.[73] Antonio Panormita's infamously obscene *Hermaphroditus* of 1425, for example, presented a vulva running freely like wine from bottles, and Aretino's sonnets for *I modi* had the juices of prostitutes flow when aroused by men.[74] Notably, the labia being parted on the left of Salviati's phallic procession (fig. 25) have below them an overturned vase already releasing plentiful fluids. These examples are of illicit sexual activity, but other erotic occasions gave rise to extravagance too. "Various liquors" fly in the climax of Johannes Secundus' sexually explicit epithalamium, composed before 1536, which stressed the difference between the couple's seed, as did medical discourse. Both husband and wife, "wet, will exude streams of different fluid," and children quickly result.[75] The emphasis works to shut down the potential for a homoerotic reading of two ejaculating bodies in concourse in the bedchamber, a further reason perhaps for both the attraction of the theory of an homology between male and female bodies and its increasing marginalization, then demise.

Quantification and comparison

The very gods first asked a question that was long reiterated in medical texts and beyond. Having been transformed into a woman for seven years, the blind male prophet Tiresias was asked by Zeus and Hera which sex enjoyed coitus more. His answer, women, infuriated Hera but intrigued men for millennia.[76] The question is almost meaningless in modern Euro-American societies because we are now trained to think in terms of incommensurable differences between a canonical system of only two defined sexes. On the other hand, the ancient but influential teleological notion that all body parts must have a purpose still leads

[73] Fernel, *Physiologia*, pp. 554–57, hereafter quoted from p. 565.

[74] Antonio Panormita, *Hermaphroditus*, trans. Eugene O'Connor (Lanham: Lexington Books, 2001), pp. 35, 131; Talvacchia, *Taking positions*, pp. 215, 217 for Aretino.

[75] *Sylvae*, 8.124–34, trans. in David Price, *Janus Secundus* (Tempe, AZ: Medieval and Renaissance Texts and Studies, 1996), p. 46.

[76] Apollodorus, *Library*, 3.6.7; Hyginus, *Fabula*, 75; Ovid, *Metamorphoses*, 3.316–38. The tale was often cited in medical texts, for example, Marinelli, *Thresor*, p. 62; Jean Liébault, *Trois livres des maladies et infirmitez des femmes* . . . (Rouen: Jean Berthelin, 1649), p. 525; Sharp, *Midwives book*, p. 67; Cadden, *Sex difference*, pp. 150–62.

some to ask today about the use of female orgasm because "it does not appear to serve any useful biological function."[77]

Some medieval theorists proposed that female pleasure was not as great in quality and intensity as that experienced by men, but greater in quantity because they were forever lustful, a misogynist trope disseminated in such genres as medieval fabliaux and Renaissance jokes.[78] While the one-seed theory endowed men with exclusive potency, the schema of two seeds carved out a different kind of space for male superiority. Whereas a woman's pleasure was doubled, since it was supposed that she enjoyed both "the pleasure of emitting and of receiving emission" as an eighteenth-century erotic text succinctly stated the still conventional case, a man's voluptuousness was more intense and paradigmatically masculine.[79] Tiresias' question was one frame by which medical knowledge was eroticized and privileged, because it presented the revelation of female "secrets." The alluring impossibility of answering the question precisely did not stop du Laurens from tackling it, nor Crooke from translating the response in 1615:

> Indeede the woman conceiveth pleasure more waies, that is in the avoyding [i.e., release] of her owne seede and also in the attraction of the mans: . . . but the pleasure of the man is more intense, partly because his seede is more hot and spirituous, & partly also because it yssueth with greater violence and with a kinde of Almaine leape or subsultation.[80]

The differing modes of quantification depend upon terms and values established centuries earlier. Albertus Magnus had put learned opinion thus: "Quantitatively, pleasure is greater in women, but intensively it is greater in men."[81]

Projective emission was a core marker of masculinity. Yielding sexual secretions and simply receiving male semen with presumed delight, a woman necessarily, so it was thought, had to have a pleasurable orgasm. Distinguishing between kinds of pleasures enabled authorities and readers to mistake almost any coital situation as innately pleasing to a woman, and to understand any less overt signs as simply a matter of her lesser intensity rather than the absence of orgasm. After all, women often "ejaculated" or released semen directly into the womb, without providing much or any external sign.

77 A. Zee, "On fat deposits around the mammary glands in the females of Homo sapiens," *New Literary History* 32 (2001), 203.

78 Jacquart and Thomasset, *Sexuality and medicine*, pp. 81, 213 nn. 104–05; Baldwin, *Language of sex*, p. 233; Barbara C. Bowen (ed.), *One hundred Renaissance jokes: an anthology* (Birmingham, AL: Summa Publications, 1988), p. 32 (a Florentine collection of *c.* 1480).

79 The quotation from *The battles of Venus*, said to be "translated from the posthumous works of Voltaire" when printed in 1760, is from Pisanus Fraxi [Henry Spencer Ashbee], *Index librorum prohibitorum* (1877), rpt. as *Bibliography of prohibited books* (New York: Jack Brussel, 1962), vol. I, p. 122. In medical literature see, for example, Lemnius, *Secret miracles*, p. 19.

80 Du Laurens, *Historica anatomica*, p. 385; Crooke, *Mikrokosmographia*, p. 288.

81 Wack, *Lovesickness*, p. 119.

Peter of Spain's thirteenth-century commentary on Constantinus Africanus' earlier attempt to analyze coitus was notable for its enumeration of the details of male delight. It succinctly outlined the factors still taken into account by later writers. Crediting an Arabic text, Peter reported that male desire was greater than women's because it consisted of four elements: "imagination of the desired thing, an imbalanced complexion that stimulates, elevating windiness, and copious seed."[82] The integrated psychosomatic scheme was followed by a list of what caused sexual pleasure in general, for both men and women. The four elements consisted first of the extreme sensitivity of the genitals, then of somatic delight the body takes in action. (For the woman, such action included "expelling the fetus," notably a motion not associated with the event of intercourse, nor with physical pleasure by most women.) The third cause was "the passage of seminal moisture through the member, for it induces a certain tickling and pleasurable motion. The fourth cause is the rubbing of sensitive members against each other, which results in a temperate heat." By these criteria, the male body obtained greater qualitative pleasure.

The "masculine member is more sensitive," and men "emit more and are more consumed in intercourse." The danger of exhaustion was thus turned into a positive sign of the superior quality of masculine pleasure. Showing no awareness of or interest in the clitoris, like nearly all European medical and religious texts before the mid-sixteenth century and many thereafter as well, Peter found little evidence for the nerve-filled nature of female genitalia or uterus. The male body was more perfect, more heated, more active, more sensitive, more copious in the output of semen that was more refined and informed with *pneuma*, more sudden in emission and more drained by it.

Motion and friction are not located specifically in or near the uterus and the male member may as well be engaged in sexual action with any sensitive part of a female or male partner. Although authors dared not mention it, engagement with one's own hand or someone else's anus, thigh or armpit (male or female) implicitly entailed a similar psychosomatic process of erotic pleasure for men. Crucially, friction generated not only pleasure but also heat that helped concoct semen. Gratification resulted from motion, friction, tactile sensitivity and then release, which was not exclusively attainable through single-minded penetration of a uterine system.

The penile shaft did not feature in Peter's account. Testicles were the very motivator of desire in debates about lovesickness, because their "fullness stimulates intercourse" and some said that "love is therefore a disease of the testicles."[83] Other medical authors followed more or less the same sense of

[82] Ibid., pp. 244–45 with parallel Latin, lines 198–200. The following is drawn from pp. 244–47. For other texts, see Cadden, *Sex difference*, pp. 158–60.

[83] Wack, *Lovesickness*, pp. 221, 235–37.

causation.[84] Other than testicles and their semen, Peter's model of men's pleasure centered on the sensitive *glans*, an area more explicitly mentioned in Peter of Abano's discussion when he located a woman's pleasure at the mouth of the womb (a term commonly used for both the cervix and the vulva) because that part "corresponds to the head of the penis (*balanus*), where extreme pleasure flourishes."[85] In other accounts, the male model was applied to female bodies in such a way that they too experienced a degree of erection. Avicenna described a superfluity of female seed causing desire to attract male semen, which led to a kind of internal swelling with "spirits" or erection as the female body reached out eagerly, an idea repeated by Albertus Magnus and remaining influential in the seventeenth century.[86] The comparison was about the three factors of semen, testicles and heat, not the supposed inversion or lack of a penis. So, for Jean Liébaut's popular French book on female maladies, issued yet again in 1649, men enjoyed greater pleasure than women in the "combat venerien" for two chief reasons, that their seed was warmer and more plentiful.[87] Due to the fundamental theory of two unequal seeds, women's minor and involuntary sexual responses could be misread as orgasmic.

Changes during the Renaissance

As the effusive passages by Fernel and Rivière indicate, sexual pleasure was of increased, overt medical interest during the Renaissance, though understanding of it did not universally improve. Besides catalyzing the professionalization of gynecology, the publication of the full Hippocratic corpus in 1525 and its absorption thereafter may turn out to be a landmark in the still-to-be-written history of women's sexual pleasure. Its detailed model of female satisfaction certainly informed the lay notion of erotic delight upheld by the minor French nobleman Pierre de Brantôme in the 1580s. Comparing sex between women with sex between a man and a woman, he opined that women needed to "bathe in cool running water, which refreshes much better than still water" and that "there is a big difference between throwing water in a vessel and just watering around it and on the edge."[88] Hence, the flow of male semen within the uterus was essential for female pleasure and the latter was considered a valid pursuit in the context of his discussion of court gossip that rarely paid heed to issues regarding offspring.

84 For example, Fernel, *Physiologia*, p. 485.
85 Cadden, *Sex difference*, p. 160, citing the *Conciliator*, which was finished in 1303.
86 Avicenna, *Liber canonis*, 356r (Bk. 3, fen. 20, tr. 1, ch. 25); Culpeper, *Directory*, p. 31. For Albertus Magnus, see Ch. 4 above.
87 Liébault, *Maladies*, p. 526.
88 Brantôme, *Dames galantes*, pp. 119–28 passim. First printed in 1665–66, it circulated earlier in manuscript. The text is translated in Jeffrey Merrick and Bryant Ragan Jr. (eds.), *Homosexuality in early modern France: a documentary collection* (Oxford University Press, 2001), pp. 105, 107.

Much early modern discussion of sexual pleasure similarly sundered pleasure from reproduction. Crucially, reproduction and uterine anatomy were irrelevant in Colombo's "discovery" of the clitoris, published posthumously in early 1560. His knowledge was very probably engendered in a courtesan's chamber, not on a dissection table or in a marital bed. Strikingly, he came up with no name for the genital part (Falloppio used the Greek *kleitoris* in 1561) and one or both of Colombo's key expressions perhaps derive from his female teacher ("the seat of women's delight" and "the love or sweetness of Venus").[89] A woman whose profession was about physical and verbal skills in erotica guided his understanding of her tactile response. The clitoris joined the anatomical lexicon neither quickly nor universally, and in certain extreme cases it was compared to the penis, despite the objections of authorities like du Laurens. In the long run, knowledge of the clitoris, unable to deliver semen, probably contributed to the decline of semen-centric theory.

Overall, the teleological basis of anatomy as well as religious interests sustained an ongoing, overt focus on licit, reproductive sex. Galen, Constantinus Africanus and others had framed discussion of human generation by first justifying pleasure because it had a reproductive purpose. Those statements expanded, into a full chapter in the case of sixteenth-century authors like the anatomist Vesalius and the surgeon Paré or the early seventeenth-century translator Crooke.[90] Whereas the early Christian polemicist Tertullian and others invested in asceticism fretted about the loss of a man's soul and self-control during orgasm, Crooke noted that "the God of Nature" had ordained that "wee are transported for a time as it were out of our selves."[91] Moreover, mutual gratification within marriage more consistently featured in the rhetoric of writers like Fernel and Rivière.

Anatomists were more aware of tactile sensuality, presumably fostered by the idea of foreplay inherited from medieval medical and erotic texts. The experience of "exquisite sense" was expanded, the various parts of the male genitals particularly warranting lengthier observation. That the male genitals were composed of several "nervous" parts, that is, especially endowed with nerves and hence sensitive, had long been observed, though early modern texts are more precise and detailed, moving far beyond Aristotle's schema of a shaft of gristle topped by a fleshy head with foreskin and counterbalanced by the weight of testicles (*History of animals* (*HA*), 493a25–b2). In part, this may have been due to increased examinations and suffering caused by the advent of syphilis, and greater attention to urinary and renal problems, as well as more frequent

[89] Colombo, *Anatomica*, p. 243. It is often not noticed that the colophon in Colombo's book is dated 24 January 1559 Venetian style and hence means early 1560 new style.

[90] Vesalius, *Fabrica*, p. 520; Paré, *Génération*, in *Œuvres*, vol. II, pp. 635–37; Crooke, *Mikrokosmographia*, pp. 197–200.

[91] Crooke, *Mikrokosmographia*, p. 200.

dissections. Expanding the words of Colombo slightly, the English surgeon John Banister wrote of the prepuce that it moves "in the acte of venerie, now upward, now downeward, to the exceeding delectation of the female."[92] In response to William Harvey's evidence for the systemic circulation of blood (announced at lectures in 1616 and printed in 1628), anatomists paid more attention to blood supply; in 1641, for instance, Thomas Bartholin added to his father's chapter on the clitoris (1611) that its extensive blood supply enabled an "exquisite perception of sensation, and erection."[93] Gradually, the tactile excitation brought about by the flow of seed was re-envisaged in relation to the flow of blood, and thence semen, testicles and heat began to fade as the determining principles of male sexuality, pleasure and virility. But that was more a story of the Enlightenment, or later.

The topic of sexual delight continued to develop well beyond elite medical analysis into the growing field of erotic images and discourse, encouraged by the rise of the printing press. Ian Moulton, James Grantham Turner, Sarah Toulalan and others have observed that the period was characterized by the sheer amount of verbiage and its explicit detail about coital variety, even while disagreeing over whether the term "pornography" is appropriate for premodern materials and how much it was a discrete genre or when its core features were formulated.[94] The intersection with medical knowledge, albeit often of a popularized, outdated sort, is striking. Much of the conceptualization of pleasure focused on what was thought of as the uterine system; woodcuts illustrating that area in Charles Estienne's *De dissectione partium corporis humani* (1545) were drawn from an erotic series of prints about the *Loves of the gods*.[95] According to a passage added in 1649 to the French version of a gynecological book on women's maladies, a Parisian woman was so delighted by the painting of a naked man that she ejaculated on the spot.[96]

When analyzing seventeenth-century pornographic texts written or translated into English, Toulalan has astutely observed that supreme pleasure was

[92] Banister, *Historie of man*, fol. 88v, from Colombo, *Anatomica*, p. 240 (reiterated in Bauhin, *Theatrum anatomicum*, p. 209, translated in Crooke, *Mikrokosmographia*, p. 215); cf. the focus only on male pleasure in, for instance, the earlier Vicary, *Anatomie*, N i recto.

[93] Bartholin, *Anatome*, p. 292, translated by Culpeper as "an exact Feeling and Erection" (*Bartholinus anatomy*, p. 77).

[94] Ian Frederick Moulton, *Before pornography: erotic writing in early modern England* (Oxford University Press, 2000); James Grantham Turner, *Libertines and radicals in early modern London: sexuality, politics, and literary culture, 1630–1685* (Cambridge University Press, 2002); James Grantham Turner, *Schooling sex: libertine literature and erotic education in Italy, France, and England 1534–1685* (Oxford University Press, 2003); Toulalan, *Imagining sex*.

[95] C.E. Kellett, "Perino del Vaga et les illustrations pour l'anatomie d'Estienne," *Aesculape* 37 (1955), 74–89; elaborated in Talvacchia, *Taking positions*, pp. 161–87. Estienne's book was released simultaneously in French and Latin.

[96] Liébault, *Maladies*, p. 80.

represented as "penile penetration *with* ejaculation" because semen was central to the fantasies, providing a "Fountain of Joys" as one text put it.[97] However, to then conclude that this semen-centric priority was solely due to the medico-erotic focus on conception and a pornographic "preoccupation with the theme of fertility" misunderstands the model I have outlined here, in which semen is *the* actual cause of pleasure.[98] The penis must be of the right length so that it "reaches . . . sufficiently to provoke a womans lust and seed," as one pseudo-medical text put it, but details about impregnation did not then follow.[99] Gynecological and pornographic texts shared much the same overt, rhetorical frame within which talk about sex was conceptualized and legitimized. But both marital and illicit sex was increasingly not focused purely on reproduction as the end goal. Various means of contraception and abortion were practiced, the notion that prostitutes were barren remained widespread, and the medical opinion of Paré and others held that the fertility of male semen was spoiled by abundant sex: by such means, the pornographic representation of endless, untrammeled sex was able to ignore the risk of pregnancy.[100] In Aretino's foundational text about prostitution that served as a model for much pornographic writing for centuries thereafter, the midwife takes a central role in the final dialogue (1536) because she facilitates the art of whoredom, not because she assists in live births. Furthermore, a character's refusal to lie with pregnant women in *The isle of pines* (1668) could be read in relation to overt denial of sodomitical misuse of semen rather than an urge to fecundate anew.[101] In general, a pornographic emphasis on the uterine placement of semen is about claiming heterocentric more than parental legitimization, as well as stressing the male source of female pleasure.

Jove's golden shower of coin/semen in Titian's *Danaë* (fig. 34) is the epitome of valuable, heated material in explosive action, penetrating an enclosed chamber aided by a thrusting dark cloud but actually impregnating by way of proximity, akin to Averroes' tale of absorbed bathwater. Flushed face, upturned eyes, right fingers spasmodically clutching the sheet and left hand buried in her genitals indicate Danaë's receptive and active pleasure. Like Dürer's old hag (fig. 42), a weathered, dark-skinned servant greedily gathers the god's abundance, hungry for both wealth and the moisturizing, revivifying semen that her withered, masculinized body has too long lacked. For the enjoyment of many

97 Toulalan, *Imagining sex*, pp. 73 (her emphasis), 74.

98 Ibid., p. 32. The assumed "connection between pleasure/orgasm and conception" (p. 64) is reiterated throughout, esp. in Ch. 2.

99 Ibid., p. 72, quoting Sinibaldus' *Rare verities* of 1658 as evidence for the preoccupation with male fertility.

100 Paré, *Collected works*, p. 931; Montaigne, *Complete works*, p. 646; Noonan, *Contraception*; Toulalan, *Imagining sex*, pp. 62 n. 2, 73–74.

101 Cf. Toulalan, *Imagining sex*, pp. 98–90.

male viewers and also some women including courtesans and mistresses, such imagery assumed, eroticized and propagated the fundamental notion of women's receptive, sensual agency that was coupled with the necessity of male semen.

Dildoes and fluids

Scoffing at a *castrato* was ostensibly justified because only sperm would satisfy a woman, in the anonymous pornographic novel *L'Escole des filles* (1655).[102] In its very fascination with eunuchs, however, the ensuing dialogue indicates a more complicated literary construction of always transferable, replicable phalli serving ever-desiring women. What medicine enumerated as the two chief causes of sexual pleasure for men and women, friction and fluids, were debated in relation to the efficacy of the dildo. The apparatus was tellingly called a beardless eunuch in Thomas Nashe's poem that gave the device its English name around 1593.[103] "Eunuke dilldo, senceless, counterfet, / Who sooth maie fill, but never can begett," was lacking in full masculinity and thence safe because it could not impregnate. But the counterfeiting was chiefly described in relation to how the dildo was a glass device filled with fluid: "nourisht with whott water or with milk; / Arm'd otherwise in thick congealed glasse." Its chariot ride involves a deep journey but the focus is on passing through "clammie waies" as the tool is splashed and sprayed by female fluids. Filled with warmed liquid (hot water or milk), or with urine in the case of Aretino's dildoes at the convent, the instrument mimicked the Hippocratic requirement of providing a masculine dousing, combined with the pleasurable warmth usually imparted by an infusion of sperm from the naturally hotter, male body.

Glass was the material in Aretino's *Ragionamento* too, whose work Nashe admired. Juvenal's phalliform glass drinking vessel (2.95) or those mentioned by Pliny (*NH* 33.4) were the possible inspiration, though glass phalli explicitly served as dildoes in satirical verse penned by the humanist Filelfo in the 1430s.[104] Archaeological finds in northern Europe and England have yielded phalli of glass, complete with testicles and usually pubic hair, from the early

102 Turner, *Schooling sex*, pp. 149–52. It was translated into English by 1676–77.

103 Thomas Nashe, "The choise of valentines," in David Norbrook and H. R. Woudhuysen (eds.), *The Penguin book of Renaissance verse* (London: Penguin, 1993), pp. 253–63. Quotations are from lines 263–317. See Patricia Simons, "The cultural history of *Seigneur Dildoe* in Renaissance Italy," in Allison Levy (ed.), *Sex acts: practice, performance, perversion and punishment in early modern Italy* (Aldershot: Ashgate, 2010), pp. 77–91.

104 Martin Davies, "An emperor without clothes? Niccolò Niccoli under attack," *Italia Medioevale e Umanistica* 30 (1987), 147.

sixteenth century and later (fig. 44).[105] So too Nashe's glass dildo included the semblance of testicles, for "Sometimes he smoothlie slideth downe the hill; / Another while the stones his feete doe kill." Many glass phalli capable of holding fluids survive, one found in the cistern of a German convent in Herford, another in a late seventeenth-century cesspit now under the National Gallery, London. Most were fitted with funnels which double as mouthpieces for drinking; users had to tip it high to make the liquid flow, thereby holding an erect set of male genitals as though it rose from their mouth. Others were like a surviving example in dark green glass which has no funnel and is perforated at

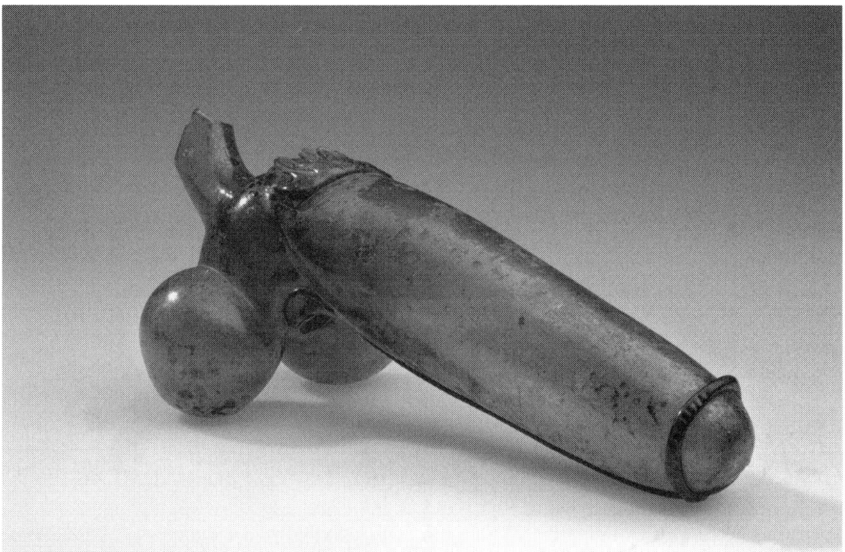

Figure 44 German, phallus glass (damaged), first half of sixteenth century, 7.2 × 18 cm, Trier, Rheinisches Landesmuseum

[105] For an intact Roman example see David Whitehouse, *Roman glass in the Corning Museum of Glass*, vol. I (Corning, NY: Corning Museum of Glass, 1997), pp. 202–03. On early modern examples see Franz Rademacher, *Die Deutschen Gläser des Mittelalters* (Berlin: Verlag für Kunstwissenschaft, 1933), pp. 56–60, 143, Pl. 9; Fritz Kämpfer and Klaus Beyer, *Glass: a world history*, trans. and rev. Edmund Launert (Greenwich, CT: New York Graphic Society, 1966), p. 280, Pl. 121; Erwin Baumgartner and Ingeborg Krueger, *Phönix aus Sand und Asche: Glas des Mittelalters* (Munich: Klinkhardt & Biermann, 1988), pp. 421–22 no. 530 (the example in Trier); V. T. van Vilsteren (ed.), *100.000 jaar Sex over liefde, vruchtbaarheid en wellust* (Zwolle: Waanders Uitgevers, 2003), p. 81; Koldeweij, *Geloof & Geluk*, p. 112; Alison Telfer et al., "Rich refuse: a rare find of late 17th-century and mid-18th-century glass and tin-glazed wares from an excavation at the National Gallery, London," *Journal of the Society for Post-Medieval Archaeology* 40 (2006), 193–95. For Sermini's reference to a *bicchiere* that may be a similar glass vessel, see Ch. 7 below.

the glans, with a hole of sufficient size for it to receive as well as dispense fluids.[106] Drinking from it mimicked oral sex, and it could have been used as a dildo. Its testicles form a base so that the container stood upright, erect on the table or shelf. In 1571 an Essex brothel-keeper was charged with serving drinks in "a glass like unto a pintle [penis] and a pair of bollocks."[107] It is likely that other such vessels were available for use in taverns, licensing raucous conversations about fluids and genitals, of the sort that may lie behind the flinging of beer at several Somerset women in the early seventeenth century.

More expense and engineering characterize an ivory dildo roughly dated to the eighteenth century, which has a pump mechanism that enabled the release of liquid (fig. 45). Inside its cloth bag, it was apparently found in the seat of a Louis XV armchair situated in a convent on the Seine near Paris. Presumably, more ordinary dildoes were less complicated or expensive and often homemade, but the material evidence of the ivory example and the potential for appropriation of glass vessels co-exists with the textual fascination about liquid-containing dildoes. Various fluids were mentioned in libertine texts, but the most common was appropriately white, warm milk.[108] The warm fluid overcame two objections about dildoes uttered by a female character in the fragment of an ancient Greek text, that they lacked heat and also yolks or chicks, a reference I believe to fecund, concocted semen though it might instead mean testicles, as Jeffrey Henderson suggests.[109] So too such contraptions would have overcome Brantôme's belief in the injurious nature of what he understood to be only dry dildoes.[110]

Whereas dildoes are in modern times regarded as primarily penetrative, earlier evidence shows that fluids were often central to the mechanism of erotic profusion. Some women were certainly executed in early modern Europe for using dildoes with other women, and modern scholars have understood this as punishment "for usurping the penetrative male role."[111] As far as I know,

[106] Erwin Baumgartner, *Glas des späten Mittelalters: Die Sammlung Karl Amendt* (Düsseldorf: Kunstmuseum, 1987), p. 104 no. 126. A delftware phallus drinking vessel, perforated at the glans, and having a cup above the testicles, probably of the late seventeenth or early eighteenth century, has been unearthed in London: Sadie Watson and Jacqueline Pearce et al., "Taverns and other entertainments in the City of London? 17th- and 18th-century finds from excavations at Paternoster Square," *Journal of Post-Medieval Archaeology* 44 (2010), 190–92, 203, including Geoff Egan, "Phallic vessel comparanda in other materials." I am grateful to Jacqui Pearce for an advance copy of this article.

[107] F. G. Emmison, *Elizabethan life: morals and the Church courts* (Chelmsford: Essex County Council, 1973), p. 21.

[108] Harold Love (ed.), *The works of John Wilmot, Earl of Rochester* (Oxford University Press, 1999), p. 304 (the play *Sodom* of the 1670s). Rochester's authorship is disputed. For an "Annis-water Robbin" see Henry Neville, *Newes from the new exchange, or the commonwealth of ladies* (London, 1650), p. 7. Warm milk filled glass dildoes in *L'Escole des filles*: Turner, *Schooling sex*, pp. 151–52.

[109] Henderson, *Maculate muse*, pp. 126, 178.

[110] Brantôme, *Dames galantes*, pp. 119–28.

[111] Ian Frederick Moulton, "The illicit worlds of the Renaissance," in Guido Ruggiero (ed.), *A companion to the worlds of the Renaissance* (Oxford: Blackwell, 2002), p. 498.

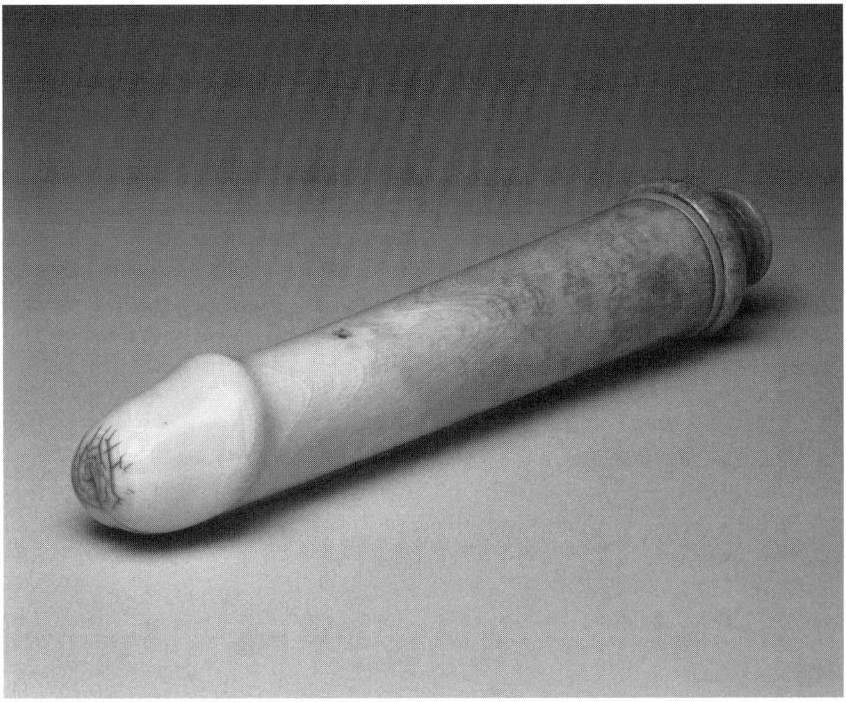

Figure 45 French (?), dildo with a contrivance for simulating ejaculation, eighteenth century, ivory, length, 205 mm, diameter 42 cm, London, Science Museum

however, the cases are not described in those terms, but as fraudulent (the penetrated woman was often represented as deceived, as was the case with Hetzeldorfer's partners) and "unnatural" like sodomy. Penetration is not invariably involved in male sodomy charges, and the use of dildoes between women can also be understood differently, as the mimicry of a delivery system in which semen was unnaturally used, in this case by being absent (or falsely imitated in "wet" dildoes). Beyond the legal realm, the fluids emitted by an instrument, like those of eunuchs, catered to the Hippocratic dousing model but were not literally bearers of male seed. They thus could be imagined to provide more pleasure than the dry models, while still not threatening the supremacy of non-castrated male bodies that alone produced actual semen. But the medical logic that had long tended to conflate semen (male and female), impregnation, pleasure and orgasm was beginning to come asunder. On the one hand, the medical priority for semen bestowed upon men everything that satisfied women so that a highly masculinist model of privilege still held. On the other hand, dildoes were designed, represented and used with such satiation in mind that the male body was less necessary. Fake fluids were meant to increase a woman's pleasure, and the simulacrum was often pictured in male-authored texts as an enticing rather than threatening device because men, but perhaps not all women, regarded them as essentially masculine yet merely imitations. During the Renaissance, female pleasure, as construed by the medical establishment, was slowly being severed from procreation. What I have termed "semenotics," or Turner "the spermatocentric model of pleasure," was what he calls a "new science of fluid mechanics" in that the Greek revival in medical discourse enabled a fuller understanding of Hippocratic and humoral theories.[112] Male semen had more than reproductive purposes, being the bearer of erotic, nourishing and, as we will see in the next chapter, curative properties.

[112] Turner, *Schooling sex*, pp. 141, 145.

7 Fertility and beyond

The way in which bodies were described by medical discourse was influenced by larger cultural habits of symbolic thinking but so too somatic metaphors had an impact on general patterns of thought and corporeal habits. Two striking types of medical metaphor are discussed here, in both their professional and lay contexts because the overlap was considerable. One presented male semen and semen-centric activity as delivering a "cure" to women, whose wombs were moistened and channels opened, their wombs purged, their health restored. The other metaphorical field relied on similar ideas but was more expansive, applying agricultural and gardening activities and words to sexual situations. In each case, pregnancy, even licit marital reproduction, was not always the expected outcome.

Many factors have to be taken into account, of course, such as context, function and local habits, the influence of convention and classical heritage, the adoption of an ironic or comedic voice or the ideological advancement of a group's self-interest. Whereas Valeria Finucci focuses on masculine anxieties regarding fatherhood by studying canonical Italian literature of the sixteenth century from a psychoanalytical point of view, for example, Elizabeth Foyster's consideration as a social historian of husbands, bachelors, adulterers and friends in seventeenth-century England finds that fatherhood was an important but not sole mode by which male honor was obtained and defended.[1] Since nearly half the patrician men in fifteenth- and sixteenth-century Venice did not marry, their culture and polity embraced pleasurable abundance that was not always reproductive.[2] This chapter, by taking a broad overview of European medical, literary and visual material urges caution against a current tendency to assume pronatalist or exclusively hetero-centric readings of much premodern evidence regarding sexual theory and practice.

Curative semen and sex

The semenotic factors of heat and moist semen were considered vital not only to the definition of masculinity but also to *women's* health. Brantôme had scant

[1] Foyster, *Manhood*; Finucci, *Manly masquerade*.
[2] Hacke, *Women, sex and marriage*, pp. 168–69, with further references.

medical knowledge, yet he understood that women's health was best served by male semen rather than the ministrations of fellow women, dry dildoes, pessaries or clysters. His belief that women had to be "well cleaned inside there by men's natural members" was credited to reports from surgeons.[3] His informants were referring to the Hippocratic belief that women's vessels needed regular clearing. Further, it was only "cool running water" and "throwing water in a vessel" that properly assuaged women's passion. His ultimate source was the Hippocratic text on seed, which spoke of male fluid extinguishing female fire, and also stated that if women

> have intercourse with men their health is better than if they do not. For in the first place, the womb is moistened by intercourse, whereas when the womb is drier than it should be it becomes extremely contracted, and this extreme contraction causes pain to the body. In the second place, intercourse by heating the blood and rendering it more fluid gives an easier passage to the menses; whereas if the menses do not flow, women's bodies become prone to sickness.[4]

Hippocratic theory was put succinctly in the oft-reprinted and translated *Secrets of women*: "sperm has the power of humidifying and heating."[5] Whether or not he read this book on women's "secrets" (a copy had been released in Lyon in 1580, a few years before he began writing), Brantôme knew that sexual intercourse with men was "better than the suppositories that doctors and surgeons use," along with medicinal waters to be used for internal cleansing and moistening.[6] Medical theory was easily deployed to support claims for the superiority and centrality of the semen-laden male body.

Notably, physical penetration was not the central issue in the Hippocratic model, and the two therapeutic elements of intercourse were moisture and heat, supplied by warm semen and friction. Women's uterine health was dependent on male bodies; in exceptional cases, like widows, other medicinal strategies sought the same result of releasing a woman's seed or excess blood (menses). The very definition of coitus from the male perspective was largely semenotic in medical literature, since it was more about releasing seed, cleansing, humidifying, purging and heating than entering, breaching or parting flesh. While we have little direct evidence about women's point of view, in cases such as Beatrice de Planissoles or Isabella De Moerloose, discussed in the previous chapter, desire was also cast in the basic terms of male and female "seed" or body fluids.

[3] Brantôme, *Dames galantes*, p. 125, trans. in Merrick and Ragan (eds.), *Homosexuality*, p. 106 (hereafter quoted from pp. 105, 107).

[4] "On generation," in *Hippocratic treatises*, p. 3. [5] Lemay, *Women's secrets*, p. 147.

[6] Brantôme, *Dames galantes*, p. 125; Merrick and Ragan (eds.), *Homosexuality*, p. 106.

Furthermore, to frame the coital "cure" as a treatment for sexual deprivation, as might be done today, is a common, Freudian misunderstanding.[7] Sexual action was considered a physiological rather than psychological process because it was curative in relation to a physical, complexional and semen-centric system of heat and fluids. The parallel between the modern understanding of sexual release from repression and the premodern notion of sexual "cure," rather, is about precedent, about humoral medicine informing the Freudian model: a plethora of obstructed matter (chiefly male semen or female menses and/or seed) was released by physical therapies in the case of premodern medicine, an excess of repressed urges was managed by psychoanalytic therapies in the modern case. Another important difference is that modern medicine has tended to narrow the coital focus to penile action alone. By means of a confidential aside from a Viennese physician, in 1886 the young Sigmund Freud was told that the only solution for a woman who was ill because she remained a virgin after eighteen years of marriage was "Penis normalis dosim repetatur!," that is, repeated doses of "normal" penis, but it was implied that the treatment was impossible because the husband was impotent.[8] Freud had "never heard of such a prescription," but the insight that sex was important to one's mental and physical health had a major impact on his subsequent theories. Premodern treatment for a host of female maladies including melancholy and "hysteria" was often sexual and physical too, but less exclusively centered on penile effects.

Health was best maintained by marital ministrations, as we will see, but medical advice had to encompass cases where a woman was suffering during a husband's absence, disinterest or inadequacy, or after she had become a widow. Various remedies tended to replicate particular aspects of coitus like friction or the uterine placement of medicinal substances; the partial mimicking of the male body was thus implicitly a case of flattery by imitation. Since desire was comprehended on the basis of the male model, the build-up of seed was regarded as fundamentally driving the desire of both women and men. But female bodies accumulated extra superfluities that needed to be released through menstruation, and the growing genre of gynecological literature in concert with the revivification of the Hippocratic and Galenic traditions devoted much attention to ensuring proper evacuation.

Hence, as a health measure, a degree of female desire and agency was often recognized. Some medical texts reiterated Galen's advice that widows purge seed by means of tactile genital treatment from midwives.[9] The misogynist

7 See the useful remarks by King, *Hippocrates' women*, pp. 220–21; Helen King, *The disease of virgins: green sickness, chlorosis and the problems of puberty* (London: Routledge, 2004), p. 79.

8 Sigmund Freud, "On the history of the psycho-analytic movement," in *Standard edition*, vol. XIV, pp. 14–15.

9 Galen, *Affected parts*, p. 185. See, for example, Nicolaas Fonteyn, *Syntagma medicum de morbis mulierum* (Amsterdam: Johann Jansson, 1644), translated as Nicholas Fontanus, *The womans doctour* (London: John Blague and Samuel Howes, 1652), p. 6.

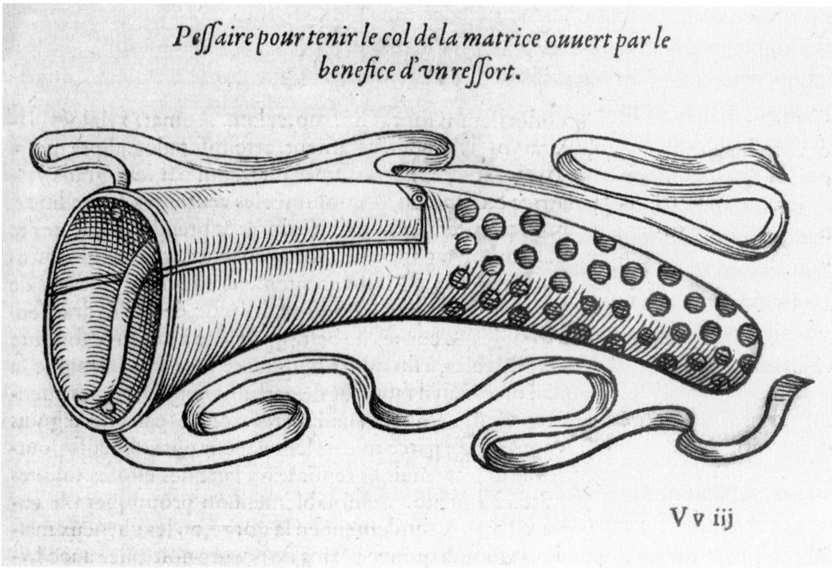

Figure 46 Ambroise Paré, vaginal applicator, in *Les oevvres de m. Ambroise Paré ... Auec les figures & portraicts tant de l'anatomie que des instruments de chirurgie, & de plusieurs monstres. Le tout diuisé en vingt six liures ...* (Paris: Chez G. Buon, 1575), p. 785

voice in Boccaccio's *Corbaccio* complained about women hiding dildoes, those "horrible instruments they employ to take away their superfluous humors."[10] The medieval gynecological manual the *Trotula* advised that certain medicines be delivered via a "pessary in the shape of the male member."[11] That very shape was adopted in 1573 by the French surgeon Paré, Brantôme's contemporary at the Valois court, when he first published his design for a vaginal applicator (fig. 46).[12] The penile instrument was, like the penis itself, the delivery system; the medicine inside the hollow implement, like male semen, was the material of the therapy.

Medicine and marriage

Of necessity, treatments by midwives, self-administration, dildoes, pessaries and syringes were without men and non-reproductive, and may have entailed

[10] Boccaccio, *Corbaccio*, p. 24. The use of such devices was called a "peccato sodomitico" in Arnaldi de Villanova, *Practica medicine* (Venice: Baptista de Tortis, 1494/95), n.p. (3.9).

[11] *"Trotula,"* p. 77.

[12] See Simons, "*Seigneur Dildoe*," and, for another example, Winfried Schleiner, *Medical ethics in the Renaissance* (Washington, DC: Georgetown University Press, 1995) p. 120.

pleasure. From the time of Hippocrates, however, most authors advised that the best option for treating female ailments was male attention, so the patient was to have intercourse with her husband, or marry in order to do so.[13] It was an easy prescription that also ensured a stable, reproducing polity and the idealized continuation of a domestic hierarchy with the wife theoretically dependent upon the husband for her very health. The physical effects are especially clear in Nicolaas Fonteyn's recommendation regarding the cure of numerous female maladies attributed to retention or stoppage of menses and seed. He concluded that "Wives are more healthfull then Widowes, or Virgins, because they are refreshed with the mans seed, and ejaculate their own, which being excluded, the cause of the evill is taken away. This is evident from the words of Hippocrates, who adviseth young Maids to marrie, when they are thus troubled."[14] The unequal two-seed model presumed that female pleasure derived from both the reception of male semen and the release of her own seed, and that basic process explained why coitus was considered gynecologically curative.

The Hippocratic *Diseases of young girls*, first printed in 1525, had indeed advised for virgins with blocked menses that "they should marry as quickly as possible. If they become pregnant, they become healthy ... Among those women who have regular intercourse with a man, the barren suffer these things."[15] No explanation was given regarding how pregnancy was efficacious.[16] The Hippocratic corpus itself was inconsistent, ascribing to women reproductive seed in *On generation / Nature of the child* but in *Diseases of women* emphasizing blood/inert menses, as did Aristotle. The short tract on premarried girls was concerned only with blood and when taken up in the sixteenth century that material remained the focus for a newly named "virgin's disease," an illness with a host of symptoms including malaise and a greenish tinge to the skin (hence "green sickness" as an alternative name) and which indicated three treatments, marriage, bloodletting and medication. The "virgin's disease" came into existence upon the publication of Johann Lange's account of it in 1554, in which he first advised a worried father to treat his daughter Anna

[13] Speaking primarily of young unmarried women and widows, the author and a commentator on *Secrets of women* allowed them to "use men" in order to expel "corrupt and poisonous menses": Lemay, *Women's secrets*, p. 132. The author may be recalling a remedy proposed for men suffering from lovesickness, which often allowed them to expel their pent up humors/semen through sex with women other than their unattainable object of obsessive desire.

[14] Fontanus, *Womans doctour*, p. 4.

[15] Rebecca Flemming and Ann Ellis Hanson, "Hippocrates' *Peri Parthenión* ('Diseases of young girls'): text and translation," *Early Science and Medicine* 3 (1998), 252.

[16] King, *Disease of virgins*, pp. 11, 51, 52, 53, 58, 70, 79, and see 79–83 for "'Marriage is a sovereign cure.'" King suggests a specifically Protestant interest in the marital cure for green sickness (pp. 4, 140), whereas I focus on a tradition that began before the Reformation and extended into popular culture.

by bloodletting and followed with a close paraphrase of the Hippocratic passage on prompt marriage.[17]

However, the current scholarly tendency to focus on early modern medicine's emphasis on marriage and generation needs to be balanced by a consideration of other evidence. In one strand of medical thinking influenced by certain aspects of the Hippocratic corpus, marriage was curative. On the other hand, the cure for a range of womanly symptoms that was traced back to the retention of either menses or seed did not necessarily involve pregnancy. Despite citing the Hippocratic work on virgins, for instance, a popular gynecological manual issued during the sixteenth and seventeenth centuries concentrated on treatments by bloodletting and recipes.[18] Seed and blood were not always carefully distinguished, in part because for many authors female seed was equivalent to the blood of menses. Those rare comments that suggested why the Hippocratic therapy of marriage worked to instigate menstruation pointed to the opening up of the vessels, which the *Diseases of women* attributed to the process of childbirth.[19] However, pregnancy was often not mentioned in early modern texts, whereas sexual activity was, and the "opening" also fits the logic of both *Diseases of women* (1.2) and another Hippocratic text, *On generation* (3), in which the moisture of male semen counteracted painful uterine contraction. In addition, impregnation was not a definitive remedy for all those patients who were already mothers, widows or menopausal.

The general advice to marry was common, and sometimes the legality of the subsequent coitus was also stressed.[20] At other times the emphasis was on lusty sex, described by Paré as "often and wanton copulation with her husband," for

17 King, *Disease of virgins*, p. 48. On green sickness, see also King, *Hippocrates' women*, pp. 188–204; Gail Kern Paster, *Humoring the body: emotions on the Shakespearean stage* (University of Chicago Press, 2004), pp. 89–99 (which concentrates on the early modern text and refers to "Lange's sex-positive thinking").

18 Marinelli, *Thresor*, p. 8. First published in Venice in 1563 in Italian, the book was translated into French by 1582, and was expanded in subsequent editions by Jean Liébault, with a title claiming it was from the Latin of an unnamed text. The passage remains the same in *Trois livres*, p. 8.

19 Hanson (trans), "Hippocrates: *Diseases of women* 1," 570, 572. It was self-evident to Nicholas Sudell, *Mulierum amicus: or, The woman's friend* (London: J. Hancock, 1666), 10: the cure was "Carnal Copulation, . . . the vessels of the womb becoming thereby much enlarged, &c." See also King, *Disease of virgins*, pp. 79, 126.

20 For example Lemay, *Women's secrets*, pp. 131–33; Ferrand, *Maladie d'amour*, p. 207; Ferrand, *Erotomania*, p. 276; Lemnius, *Secret miracles*, p. 18; Marinello, *Medicine*, fols. 123v, 176r, 177r (noting the afflictions of nuns and widows), fols. 175v–76r, 180r; Bunworth, *Doctresse*, p. 34; Sharp, *Midwives book*, pp. 200, 235, 240; Robert Burton, *The anatomy of melancholy*, ed. Floyd Dell and Paul Jordan-Smith (New York: Farrar & Rinehart, 1927), p. 355 (the sixth, posthumously published edition of 1651). See also Ilza Veith, *Hysteria: the history of a disease* (University of Chicago Press, 1965), pp. 11, 13, 116–18, 126, 267; Jacquart and Thomasset, *Sexuality and medicine*, p. 176; Laurinda S. Dixon, *Perilous chastity: women and illness in pre-Enlightenment art and medicine* (Ithaca: Cornell University Press, 1995), pp. 44, 49, 112, 159–67, and 151–53 for Abraham Bosse's etching about clysters.

thus she would be instantly revived.[21] Daniel Sennert's *Practical physick* of 1664 blamed "the Virgins Disease" (chlorosis) on "stoppage of terms" (menses) and the subsequent gathering of bad humors, and cited Hippocrates when advising marriage.[22] This professor at Wittenberg knew that "Venery is good" because it "heats the womb and the parts adjacent, opens and loosens the passages, so that the Terms may better flow to the Womb," effects that arise from the conceptualization of sexual activity in terms of heated semen, friction and motion. Notably, this common thinking did not require pregnancy and thus sexual pleasure was being separated from procreation. Echoing Fonteyn's belief that "*Venerey* is exceeding wholesome" for widows, Sennert is sex-positive, but again for medicinal and physical rather than psychological reasons.

Vernacular medical advice books repeated the simple formula. "If the Patient be a Maid, a Husband is the best Medicine" for suffocation of the womb, said Alessandro Massaria, professor at the University of Padua, in *De morbis mulierum* published posthumously in 1600.[23] Two years after being published in an English translation, the wording was repeated in medical advice at the back of Sarah Jinner's cheap almanac and prognostications for 1659.[24] What she did not pass on, however, was a passage kept in Latin by Massaria's translator. One treatment for "suffocation of the womb" was the Galenic vaginal massage by another woman's finger dipped first in scented oil. But Massaria added that, if the patient were married, her husband could instead anoint his penis with warmed oils and then copulate with his wife, whose womb would immediately descend from its improper position.[25] This prescription was informed by the sense of the uterus being voracious for male sperm, which would depart from the upper part of the body where it had caused breathing difficulties and other symptoms and return to its rightful place, ever eager to receive semen, as Leonardo's drawing had indicated (fig. 29).

The knowledge of a marital cure was also disseminated by way of genres such as jokes, riddles, carnival songs, short stories, chapbooks and court gossip. Before Galen, one of Martial's satirical epigrams had a woman use "hysteria" as the reason why she thought "being fucked is a necessity" (11.71). The aging husband, however, was not up to the task and "straight away the men doctors approach and the women doctors retire," meaning that female friends and

21 Paré, *Œuvres complètes*, vol. II, pp. 759, 767; Paré, *Collected works*, pp. 945, 948. Also, for example, Lemay, "Guainerius," p. 323; Lemnius, *Secret miracles of nature*, p. 18.

22 Daniel Sennert, *Practical physick* (London: Peter Cole, 1664), pp. 100, 105–06.

23 Alessandro Massaria (d. 1598), *Praelectiones de morbis mulierum* ... (Leipzig: Abraham Lamberg, 1600), republished in *Practica medica* (Frankfurt: Nicolai Bassaei, 1601), translated by Turner as *De morbis foemineis*, reissued in 1686. Here quoted from the first English translation, p. 78.

24 Sarah Jinner, *An almanack and prognostication for the year of our Lord 1659* (London: J.S. for the Company of Stationers, 1659), n.p.: "a husband is the best medicine."

25 Massaria, *Woman's counsellour*, p. 75.

perhaps midwives were inadequate whereas any male "doctor" could and would readily apply the "drastic therapy" of sexual intercourse. One of Poggio Bracciolini's mid-fifteenth-century popular tales proposed a virtual maxim, that "a husband will be a wife's best doctor (*curator*)," the sort of phrasing echoed around 200 years later by the physician Massaria.[26] The notion still gave rise to notable jokes in the seventeenth century, when two of the amusing sayings recorded by Sir Nicholas Le Strange ran: "She that hath the greene sicknesse if she will be well Recovered, she must be well Covered [laid upon sexually], for cold is a nourisher of the disease," and "A widow is the consumption of love, for nothing will helpe her but a new husband."[27]

There were no qualms about extending that physic beyond the marital chamber. A monk cured a nun's burning malady with "sweet and tasty" draughts of *medicina* administered regularly from his "drinking glass" (*bicchiere*) in an Italian *novella* written by Gentile Sermini around 1425.[28] He may well have had in mind those glass vessels formed in the shape of the male genitals, referred to later by Filelfo and Aretino. "Doctors" offered their marvelously curative salve to widows in order to purge their uterine problems, applied in a suggestively insertive manner according to a sixteenth-century carnival song.[29] Other Italian satire and burlesque suggested that even the impotence of older men could be cured by sodomitical semen.[30]

A quip in an anonymous sixteenth-century comedy written in Venetian dialect might be misunderstood unless the erotic implication of doctoring is grasped. Yearning for the attentions of a foreign dandy, the young widow Angela insists that she needs medical attention for her fever. She believes that only one such physician exists, this very man Giulio, but her cynical servant Nena comments wryly that "anyone who is not amongst the castrated would do," that is, the "doctor" must have testicles. The sly allusion is to more than incompetent quackery or to a profession exclusively gendered as masculine, for testicles are represented as quintessentially medicinal containers.[31] Later in the

[26] Bracciolini, *Facezie*, pp. 144–46, also pp. 236–38 for two more tales. See also Boggione and Casalegno, *Dizionario*, p. 26 for *medicina* and *medicinare*.

[27] Nicholas Le Strange, *Merry passages and jeasts: a manuscript jestbook of Sir Nicholas Le Strange (1603–1655)*, ed. H. F. Lippincott (Salzburg: Institut für Englische Sprache und Literatur, Universität Salzburg, 1974), p. 163.

[28] Gentile Sermini, *Novelle*, ed. Giuseppe Vettori (Rome: Avanzini e Torraca Editori, 1968), vol. I, pp. 107–19. The treatment is often referred to with the verb *guarire* ("to cure").

[29] Bruscagli, *Trionfi*, pp. 282–84. [30] Toscan, *Carnaval*, pp. 240–44.

[31] Anonymous, *La venexiana*, ed. Ludovico Zorzi (Turin: Einaudi, 1982), p. 18; my translation is adjusted from Laura Giannetti and Guido Ruggiero (eds. and trans.), *Five comedies from the Italian Renaissance* (Baltimore: Johns Hopkins University Press, 2003), p. 290.

play the scenario is overt, for a recently married woman also urgently requires Giulio's attendance because he is "the only one who can cure her."[32]

Semenotic elements appear in such metaphors as "sap," "pills," "physic" and heat. An anonymous English poem with the title "A medicine for the greene sicknes" suggested the curative application of the "Vir tree," a pun on the Latin *vir* for man but also recalling *verga* for penis.[33] A medicinal recipe was supplied: tree bark was "mixt white and red like milke & bloud," colored as though the sap was both milky semen and womanly blood/menses; the restorative "pretious oyle" consisted of "tickling droppes" issuing from the tree's "cave well warmed by [the woman's] heat." The curative idea also lay behind the synecdoche of "pill" for testicle, filled with healing goodness, and Pepys was using common parlance when he suggested one cold morning in December 1661 that he and his wife might "take Phisique."[34] The same language appeared in some of the chapbooks he later collected.[35] The overlay of sexual activity with women's medical cures was spread through streets, homes, taverns, ships and wherever else men and women set themselves to singing, rhyming and riddling.

The act of cleansing was cast as essentially masculine, due to the medical truism, reiterated by Brantôme, that women benefited from an opening of their passages and a purging of their excessive matter, performed primarily through male-supplied friction and heated, fluid semen. Performers playing the role of Tuscan *muratori* boasted in a carnival song that masons and plasterers "clean out" an old house; anonymous choristers gleefully used suggestively sweeping brushes to do the same in another song.[36] Latrine-cleaners in a song that was attributed to Lorenzo de' Medici (d. 1492) when it was published in 1559 cleansed women's "wells," emptied chamber pots that had "cracks" in them and repetitively applied their "plunger."[37] According to court testimony, on Christmas Eve 1609 an adulterous wife in London enjoyed the saucy talk of her

32 Anonymous, *Venexiana*, p. 88; Giannetti and Ruggiero (eds. and trans.), *Five comedies*, p. 317.

33 Moulton, *Before pornography*, p. 47. See also "On his mistrisse having the green-sicknesse," in John Mennes and James Smith, *Musarum deliciae* (London: Henry Herringman, 1655), p. 80; Pepys, *Pepys' penny merriments*, p. 66; the ballad "The maids complaint / for want of a dil doul. / This girl long time had in sickness been, / which many maids do call the sickness green," Pepys, *Diary*, vol. IV, p. 50; Crawford, "Sexual knowledge in England," p. 95.

34 Partridge, *Shakespeare's bawdy*, p. 160; Williams, *Dictionary*, pp. 1029–30; see also pp. 355–56 (cure), 621–24 (green sickness), 713–14 (injection), 1018–19 (physic, including Pepys), 1019–20 (physician), 1464 (uterine fury); Williams, *Glossary*, pp. 146 (green sickness), 210 (mother).

35 Pepys, *Pepys' penny merriments*, pp. 70, 107, 237.

36 Bruscagli, *Trionfi*, pp. 227–29, 421–23. See Toscan, *Carnaval*, pp. 1052–54 for "conciare" and "acconciare"; Boggione and Casalegno, *Dizionario*, pp. 140–43 for cleaning, including sweeping.

37 Anton Francesco Grazzini, *Tutti i trionfi, carri, mascherate o canti carnascialeschi andati per Firenze dal tempo del Magnifico Lorenzo de' Medici fino all'anno 1559* (Lucca: Pel Benedini, 1750), vol. I, pp. 21–22.

lover, who said to her "I hope I have skoured yow now, I hope so quoth she . . . and laughed at it."[38]

It was often the case that an apparent, virtuous meaning assigned to an object or action could be reversed. Cleaning thus bore a sexually illicit subtext; in ancient Greek to sweep out or debug alluded to deflowering a male or female virgin.[39] In several European vernaculars, to sweep also meant to screw, chiefly due to the repetitive back and forth motion, but the slang was also informed by the medicinally beneficial result of clearing away excess, stale matter.[40] To brush or use the curry comb had sexual connotations in German, picked up in Hans Baldung Grien's depiction of the witches' Sabbath where the small broom in the foreground is incongruous amidst the decay and seems, like sexualized details such as phallic sausages and the women's nakedness, to accentuate libidinal excess (fig. 59). The emblematic small whisk broom on the sleeve of an over-decorated woman in one of Urs Graf's ink drawings dated 1518 satirically notifies the viewer that she is adept at sensual stroking.[41]

Ludovico Sforza's many emblems included just such a brush or *scopetta*, drawn in an allegory of Milanese justice by Leonardo in the late fifteenth century. This device is "a small besom brush for clothing etc., with which Ludovico saw himself dusting off all Italy according to one of his *imprese*."[42] Given the alternative meaning of the object, however, the brush off Ludovico envisaged was as much sexual as moral. With this ostensibly moralizing emblem, on another level the Milanese lord was threatening to screw any dirty scoundrel who tried to mess with him. The aggression of his statecraft was furthered by the implication that thus he would symbolically sodomize his opponents.

The metaphor of cleansing was plausible in moments of intimacy as well as public songs and quips, and extended from medical to satirical discourse. Alessandro Benedetti's anatomical text of 1502 compared the rough sides of the womb to walls prepared for the adhesion of cement by scraping.[43] Building metaphors were particularly apposite when applied to the architect Sir Christopher Wren. According to English satire against the courtier circulating in the late

38 Gowing, *Domestic dangers*, p. 247. 39 Henderson, *Maculate muse*, pp. 174–75.

40 Flemish and Italian usage of "to sweep" in the sexual sense is noted in Charles Harbison, "Sexuality and social standing in Jan van Eyck's Arnolfini double portrait", *Renaissance Quarterly* 43 (1990), 285 n. 100; see also Toscan, *Carnaval*, p. 1746 and passim (scopa); Aretino, *Ragionamento*, p. 46 ("scardassare il pelo").

41 Christian Müller, *Urs Graf: Die Zeichnungen im Kupferstichkabinett Basel* (Basel: Schwabe & Co., 2001), p. 180, Pl. 19 (signed and dated 1518); for another example, held by a naked woman, see p. 118; and pp. 149–50 for a naked woman holding a curry comb, about to "fleece" an old, importunate fool. In 1517 he signed a more personal drawing, portraying a woman, with a signature that incorporated a comb and a curry comb: pp. 173–74.

42 Martin Kemp, *Leonardo da Vinci: the marvellous works of nature and man* (London: J. M. Dent & Sons, 1981), p. 165.

43 Benedetti, *Anatomice*, p. 176.

1680s he found that his marriage "wanted repairs" and that he would restore a lady at court because he "has orders to new white her," that is, apply another layer of seminal whitewash.[44] Purgative and white, the various plasters or paints splashed around through the centuries in semen-centric rhetoric were endowed with special properties of renewal.

For a writer like Aretino, whose erotic focus was primarily penetrative, the medical metaphor of a cure was also efficacious. In one of his sonnets for *I modi*, a prostitute urges the man on: "touch me to the marrow of my bones with your oh-so-venerable cock, which cures cunts of their jitters."[45] The "cure" was purely sexual, and somewhat comic, for it was literally eradicating *tosse*, defined by Florio as "a cough, a coughing," a spasmodic urge that was not particular to women or their health. Laughter, another expulsive act of *pneuma* like coughing and ejaculation, was similarly likened to orgasm. Given the relationship between humor and obscenity or what Cicero characterized as ugliness, it is not surprising that some sixteenth-century pharmacy jars bear overtly sexual images. The curative nature of the drug stored within was probably signaled by the external image, such as a woman lifting up her dress to exhibit her genitals to an awaiting, winged phallus with enlarged testicular haunches in the case of a central Italian albarello of the early sixteenth century.[46] The jar probably housed pessaries to "cleanse" female clients, or drugs to be inserted into the sort of phallic device illustrated by Paré (fig. 46).

In some tales, a visiting healer enables a wife to commit adultery under the husband's nose, a man who is ironically a physician in a fifteenth-century story by Masuccio Salernitano.[47] The wife appropriates his professional language, referring to the Hippocratic metaphor when her pleasure is likened to "a flood of water extinguishing a little fire" and remembering a dictum of Avicenna's when thinking that she had been "totally freed from the incurable pangs of the Mother [hysteria] by the opportune remedy."

Medical knowledge and cultural humor colluded in the representation of youthful, urbane masculinity managing its expenditure of valuable, curative

44 *Poems on affairs of state: Augustan satirical verse, 1660–1714*, vol. V: *1688–1697*, ed. William Cameron (New Haven: Yale University Press, 1971), p. 134.

45 Talvacchia, *Taking positions*, p. 205 (translation adjusted). For *tosse*, see Florio, *Queen Anna's new world of words*, 570; Toscan, *Carnaval*, pp. 801, 1760 and passim. For "laugh," see Ch. 2 above.

46 For an illustration see Catherine Hess, "Pleasure, shame and healing: erotic imagery on maiolica drug jars," in Allison Levy (ed.), *Sex acts: practice, performance, perversion and punishment in early modern Europe* (Aldershot: Ashgate, 2010), pp. 20–21, fig. 13 (in the Museum für Kunst und Gewerbe, Hamburg).

47 Masuccio Salernitano, *Il novellino*, ed. Salvatore Nigro (Milan: Biblioteca Universale Rizzoli, 1990), pp. 140–41, 143, 147; *De la Saineresse*, in *Cuckolds, clerics, and countrymen: medieval French fabliaux*, trans. John Du Val, ed. Raymond Eichmann (Fayetteville: University of Arkansas Press, 1982), pp. 106–09.

semen, in contrast with the figural type of the incompetent, cuckolded duffer. It was a medical truism that complexional vigor waned with age, and that "the semen of man in his youth is strong; in old age, ill-health, and lechery it becomes impure."[48] If there was amongst men an ever-present fear about satisfying insatiable female demand, there was nevertheless a counterbalancing assurance that women's need was properly directed at just what only men could offer. The ever-young, sexually active, semen-bountiful, assertive man faced the challenge of female desire, finding it enticing as well as threatening. "Anxiety" and inadequacy were displaced onto other men. Courageously, driven by a naturally heated state, potent men might risk dessication but they were eradicating female hunger with a thorough dousing. It was in their power to deliver doses of male semen, the paradigmatic, regenerative source of female pleasure and health.

Sex in the field

In European medical literature the most common of all metaphors about reproduction represented the womb as a field. The male genitals were thus likened to a farmer, the yeoman, the sower of seed (*semen* in Latin), the ploughman, the tiller, the irrigator, all active, essential occupations by which the receptive land prospered under male oversight. Semen-centric features played an important role within this metaphorical cluster. Unaware of or underestimating the conventional force of agricultural metaphors, some scholars have found historically or geographically specific or exclusive significance, more than is warranted, in early modern reiterations of the trope. Only after this broad cultural pattern is understood might more focused studies reveal local or regional particularities. Whether in England or France, Germany or Italy, the cultural heritage from antiquity informed early modern rhetoric. Greek allusions to the female body as land or a furrow to be seeded, ploughed and irrigated went beyond the medical sphere. Plato, for instance, thought the etymology of Artemis' name indicated that the goddess of chastity "hates the plough."[49]

Literary and medical analogies were repeated, perhaps instigated, at the level of obscenity and humor, where hard labor and violent action were more evident. Thus, in Greek phraseology coitus was from the male point of view about breaking up the ground, stirring and hoeing the earth, digging into it, and stripping it of fruits, a set of assertive images that was not only about reproductive sex but sometimes applied to sex with a younger, less powerful male

[48] Benedetti, *Anatomice*, p. 160; Lind, *Studies*, p. 97.

[49] John Winkler, *The constraints of desire: the anthropology of sex and gender in ancient Greece* (New York: Routledge, 1990), pp. 125, 231 n. 21. See also Page duBois, *Sowing the body: psychoanalysis and ancient representations of women* (University of Chicago Press, 1988).

partner.[50] The sexualized ploughshare, field, garden or meadow featured in ancient and medieval Latin too.[51] Late medieval badges featuring ploughs may have unrecognized sexual connotations.[52] "Plough, for God's sake," the figure of Genius exhorted the barons around 1275 in the *Roman de la rose*, "plough and restore your lineages."[53] The genital connection was clear in Florio's dictionary, for *vomere* or *vomero* meant "the plough that pierceth the ground, as *Vomitare*. Also taken for a mans privities"; the referred verb *vomitare* (and also *vomire*) signified "to vomit, to cast, to spue, to perbreake, to cast up."[54] The piercing and churning of the ground with a ploughshare was linked with the subsequent ejaculatory casting forth of seed.

Clearly, the plough is a penetrative, violent tool, cutting through the virginal field in Ovid's *Metamorphoses* (7.119). But it is striking that ploughing was chiefly a preparatory act, ejaculation and insemination the end result. That was the focus when Lucretius admonished women not to move during sexual intercourse, because otherwise "she turns the [plough]share clean away from the furrow and makes the seed fail of its place" (4.1273–74). The female furrow is more uterine than genital, and the plough is aimed at planting seed in that inner ground. The purpose of the disturbing plough is clearest in a passage from Plutarch's musings about offspring. Following the Hippocratic model, menstruation was regarded as a process that cleansed the womb, readying it for impregnation: "it is Nature's custom and care to discharge the blood at monthly periods by opening canals and channels for it, to lighten and cleanse the rest of the body and in season to render the womb fertile ground for ploughing, as it were, and sowing."[55] As we have seen, Hippocratic theory posited that coitus opened up obstructed "channels"; in that sense, breaking up the ground and forming furrows with a plough were male functions aimed at readying the womb, into which seed was cast.

Building on such impeccable ancestry, the rustic metaphor was reiterated in the important text from southern Italy in the first half of the twelfth century that recorded the dissection of a pig. The uterus "is also nature's field (*ager naturae*), which is cultivated that it may bear fruit; in which, when seed is sown, it remains

[50] Henderson, *Maculate muse*, pp. 46, 65, 166–68, nos. 283–87, 292, 294; Adams, *Latin sexual vocabulary*, pp. 83, 84, 113.

[51] Lucretius, *De rerum natura*, 4.1107, 1273–74; Virgil, *Georgics*, 3.135–36; Adams, *Latin sexual vocabulary*, pp. 24–25, 82–85, 154–55; Jacques André, *Le vocabulaire Latin de l'anatomie* (Paris: Les Belles Lettres, 1991), pp. 184, 186.

[52] Examples include van Beuningen and Koldeweij (eds.), *Heilig en Profaan*, p. 241; Koldeweij, *Geloof & Geluk*, p. 121.

[53] De Lorris and de Meun, *Roman de la rose*, vol. III, p. 91 (lines 19671–72); de Lorris and de Meun, *Romance of the rose*, p. 324.

[54] Florio, *Worlde of wordes (1598)*, p. 496; Boggione and Casalegno, *Dizionario*, p. 233, and pp. 119–28, 228–33 for metaphors of agricultural implements and labor, including irrigation.

[55] Plutarch, *Moralia*, 495d–e (*De amore prolis*, 3).

as on good ground and through the cooperative action of natural warmth, and the mediation of vital spirits, it becomes implanted like a germinating seed."[56] Around 1363, the cleric and papal surgeon Guy de Chauliac focused on seed when comparing the two sexes. Seed was the basis of his model, here quoted from the Middle English translation of his Latin:

> Sperma forsothe is the seed or burgenynge of mankynde. In men it is throwen oute (*extra*), in wommen it leveth withynne (*intra*) . . . The matrice forsothe is the felde of mannes generacioun (*ager generacionis humane*) and by consequent it is a receyuynge member . . . It is large forsothe as the yerde turned ayen or putte withynne, in 7° De Utilitate Particularum [sic: Book 6 of Galen's *On the usefulness of the parts*] . . . The yerde forsothe is the tilier of mankynde (*agricultor nature humane*).[57]

Aristotelian initiative, caloric extrusion, anatomical inversion and semenotic projection all worked in conjunction with agricultural metaphor.

But in neither rural labor nor cultural practice was the plough the sole implement used in the field. Adam was destined to toil in the ground raising crops, Eve to bear children in pain (Genesis 3.16–18), duties often supplemented pictorially in Adam's case by the wielding of a hoe or shovel and in Eve's example by the domestic work of spinning. Jacopo della Quercia's representation of the first parents' labor, part of the cycle of Adam and Eve carved in marble reliefs around 1425–38 for the portal of S. Petronio in Bologna, especially brings out the symbolism of uterine spindle and sexual spade (fig. 47). In line with his left thigh and genitals, Adam grips the shaft and thrusts his pointed tool towards the cultivated, furrowed ground that has already yielded two sons.[58] Adam's sturdy body, determined activity and flying cloak accentuate his ordained labor and his quintessentially masculine force acting on the exterior world. Eve, in contrast, stands passively, rooted to the spot by the infants clinging to her legs, one of whom reaches up to emphasize her receptive body. Her uterine, maternal nature is further signaled not only by her round spindle but also the cloth bunched before her womb, possibly holding the seed that will be cast on the fertile, tilled ground.

The same notions were conveyed in the popular cultural tradition, by such means as song, or love magic. In June 1500, an itinerant minstrel pleased the

[56] Corner, *Anatomical texts*, p. 53. Also from twelfth-century Salerno, the *Trotula* text about women's bodies spoke of seed and fields (p. 71).

[57] Guy de Chauliac, *The Cyrurgie of Guy de Chauliac*, ed. Margaret S. Ogden (Oxford University Press, 1971), pp. 67, 69; Guy de Chauliac, *Inventarium*, vol. I, pp. 52, 54.

[58] Luciano Bellosi et al., *La basilica di San Petronio in Bologna* (Milan: Silvana Editoriale, 1983), vol. I, pp. 188–89. Adam's hoe and Eve's spindle are also prominent in a pair of drawings by Antonio Pollaiuolo dated to the late 1470s or early 1480s: Alison Wright, *The Pollaiuolo brothers* (New Haven: Yale University Press, 2005), pp. 184–88. The hoe is tellingly between Adam's legs in Robetta's engraving of the postlapsarian family: Paolo Bellini (ed.), *Catalogo completo dell'opera grafica del Robetta* (Milan: Salamon e Agustoni editori, 1973), pp. 30–31.

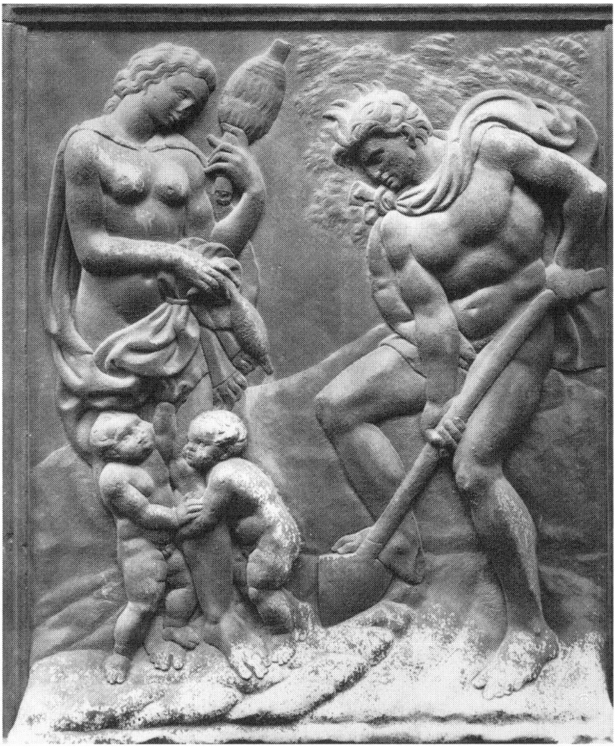

Figure 47 Jacopo della Quercia, *Adam and Eve at their labors*, *c*. 1425–38, marble, Bologna, S. Petronio

Venetian chronicler Marin Sanudo, who recorded the youth's opening lines: "Take her now, country boy, / The girl in the petticoat, / You will make her work hard / With a hoe and rake."[59] The song's lad works her over like a field, tilling with rake and hoe, aerating soil or, in Hippocratic terms, opening up channels. It was telling that the ploughshare, the hoe and the shovel were tools close to hand and appropriated by the village healer and love magician Apollonia Madizza to cure impotent men. In 1591 this practitioner from the Friuli region told the Venetian inquisition that she had some of these items placed under the bed of the afflicted, a typical case of sympathetic magic.[60] A set of Italian ditties, reported by Brantôme in the 1580s, which staged a confrontation between husband,

59 Sanuto, *Diarii*, vol. III, col. 392; trans. in Sanudo, *Venice città excelentissima*, p. 343 (which gives "jumper" for *guarnel*). Since one word for hoe (*marrone*) elided with *marone* (chestnut), testicular references were possible in word play: Prizer, "*Facciamo*," p. 197.

60 Ruggiero, *Binding passions*, pp. 168–69.

adulterous wife and her lover, had her complain, and the men respond, about the cultivation and "pruning" of her vineyard.[61] Whether by way of ongoing oral culture or cultural reinvention, classical metaphors lived on as efficacious symbolic objects and metaphors in amorous quips and rituals.

While a plough initially turned over the soil and prepared it for sowing or planting, farmers used a harrow to break up larger clods, a function taken over on occasion by the dragging of a heavy log. That activity pictured in an engraving attributed to Israhel van Meckenem, however, is not an everyday view (fig. 48). According to Malcolm Jones, the late fifteenth-century print visualizes the proverbial notion that a man deceived or rejected by his wife or mistress has wasted his labor, a mocking idea stressed by the scroll inscribed "al verlaren aerbeit" (all wasted effort, or trouble in vain).[62] Knowledge of agricultural metaphors, combined with the man's appearance, enables the drawing forth of further nuances. Any strained exertion would illustrate Jones' sense, but the selection of toiling with the earth adds an explicitly sexual element to the ridicule. A thirteenth-century poem sometimes attributed to Dante urges the avoidance of Eros: "otherwise, you are ploughing a bad field / in which good grain will not grow; / indeed, whoever sows there / will lose his seed."[63] In the print, the man's loss of seed/semen has dried him out and all his masculine labor has been in vain. As Galen had observed, after sexual intercourse the body of a strong youth "is changed to thinness," a condition exacerbated in the case of the depicted character because the exercise has been excessive.[64]

The efforts of Meckenem's figure are expended on uneven but sprouting ground, as though he has misdirected his efforts on a fertile yet untamed "field." His cheeks are sunken, his frame lean, the legs thin, his back bent, all signs that little strength remains and that his masculine resources are spent. A dandy endowed with a tasseled cap, fancy sleeves, hose, soft courtly shoes and a large, elaborate sword, the man is no ordinary peasant but a wastrel who has cast his seed inappropriately and too often. The valuable resource of semen is depleted; the sheathed sword hangs limp; no purse is in sight. Dried out, sodomite or womanizer or both, his erotic effort at clearing the ground results only in corporeal as well as monetary and social loss, for he exists alone and emasculated in a deserted spot.

61 Brantôme, *Dames galantes*, 179–80.

62 Malcolm Jones, "'Fiddlers on the roof and friars with foxtails': observations on/occasioned by David Teniers' *Netherlandish proverbs*," in Wolfgang Mieder (ed.), *The Netherlandish proverbs: an international symposium on the Pieter Brueg(h)els* (Burlington: University of Vermont, 2004), pp. 164–94, esp. p. 170. A unique copy of the print was last recorded in 1926: Koreny, *Israhel van Meckenem*, vol. XXIV, p. 183 no. 476, vol. XXIV A, Pl. 476.

63 *"The fiore" and the "Detto d'amore,"* pp. 514–17.

64 Galen, *Hygiene (De sanitate tuenda)*, trans. Robert Montraville Green (Springfield, IL: Charles Thomas, 1951), p. 134.

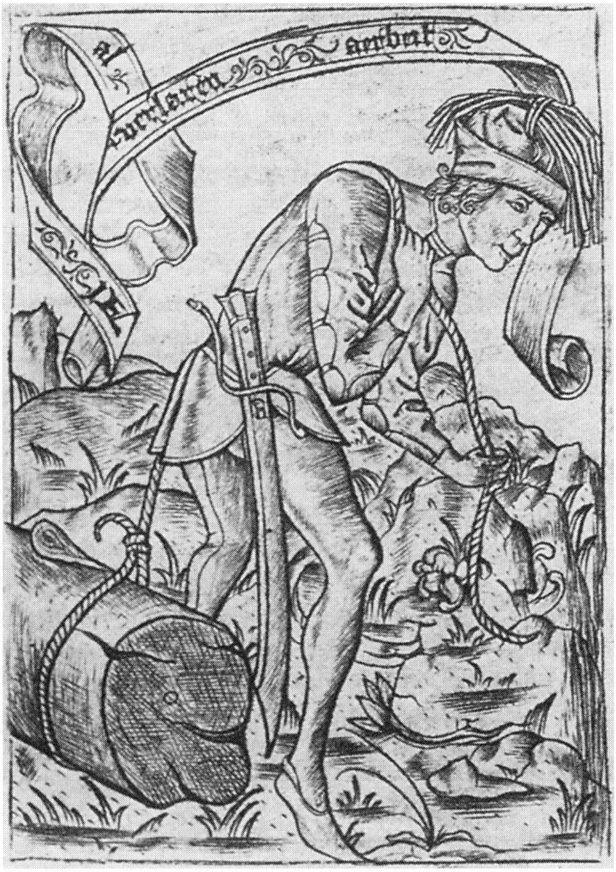

Figure 48 Israhel van Meckenem, *"All wasted effort,"* *c.* 1500, engraving, 102 × 70 mm

The log-dragger has fallen into a lowly rustic state, without the tools fashioned and forged by the latest technology that more often appear in sexual metaphors. Implements such as a large knife and a shovel with a notably firm shaft that never strayed from its purpose enabled a man to tend a woman's "garden," according to Ruzante's carnival monologue, the *Lettera giocosa*. The short piece was probably performed on February 4, 1524, when the Venetian *compagnia* of the *Ortolani* (Gardeners) paraded in a masked pageant around Piazza San Marco accompanied by musicians and brandishing various farming equipment such as hoes, shovels, blades, plough shares and rakes, all items with sexual connotations.[65] The carousers included finely dressed noble youths, while the costume of others (including some of the aristocrats?) represented the wearers as mere peasants. Sometimes the agricultural metaphor was amusingly reversed: phalli are the crop to be sprinkled with water by a maiden on an ancient Greek vase or tended as plants by gardeners, some holding shovels, on late medieval badges.[66]

Country folk and landowners alike found inspiration in their surroundings for the construction of erotic language. According to Piovano Arlotto, a fifteenth-century Florentine priest and raconteur, an abashed young Tuscan peasant confessed to him that at the age of fifteen he had committed an unpardonable sin: "I took my beater for a stroll and I gave him fodder in such a way that I took great pleasure from it many, many times."[67] The *battisteo* was a thresher, hand fed a special kind of masturbatory nutriment, and the man's represented choice of language had nothing to do with the fertility of his crops or his potential fatherhood. On some badges and in certain phrases, a bird pecks avidly at the seed-issuing head of a phallus or at a woman's "granary," a suggestively repetitive (and, in the former case, homoerotic) action about satiating hunger, which nevertheless destroys the kernel's reproductive capacity.[68]

Husbands had to reap the harvest. A dissatisfied, adulterous wife in Boccaccio's *Decameron* accused her spouse of neglecting his duty, which had been "to tend my little field" and bring in a harvest.[69] Hence, when a woman's pregnancy incited the comment that "a good ploughman's found a good field," as Erasmus put it in 1523, it was a well-understood sexual euphemism, one that appeared in law courts and cheap pamphlets as much as learned Latin or vernacular literature.[70] Boncompagno (d. 1240), a teacher of rhetoric at the University of Bologna, wittily applied the medical metaphor in a Latin letter supposedly written by a wife complaining about her husband spending more than two years away at his studies: "I am a woman, and young, so that every day I get depressed, because rain and dew never light upon my field."[71] One of a husband's key duties was "irrigation."

[65] Ruzante, *Teatro*, pp. 1246–49, 1590–95; Ronnie Ferguson, *The theatre of Angelo Beolco (Ruzante): text, context and performance* (Ravenna: Longo Editore, 2000), pp. 29–31. The shovel handle is a clear genital reference in Bibbiena, *Calandria*, p. 62.

[66] Johns, *Sex or symbol?*, Pl. 5; Jones, *Secret middle ages*, p. 254.

[67] Piovano Arlotto, *Facezie, motti e burle*, ed. Chiara Amerighi (Florence: Libreria Editrice Fiorentina, 1980), p. 59. In a variant, the peasant "led his horse by hand": Poliziano, *Detti piacevoli*, p. 87. The motion of winnowing serves for a sexual analogy in anonymous, *Venexiana*, p. 66.

[68] For example, Giovanni Sercambi, *Novelle*, ed. Giovanni Sinicropi, 2 vols. (Bari: Laterza, 1972), vol. I, pp. 98, 138; Boggione and Casalegno, *Dizionario*, pp. 174–75.

[69] Boccaccio, *Decameron*, p. 174. See Toscan, *Carnaval*, pp. 1427, 1662, 1674 and passim (*arare*, *campo*).

[70] *Collected works of Erasmus*, vol. XXXIX: *Colloquies*, trans. Craig Thompson (University of Toronto Press, 1997), p. 319.

[71] Peter Dronke, *Medieval Latin and the rise of the European love-lyric*, 2nd edn. (Oxford: Clarendon Press, 1968), vol. II, p. 483. The metaphor of rain is also used, for example by Ebreo (see Introduction, above) and in Erasmus, *Institution of Christian matrimony*, p. 237.

At the level of everyday speech we have a rare record of coitus interruptus which was occasioned when an Englishwoman complained to a court about her husband: "what seed should be sowen in the right ground he spent about the outward part of her body."[72] At the level of inexpensive print, a ritual of love magic to attract a man, preserved in an English chapbook of the 1680s, has the hopeful woman casting seed from her apron and intoning "Hempseed I sow; Hempseed I sow; / He that must be my true love come after me and mow."[73] Holding seed close to her womb, the suitor herself sowed the field but the implement that will close the agricultural cycle and bring in the harvest was the masculine scythe.

Fueled by the printing press, the rural tropes were powerfully present in the fiction, poetry and medical discourses of sixteenth- and seventeenth-century Europe. In medical literature from ancient to early modern times and beyond, in Latin and numerous vernaculars, men were farmers tilling the feminine "field of nature."[74] Giovanni Marinello's popular, vernacular book on women's illnesses of 1574 noted that semen was to be spilled or scattered (*spargere*) into the "campo della donna," extending the metaphor to the discussion of causes of sterility when observing that the ground might be as hot and arid as Ethiopia.[75] Sharp's *Midwives book* of 1671 thus repeats a very standard trope: "Man in the act of procreation is the agent and tiller and sower of the ground, woman is the patient [i.e., passive] or ground to be tilled" and "the womb is that field of nature into which the seed of man and woman is cast."[76] In more vivid terms, the idea was echoed by a seventeenth-century woman from Glastonbury who conveyed basic Hippocratic information to a kinswoman by pointing out that "she had a good cunt and . . . if she did not [make use of it] she would do her self wrong, for if ground were not tilled and manured it would be overgrown with thorns and briars."[77] The curative function of semen and friction is at play in her imagery, and marriage was not the context, for she was trying to recruit the maiden into prostitution. Common to much of the theme, put to vivid use in medical and poetic literature but also everyday speech, is the ploughing and clearing of the

72 Quaife, *Wanton wenches*, pp. 172–73.

73 Pepys, *Pepys' penny merriments*, p. 67. For the sickle or scythe (*falx*) in medieval Latin, see Adams, *Latin sexual vocabulary*, p. 24. Using the hoe, or mowing with a scythe, feature in Renaissance carnival songs: Prizer, "*Facciamo*," pp. 187, 189, 197.

74 Latin examples include Berengario, *Isagogae breves*, fol. 20v; Fernel, *Physiologia*, p. 568; Bauhin, *Theatrum anatomicum*, p. 221. English examples include Vicary, *Anatomie of mans body*, M iii recto, N i verso; Crooke, *Mikrokosmographia*, pp. 200, 221, 258, 270, 271; Williams, *Dictionary*, pp. 782–83. For French examples see Villon, *Poems*, pp. 4, 114 (1460s); Paré, *Œuvres complètes*, vol. I, p. 161, vol. II, pp. 636, 641; Montaigne, *Essais*, vol. III, p. 856; Duval, *Hermaphrodits*, p. 39.

75 Marinello, *Medicine*, fol. 54r–v. Dry, arid soil was also a metaphor for sterility in Joubert, *Popular errors*, pp. 122–23.

76 Sharp, *Midwives book*, pp. 32, 53 (see also pp. 23, 52, 75 for similar language).

77 Quaife, *Wanton wenches*, p. 149.

channels and underbrush of a woman's field, as much for her health as for the production of children.

Gardens, flowers and fruits

When the scene moves to gardens, abundance is rife but so too does pleasure become more evident. From ancient Greek to Renaissance Italian and Restoration English, female genitals were gardens to be cultivated, yielding fruits and flowers.[78] Roses in particular were metaphors in anatomical and poetic literature alike, symbolizing the maidenhead to be deflowered and female parts like the cervix or the genitalia (chiefly female, with an occasional reference to the male prick of the thorns), as well as Venus, goddess of desire.[79]

The imagery was commonplace. The beloved in *Song of Songs* dwelled in "a garden inclosed . . ., a spring shut up, a fountain sealed" (4.12), for instance; the abode of the goddess of desire, Venus, was filled with streaming fountains and flowery meadows according to Claudian's wedding poem for Honorius Augustus (*c.* 400 CE).[80] Mild but suggestive rural metaphors readily featured in the gardens and fountains of love that populated medieval and Renaissance poetry, manuscripts and prints, eventually enhancing the erotic potential of the pastoral mode, a genre revivified during the Renaissance. Fecund imagery was as much amorous as strictly marital for marriage was more the backdrop than the end point of much literature. Most of the poems, *novelle* and comedies in which erotic euphemisms and overt metaphor flourished focus on plots concerning adultery or pre-marital sex. The metaphors – such as an aroused man "feeling himself growing like the grass in the meadow" – did not require a Latinate knowledge of the pastoral genre set in idyllic fields.[81] Priapus, after all, was the guardian since ancient times of gardens and crops, and a whore's genitals could easily be cast as a *petit jardinet*, as the French poet François Villon did satirically in the early 1460s.[82]

[78] For example, Henderson, *Maculate muse*, pp. 46, 135–36; Adams, *Latin sexual vocabulary*, pp. 84, 113, 229; Fernel, *Physiologia*, p. 84; Florio, *Worlde of wordes (1598)*, p. 163; Vesling, *Syntagma*, pp. 77–78; Williams, *Glossary*, pp. 95, 128–29, 135, 240, 262–63; Williams, *Dictionary*, pp. 378, 517–19, 560–62, 1059–60, 1170–72; Jones, *Secret middle ages*, pp. 263–64.

[79] Examples are legion. See, for example, Culpeper, *Directory*, p. 25; Sharp, *Midwives book*, p. 43; Jacquart and Thomasset, *Sexuality and medicine*, pp. 32, 37, 204 n. 71; Rubinstein, *Dictionary*, p. 224; Guy de Tervarent, *Attributes et symbols dans l'art profane: dictionnaire d'un langage perdu (1450–1600)*, 2nd edn. (Geneva: Droz, 1997), pp. 377–78; Williams, *Dictionary*, pp. 1170–72.

[80] Claudian, *Epithalamium of Honorius and Maria*, 49–96; Williams, *Dictionary*, pp. 580–82.

[81] Bandello, *Novelle*, vol. II, p. 303.

[82] Villon, *Poems*, p. 59; Giancarlo Fiorenza, "*Priapea* and the poetic garden," in his *Dosso Dossi: paintings of myth, magic, and the antique* (University Park: Pennsylvania State University Press, 2008), pp. 87–92.

While reproduction informed much imagery, it was not ubiquitous. The most common metaphor for the embryo was fruit; the bride too was newly ripened fruit (especially apples), to be picked or harvested. In the words of Plato's *Timaeus*, men, "culling as it were the fruit from trees, . . . sow upon the womb, as upon ploughed soil, animalcules" that develop eventually into human beings.[83] The language of arboreal propagation recurs in the Bible. Every tree that did not bear good fruit, that is, children, was axed and burned (Matthew 3.10; Luke 3.9); yet that very phraseology was mocked in Aretino's comedy *Il marescalco* (1533), in which the plot's central dilemma is solved at the end by a male–male wedding.[84] All the characters are satisfied, but the "fruit" of children will not result despite the urging of a tiresome pedant.

Celebration of fecundity was not only about licit offspring but also marked sensual pleasure, feminine willingness and availability, and the regular exercise of virility. Such is the scenario in an engraving attributed to an anonymous Italian (possibly Venetian) designer (fig. 49), replete with typical features of amorous gardens, including the flowing fountain, idyllic enclosure far from urban cares, and the focus on bird song and music.[85] Around the same time, in conventional poetic vein, Lorenzo de' Medici defined gardens as loci of sensual delight and their abundance was a metaphor for proximity to the object of his desire: "paradise ... means nothing other than a most agreeable garden, abounding with pleasant and delightful things, with trees, with apples, with flowers, with fresh and flowing waters, songs of birds, and in effect with all the amenities that the heart of man can think of. And thus it is proved that paradise was where such a lovely lady was."[86]

Source of life and refreshment, fountains are common in amorous gardens, where they can also signal Hippocratic attention to the necessary moistening of female bodies. As the French nobleman Brantôme put it in the 1580s, aroused women need to "bathe in cool running water" and the irrigation must run deep, reaching into the uterus because "there is a big difference between throwing water in a vessel and just watering around it and on the edge" and this medical subtext may add to the voyeuristic pleasure offered by numerous visual and

83 Plato, *Timaeus*, 91c–d; also, for example, Aristotle, *GA*, 765b30; Plutarch, *Moralia*, 495e; Thornton, *Eros*, pp. 143–44. In *Timaeus*, 86c, retained male seed builds up pressure as though "it were a tree that is overladen beyond measure with fruit." For apples associated with women or their virginity, as well as breasts and sexual pleasures in general, see Williams, *Dictionary*, pp. 28–30, and more generally 560–62 (fruit).

84 Aretino, *Commedie*, pp. 48, 92, 101.

85 Zucker, *The illustrated Bartsch 24 Commentary part 3*, pp. 207–09; Gert Jan van der Sman, *De eeuw van Titiaan: Venetiaanse prenten uit de Renaissance* (Zwolle: Waanders Uitgevers, 2002), p. 26.

86 *The autobiography of Lorenzo de' Medici the Magnificent: "A commentary on my sonnets,"* trans. James Wyatt Cook (Binghamton: Medieval and Renaissance Texts and Studies, 1995), p. 89 (with parallel Italian).

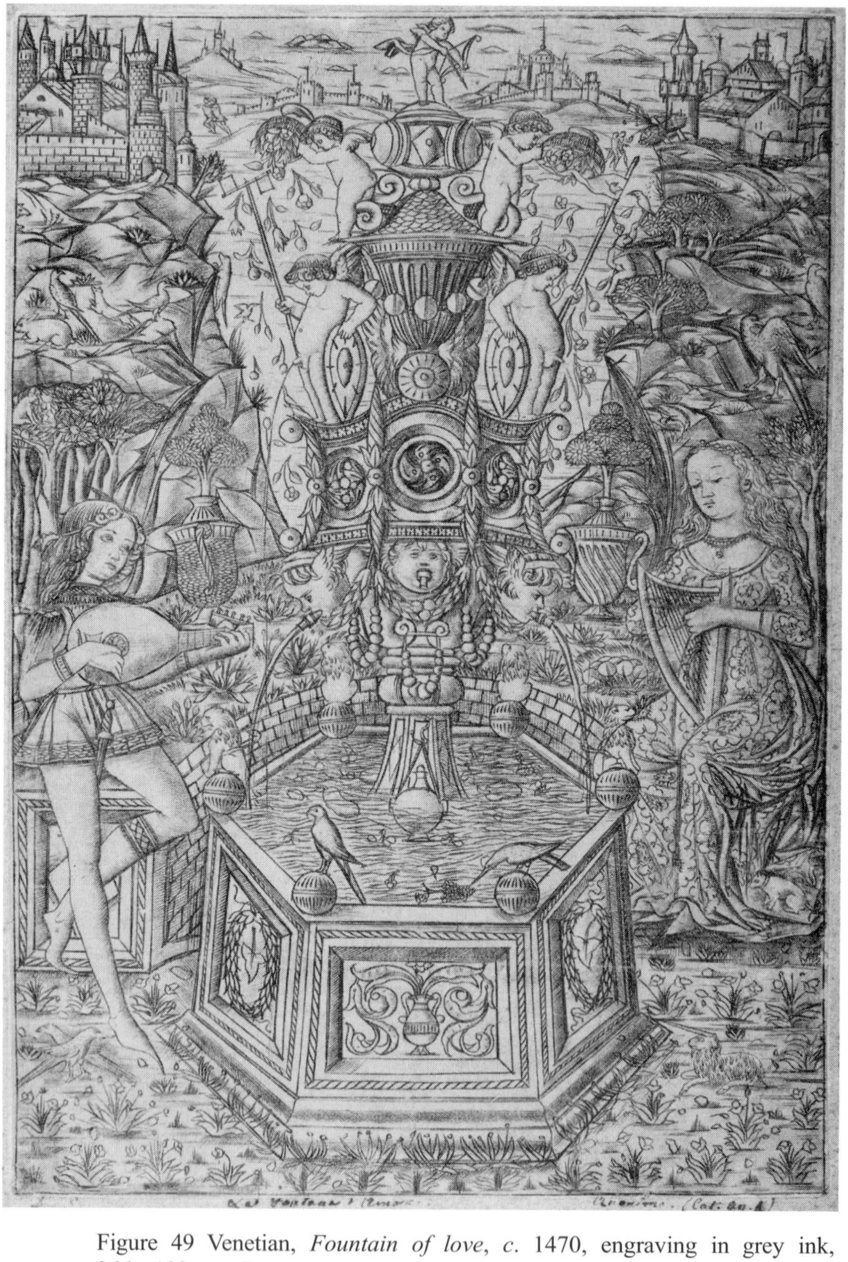

Figure 49 Venetian, *Fountain of love*, *c.* 1470, engraving in grey ink, 266 × 183 mm, Bassano del Grappa, Museo Civico, Collezione Remondini

poetic images of nymphs bathing in secluded pools.[87] The liquids emitted from the genitals of statues of charming putti, pissing water in garden fountains and interior wall fountains or issuing wine in tableware figures and public fountains, were often ambiguous, alluding to the erotic and witty connotations of fluid refreshment that might be water or wine, urine or semen.[88] Jerome Duquesnoy's bronze *Mannekin-Pis* of 1619 in Brussels (fig. 50) is the most famous surviving instance of the type, confidently and merrily dispensing precious water to the populace whose cohesion was facilitated by both the water and the joke. Similar sculptures of male infants instead bestowed wine during civic celebrations of such events as entries, the projecting stream providing free drink as well as amusement while connoting magnificence, largesse and abundance.

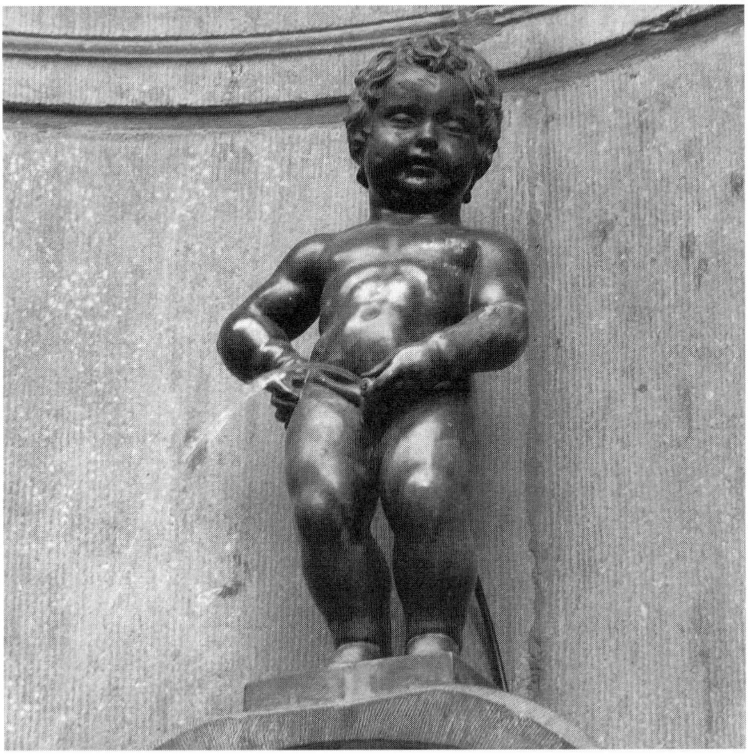

Figure 50 Jerome Duquesnoy, *Mannekin-Pis*, 1619, bronze, Brussels

[87] Brantôme, *Dames galantes*, p. 123, trans. in Merrick and Ragan (eds.), *Homosexuality*, p. 105.

[88] See Catherine Emerson, "Are you taking the piss(e)? Early appearances of the urinating boy in the Low Countries and northern France," in Adrian Tudor and Alan Hindley (eds.), *Grant risee?*

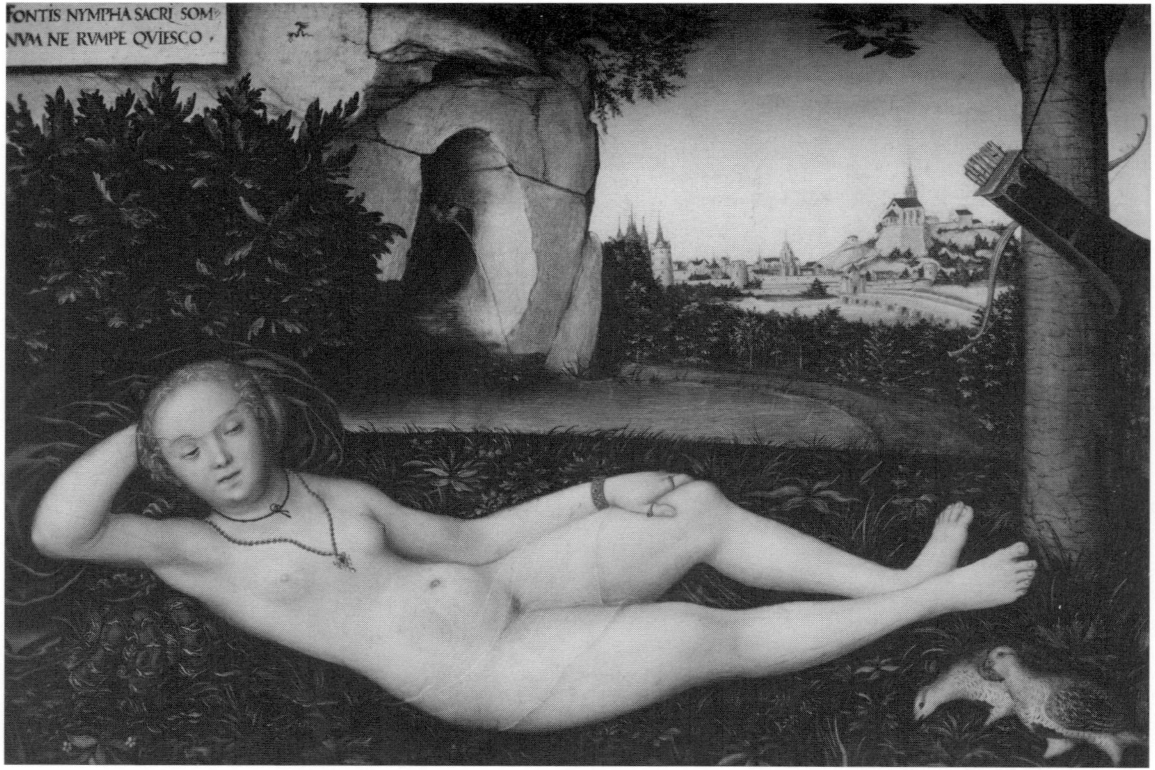

Figure 51 Lucas Cranach the Elder, *Nymph of the spring*, after 1537, oil on panel, 484 × 728 mm, Washington, DC, National Gallery of Art, Gift of Clarence Y. Palitz

Erotic fountains feature in a series of popular paintings by Cranach and his workshop depicting a *Nymph of the spring* (fig. 51).[89] The reclining, naked female figure is situated near a secluded pastoral fountain, the images thereby demonstrating pictorial deftness with a classicizing as well as sensual theme. Cranach's consummate skill in creating the illusion of transparent veils was transferred to the challenge of painting streams of clear water. In a sense the flowing fluid stands in for male presence, as it did for Brantôme. That allusion to male bodily release is complemented in the Leipzig example by a seated faun or satyr clutching a sharp stick atop the fountain's Corinthian capital. In other cases, the arc of water falling from the fountain in the background draws attention to the foreground figure's erogenous zones and in examples such as the paintings in the Thyssen-Bornemisza collection, Besançon and Washington DC that arc, if extended, would arrive at her genitals.

The Italian print's embroidery-like profusion of vegetal detail and pattern (fig. 49) increases the impression of paradisal fecundity in that fountain's setting. As is so often the case, sexual longing rather than marital fertility is the primary focus of the courting young couple, who come to musical harmony in a garden of desire and universal plenitude. With a unicorn below her feet, the damsel remains virginal, for the moment. Much of the detail works as sexual double entendre, from the birds symbolizing the male genitals or two monkeys in trees (denoting lust) to the peeing putti, their vulval shields and the kinds of musical instruments being fingered. The youth embraces the rounded body of a feminized lute, the damsel plucks at the strings of a harp. Playing with words about musical strings brought to mind a penis able to relax and then tighten, but women's sexual arousal was taken into account too.[90] The abbess in Aretino's licentious convent "was dying to rub the boy's bow over her lyre."[91] The Italian *lira* meant not only a musical instrument but also a furrow; Florio's definition of the verb *lirare* (1611) meant to play the lyre or "to rake or harrow the ground that is sowed to hide the seede in it." It was thus an alternative for the classic metaphor of "ploughing" a woman, and the musical action clearly refers to friction and motion but not penetration. In the case of the anonymous engraving, such sexual innuendo has the damsel preparing her own ground in a sense, for the harp firmly lodged between her legs was another metaphor for female genitals, while her wooer's penile knife is stiff at his own groin.

Two putti piss "water" into the fountain's basin, but this act was often understood as the casting of semen into a womanly vessel. Above them two

The medieval comic presence, La Présence comique médiévale: essays in memory of Brian J. Levy (Turnhout: Brepols, 2006), pp. 31–48; Simons, "Bodily fluids," 331–73.

89 The earliest painting was executed in 1518, the later ones were produced after 1537. See Friedländer and Rosenberg, *Cranach*, pp. 93–94, 121, 150, nos. 119–20, 259, 402–04; Brinkmann (ed.), *Cranach*, pp. 55–57, 330–33.

90 Adams, *Latin sexual vocabulary*, pp. 21, 22, 25; for example, *Priapea*, 6.5–6; 68.15–16.

91 Aretino, *Ragionamento*, p. 40, and 143 for harp; *Dialogues*, pp. 36, 110.

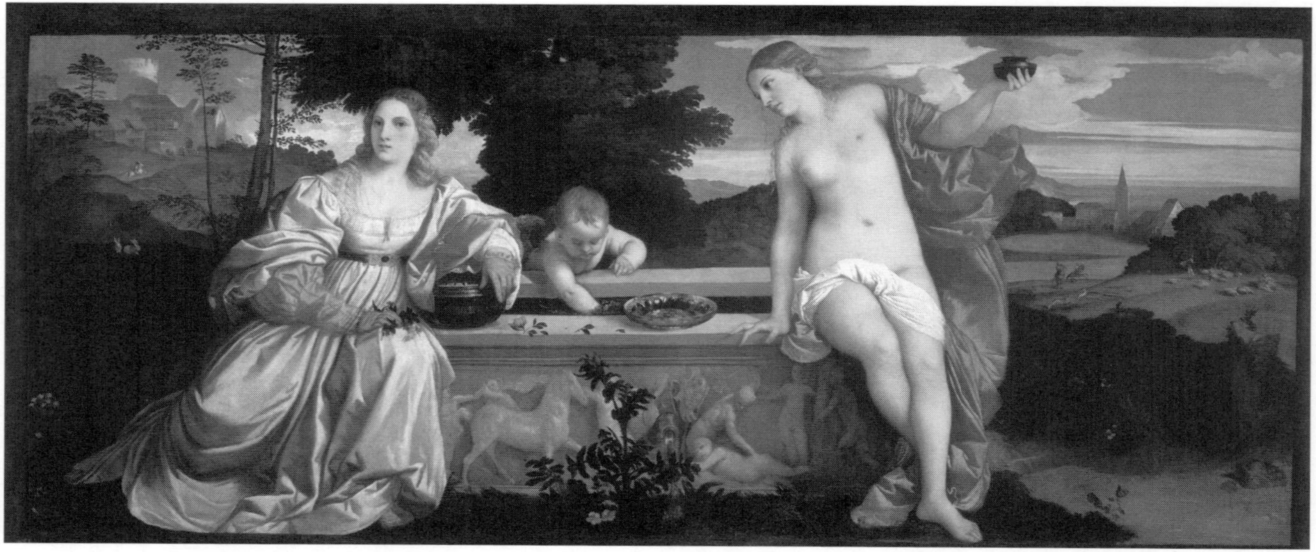

Figure 52 Titian, *"Sacred and profane love,"* *c.* 1514–15, oil on canvas, 118 × 279 cm, Rome, Galleria Borghese

winged infants upturn baskets to let loose a stream of flowers and buds; the mixing of these two elements metaphorically indicates sexual intercourse. As with the anatomical terminology, flowers usually connoted femininity, and their plucking signified the loss of virginity and the sexual possession of a woman.[92] Scattered by ladies from the ramparts of mock castles during public performances of sieges, as we have seen in Chapter 1, flowers were also contradictory signs of erotic welcome, bestowing on the masculine knights a reward that referred to their ultimately successful entrance through the ostensibly defended "portal." Moreover, "flowers" was sometimes used as a euphemism for menstruation and, since the menses were often conflated with female seed the shower of red buds refers to a willing female response.[93]

Associating female genitals and seed with floral imagery was an influential practice in the *Roman de la rose*, in which "plucking" the beloved's virginal "rose" was the male hero's ultimate goal, after which he immediately awoke. In the last page or so of the lengthy poem, written around 1275, the hero "scattered a little seed on the bud when I shook it, when I touched it within in order to pore over the petals . . . I so mixed the seeds that they could hardly be separated; and thus I made the whole tender rosebush widen and lengthen."[94] (Leonardo later drew the cervix precisely opening and elongating as it reached toward male semen; see fig. 29.) The Italian version of the popular poem, *Il fiore*, has the lover boast that "I succeeded in deflowering the Flower, / and with the seed that I had carried, / after the ploughing, so came the sowing. / The seed of the Flower had descended (*era cascata*); / I mixed the two of them together / such that much good fruit has issued forth."[95]

Coitus was described as the mingling of fluids and other metaphorical items. *Il fiore*'s cascade of falling female seed resembles the engraving's floral stream falling alongside jets of male fluid, and the mixing occurs in the basin of the fountain, itself an architectural representation of phallic erection inserted into a uterine vessel. Cupid aiming his bow stands atop the fountain in the engraving, but in Titian's updated treatment of a similar theme in the painting of *c.* 1514–15 first called *Sacred and profane love* only in 1792 (fig. 52), he participates more actively in the erotic union by stirring the waters

92 For urination, see Simons, "Bodily fluids," 331–73. On flowers and gardens see, for example, Kleinhenz, "Texts, naked and thinly veiled," pp. 83–109; Williams, *Dictionary*, pp. 517–19 (flower, especially meaning either virginity or menses), 580–82 (garden), 1170–72 (rose); Camille, *Medieval art of love*, pp. 23–25, 73–81, 107–11.

93 Joubert, *Popular errors*, p. 99; Boggione and Casalegno, *Dizionario*, pp. 500–1; Ch. 6 above.

94 De Lorris and de Meun, *Roman de la rose*, vol. III, pp. 152–53 (lines 21689–712); De Lorris and de Meun, *Romance of the rose*, p. 353.

95 *"The fiore" and the "Detto d'amore,"* p. 495. For other references to sexual ploughing, see pp. 53 and n. 3, 165, with a discussion about ploughing and deflowering in the Introduction, pp. 15–18.

of the sarcophagus-turned-fountain.[96] Roses are held in the clothed woman's hand and one rests on the rim of the sarcophagus, beneath which a relief depicts a scene of horses and a naked man being beaten. Against this backdrop of unruly passion carved on a white marble object, water ejaculates from a polished bronze spout onto a flourishing rose bush.

In the right background, a seated couple kisses amidst a pastoral scene of a shepherd with his flock and, nearby, hunters with their dogs avidly pursue a hare. Two more hares or rabbits stand out against the green sward on the left. These animals were renowned for their licentious nature as well as symbolizing female pudenda and also fertility because they were, according to Aristotle, "abundant in semen."[97] Although the meaning of the female figures in the foreground remains debatable, the display of attractive female flesh in Titian's œuvre was always imbued with sensual import. This work was commissioned for an elite marriage, one in which the wife had been married before and was thus sexually knowledgeable, but the sources and effects of its erotic imagery were not exclusively marital. Rather than domestication or children, its focus was on desire and virility, bringing the language of romance and eros to apply to nuptial union.

Inevitably, the "fruits" of sexual union were not always legitimate children. The ubiquitous imagery of fruits and vegetables decorating early modern objects and populating the erotic lexicon since ancient times is as much about sexual pleasure and excess, if not more so. The "fruti" women are urged to take by an inscribed banderole on a maiolica plate from early sixteenth-century Deruta are leafy phalli, complete with penis, glans and testicles (fig. 43), recalling just those "fruits" of glass delivered to Aretino's bawdy nunnery or plucked by avid women from phallus trees. Too often, the overall imagery of bounty is reduced by modern commentators to no more than a theme of marital fertility, but the typical context for the metaphors is erotic, often adulterous, discourse that either ignores marriage or is explicitly located elsewhere, usually in a convent, church, garden or classical setting. The phallus tree in Massa Marittima is situated beneath a granary and in conjunction with the public water source it stands for communal abundance more than an increase in the town's population. Even Titian's canvas (fig. 52), while related to a widow's second marriage, addresses pastoral and pagan sensuality rather than the domestic or reproductive realms. In other words, it is well to remember that even the Catholic Church believed that reproduction was not the sole purpose of sex

[96] Wethey, *Titian*, vol. III, pp. 20–22, 175–79; Humfrey, *Titian*, pp. 86–87.

[97] Aristotle, *GA*, 774a30–b5; de Tervarent, *Attributes et symbols*, pp. 276 (lapin), 287–88 (lièvre); Brumble, *Classical myths*, p. 343; Williams, *Dictionary*, pp. 297–300 (cony), 645–46 (hare), 805–06 (leveret). The Latin *cuniculus* (rabbit) could be confused with *cunnus* (vulva, female genitals, hence cunt).

within marriage, and perhaps this was especially so in instances where the bride was already sexually experienced.

Numerous other meanings arise from vegetal abundance, including dynastic and national power and prosperity, political liberality and magnificence, paradisal plentitude, sensual enjoyment, anti-moralizing cheer, and artistic variety (*copia*).[98] Most of these themes resonate with erotic signification. Seed-filled and bursting figs or melons (fig. 53), like flowers newly opened from their buds, visualized fresh and ripe flesh ready for the "plucking," not just in the sense of deflowering but more broadly suggesting an eager readiness for sexual play. Rocco's homoerotic dialogue *Alcibiade* of around 1630 was lyrical about "the flowered garden" of a boy, likening the anus to a "nascent rose with tight folds, tinted with a host of colors, snow vying with purple."[99] Peaches commonly referred to either the fuzzy beards of youths or male buttocks; figs were the

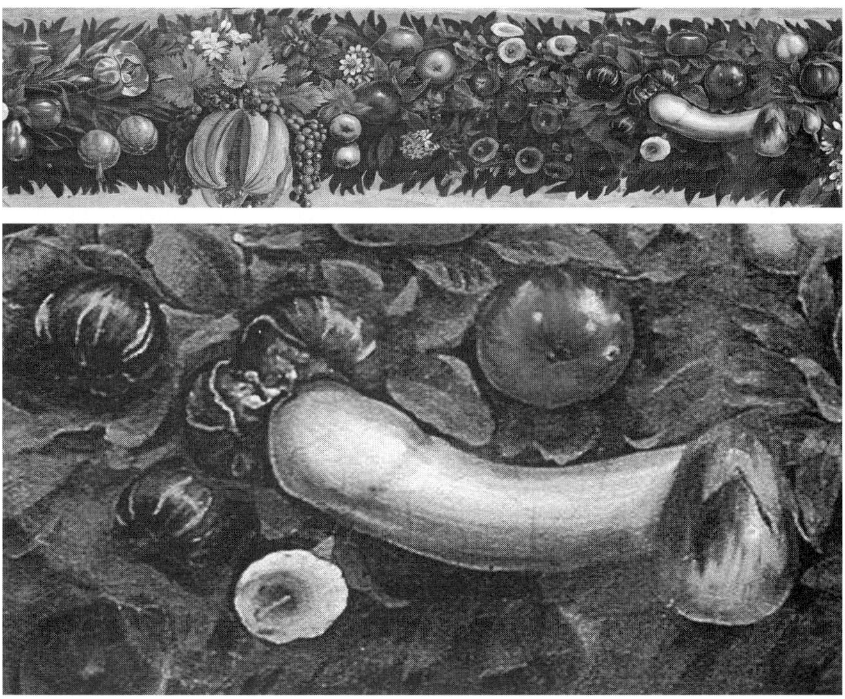

Figure 53 Giovanni da Udine, festoon above *Mercury*, *c.* 1517, fresco, Rome, Villa Farnesina, loggia

[98] On abundance see, for example, Zorach, *Blood, milk, ink, gold*.
[99] Rocco, *Acibiade*, p. 85. For the rose as the anus, see Toscan, *Carnaval*, p. 1742 and passim.

renowned Italian metaphor for a woman's genitals; a variety of gourds represented the erect male penis.[100]

Since medical theory located virility in the testicles, there was much metaphorical emphasis on masculine vegetal forms that produced prolific seed. Virility was certainly signified by the amount of children (chiefly sons) a man might produce, though men without children were not necessarily considered weak, and the parental factor was a subset of the fundamental yardstick, the profusion of semen and number of ejaculations. Eggs, a common farmyard product, were indicators of testicles and male seed, hoarded too much by a brooding, overly domesticated man who lacked vigor.[101] In German and Netherlandish images, however, a man's full basket of eggs was instead oftentimes expended on an adulterous woman, a tale accentuated in Beuckelaer's case (fig. 36) by his overt display of birds and the erect purse/genitals between his legs. An engraving by Cornelis Matsys of 1549 positions an open-mouthed jug (a uterine vessel) adjacent to a woman who receives an egg from a man's basket, the handle of which she eagerly grasps. Standing above them, his wife despairs that he "lays his eggs in the nest of another and leaves me unrequited," a reference to the woman's desire for semen rather than the penis.[102] Ben Jonson's verse for *Coryat's crudities* of 1611 draws out the monetary allusion, accompanying the image of a woman pelting a man in a gondola with eggs: she "shootes egs at him empty of Chickens, / Because shee had made his purse empty of Chiquins."[103] The latter were Venetian gold coins, emptied from the visitor's scrotal "moneybag" by a courtesan who, supposedly, had so much sex that her slippery womb was infertile.

A gourd pressing into a fig and forcing open its seed-filled interior is clearly a pictorial play on the Italian *fica* (fig) for female genitals (fig. 53). But when working in the Villa Farnesina (then Chigi) under Raphael's direction around 1517, the decorative specialist Giovanni da Udine placed a closed eggplant of similar shape at the other end of the penetrative gourd. A male testicle matched the

100 For an introduction to such imagery see Margaret Sullivan, "Aertsen's kitchen and market scenes: audience and innovation in northern art," *Art Bulletin* 81 (1999), 258–59; Linda Wolk-Simon, "'Rapture to the greedy eyes': profane love in the Renaissance," in Bayer (ed.), *Art and love*, pp. 49–53.

101 Boggione and Casalegno, *Dizionario*, p. 374; Dekker, *Humour in Dutch culture*, p. 113; Jones, *Secret middle ages*, pp. 6, 11, 168, 236–37.

102 Honig, *Painting and the market*, pp. 58, 43, 257 n. 128, fig. 8; see also her fig. 10, Dürer's engraving of *Peasants on the way to market* (1519); Silver, *Peasant scenes and landscapes*, pp. 108, 273 n. 21.

103 Patricia Fortini Brown, *Private lives in Renaissance Venice: art, architecture, and the family* (New Haven: Yale University Press, 2004), p. 159; Boggione and Casalegno, *Dizionario*, p. 374 (*uova* for testicle). This inverts the carnival practice of men throwing eggs filled with perfumed water into women's windows above, observed, for instance, in Venice in 1549: "The travels and life of Sir Thomas Hoby," ed. E. Powell (London: Royal Historical Society, 1902), p. 14. For an illustration of 1642 see *Il Carnevale Veneziano nelle maschere incise da Francesco Bertelli*, ed. Lina Padoan Urban (Milan: Edizioni Il Polifilo, 1986), pl. IV.

female vessel, each containers of seed. The cucumber appeared in bawdy imagery not only for its morphology but also because it was especially filled with seeds and quickly grew.[104] The eroticized fruits, replete with seeds like a bursting pomegranate, that tumble around the face of a smiling satyr on a maiolica dish from Venice dated to the 1540s include a pale gourd that stands out against the lushness, its long penile neck attached to a swelling sac that represents the scrotal mass.[105]

Bunches of grapes are frequently suspended amidst the ludic festoons of Agostino Chigi's loggia. Near the visual pun with fig and gourds, grapes are draped either side of a central melon as though they signify seed-laden testicles "covering" the seed-filled uterine organ (fig. 53).[106] These juicy fruits resembled dangling testicles, abounded with seed inside a layer of skin and yielded juice. According to Galen's anatomical description, the seed-preparing vessels of the male body were so twisted and elaborate that they resembled the tendrils of vines, an analogy picked up by the Renaissance anatomist Vesalius and thence reiterated by popularizers like the midwife Jane Sharp.[107] A bunch tellingly hangs to the side of the grape leaf that hides a man's genitals in a grisaille panel attributed to Luca Signorelli and usually identified as an *Allegory of abundance*.[108] One of Lot's incestuous daughters seductively, knowingly displays a succulent bunch in Jan Massys' depiction of *Lot and his daughters* (1563; Vienna Kunsthistorisches Museum), the sensual point confirmed by a nearby melon which has been cut open to reveal its vulva-like, seed-laden interior. As Dionysus' fruit, the grape was especially known as a symbol of seed-filled fecundity and pleasure. Thus Spenser's *Faerie queene* had "that gracious God of wine" conjoining himself with Philliras when "He turned himselfe into a fruitfull vine, / And into her faire bosome made his grapes decline" (3.11.43). A woman's body was a wine-press crushing juice from a male partner in one of Firenzuola's *novelle*, when a man fantasized about "discharging a loadful into her press."[109] Similarly, a man exclaims "you should

104 Henderson, *Maculate muse*, p. 125 n. 94; Adams, *Latin sexual vocabulary*, p. 27, with the addition of *Priapus poems*, p. 81; Medici, *Opere*, vol. II, p. 792; Mirella Levi d'Ancona, *The garden of the Renaissance: botanical symbolism in Italian painting* (Florence: Olschki, 1977), pp. 117, 157; Boggione and Casalegno, *Dizionario*, p. 295; Williams, *Dictionary*, p. 348 (cucumber). For onions, leeks and scallions increasing the amount of male sperm, see Sheila McTighe, "Foods and the body in Italian genre paintings, about 1580: Campi, Passarotti, Carracci," *Art Bulletin* 86 (2004), 317.

105 See Linda Wolk-Simon's entry in Bayer (ed.), *Art and love*, p. 219, no. 111 for the dish in the Victoria and Albert Museum.

106 Morel, "Priape," 13–28, figs. 1, 12–15.

107 Galen, *Semen*, p. 107; Vesalius, *Fabrica*, pp. 522, 524; Sharp, *Midwives book*, pp. 15, 16, 50.

108 For the painting in the Uffizi, dated to the early 1510s, see Tom Henry and Laurence Kanter, *Luca Signorelli* (New York: Rizzoli, 2002), p. 231, no. 106. Grapes are suggestive in *Priapea* 30.3, 42, 51.6, 53.

109 Firenzuola, "Ragionamenti," in his *Opere*, p. 109; for grape juice see Boggione and Casalegno, *Dizionario*, p. 360.

see how she squeezes the grapes in the wine-press!" in a French Mardi Gras play performed in 1512.[110] Much of the text is filled with double entendre jokes about the wife's neglected vineyard needing the attention of hoeing, deep digging and turning over of the soil. Pleasure to be had from wine doubtless increased the sensual and amusing associations of grapes.

They are one of the fruits singled out in Ovid's famous passage on impotence, which resorted to images of obstructed fluid and disused seed: "when a well is damned by charms, its water dries up; through incantations acorns drop from oaks and grapes from vines, and apples fall when no one has touched them" (*Amores*, 3.7.32–34). Each of these fruits instead appears fresh and ripe in most visual and poetic imagery. Acorns are just one instance of the cultural habit that continues to associate nuts with the testicles. In medical terminology, various elements of the genital systems were compared with nuts. Female "stones" or ovaries were smaller than the male testicles, merely akin to the size and form of a large almond, whereas large chestnuts were likened to testicles.[111] Prostates were "of the bigness of a Walnut, or very neer," and the same wrinkled nut could be called "Jove's glans" or Jove's penile head.[112]

The Latin *glans* literally meant "acorn" and the most common medical analogy, in a variety of languages, was between the acorn and the smooth head of the penis with the slight tip of an uncircumcised organ.[113] The ancient Greek βαλανοσ meant both acorn and penile glans, used in each sense by Aristotle, for example, and appearing in some Latin medical texts much later as *balanus*.[114] As Sharp explained it, visual and morphological reasons made the naming plausible: the "Nut of the Yard, when it is half covered with the foreskin, looks like an Acorn in the Cup, and therefore some call it *Glans*, which in Latin signifies an Acorn."[115]

110 Bowen, "Metaphorical obscenity," 340–41.

111 For example, Raynald, *Byrth of mankynde*, fol. 14v; Berengario, *Isagogae breves*, fol. 22r; Sharp, *Midwives book*, p. 34. See Prizer, "*Facciamo*," pp. 196–97 for chestnuts.

112 For the first quotation, see Culpeper, *Directory*, p. 17 (also Vesling, *Syntagma*, p. 64; Sharp, *Midwives book*, p. 22); for the second, Macrobius, *Saturnalia*, 3.18.3, reiterated, for instance, in *The first and seconde partes of the herbal of William Turner* (Cologne: Arnold Birckman, 1568), pt. II, fol. 23v (*glans iovis*).

113 For example: Adams, *Latin sexual vocabulary*, pp. 29, 72, 138, 228; André, *Vocabulaire*, pp. 175–76; William Denny Baskett, *Parts of the body in the later Germanic dialects*, (University of Chicago Press, 1920) p. 107 (*eichel*); Louise Vasvari, "The battle of flesh and Lent in the *Libro del arcipreste*: gastro-genital rites of reversal," *La Corónia* 20 (1991), 6–7 (Spanish, *bellota*); Rubinstein, *Dictionary*, pp. 4–5, 173; Williams, *Dictionary*, p. 966; Toscan, *Carnaval*, pp. 1451, 1701 (*ghianda*); Boggione and Casalegno, *Dizionario*, p. 290; Jones, *Secret middle ages*, pp. 267–68.

114 Aristotle, *HA*, 493a27 (as penile glans), 603b31 (as edible nuts); see also Henderson, *Maculate muse*, pp. 41, 65, 119, 120; Adams, *Latin sexual vocabulary*, p. 72; Hodges, "Ideal prepuce," 378, 395. *Balanus* is still in use in Duval, *Hermaphrodits*, pp. 44, 46.

115 Sharp, *Midwives book*, p. 31.

In the plural, generic nuts often referred to the testicles, as is done in a gilded and incised copper pendant case (fig. 54).[116] This toilette case, fashioned for a woman's belt during the first half of the eighteenth century, has a central tubular case for items like needles, tweezers and a spoon for cosmetics, and two pendulant acorn-like containers at either side probably contained perfumed herbs. As the woman moved, the case hanging near her genitals would have

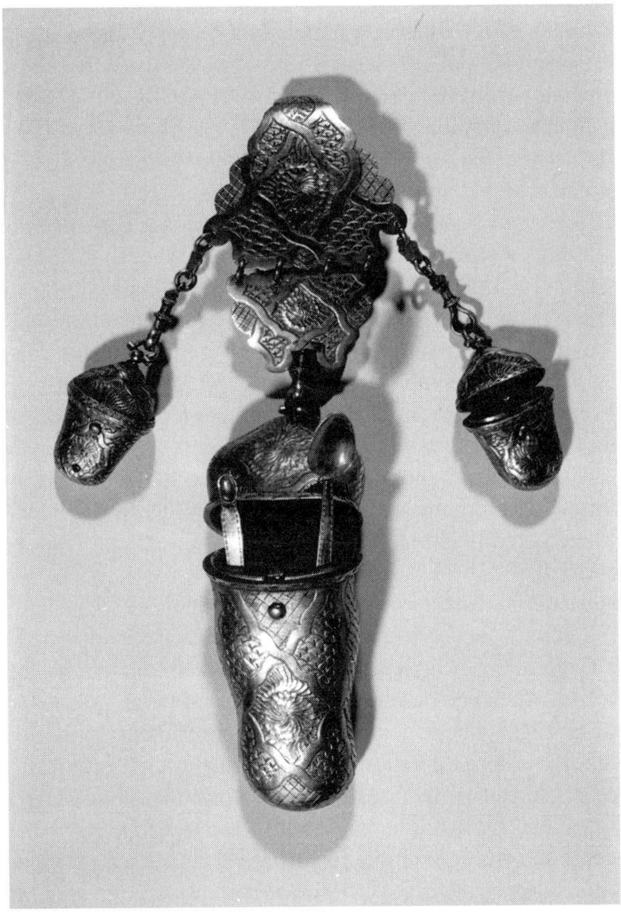

Figure 54 Pendant case, first half of the eighteenth century, gilded bronze, Venice, Museo Correr

116 *Il gioco dell'amo: Le cortegiane di Venezia dal trecento al settecento* (Milan: Berenice, 1990), p. 173. For earlier objects and images that play on acorn/glans, see Jones, *Secret middle ages*, pp. 267–68.

dangled and swayed provocatively. The brisk snapping up of the hinged element presumably created the impression of elongation akin to erection. In a sense, by wearing, moving and using the case she became mannish, rather like courtesans who were said to wear men's clothing or undergarments to attract the sodomitical interest of male clients.[117] More broadly, the wearer's display declared her to be daring, sexually knowledgeable and witty. Men's purses echoed their own testicular "bursa" and codpieces had called attention to a man's genitals; secular badges flaunting phallic or vulval animals were probably exhibited by women as well as men, female medicinal applicators made of metal mimicked the engorged penis (fig. 46) and this woman's bronze container doubled as a finely crafted, vegetal metaphor of the genital signs of the opposite sex. Perhaps, like sympathetic love magic, the case connoted the woman's desire to attract male attention. The physical double entendre also worked as the kind of joke acceptable amongst the noble class according to a character in Castiglione's *Book of the courtier*. Close-to-obscene jokes were deemed acceptable enough if they were veiled (*occulto*) because they had a superficially innocuous meaning, in this case acorns and a rounded shaft.[118]

Despite or perhaps because of Europe's growing urbanization, medical and erotic metaphors were still in large part drawn from the rural and village life of arable farming, orchard-keeping and gardening. Writers, workers, performers and image makers not only invented fresh metaphors for their age but also relied on pre-existing metaphors that they and their audiences had already learned to naturalize. Although Sharp's plough and acorn were millennia old, her particular way of writing about them was to be appreciated. Resorting to established metaphors authenticated the book's authority, for it fitted with readers' expectations and knowledge.

Eroticized agricultural images infiltrated a broad range of social language and pictures, from a church façade in Bologna to a carnival monologue in Venice, from a Mardi Gras farce in France to an Englishwoman's earthy advice to a female relative, and audience members were expected to understand the bodily, sexual references. Established medical learning contributed to the long life of such metaphors, but their adaptation beyond Latinate circles and their spread into fields like visual representations, street performances and slang indicates that the analogies and implications made sense and gelled with people's physical experiences. Daily rural practice, for instance, continued to be meaningful and to inform metaphors used in the cities. The increasing interest in the pastoral genre of literature and visual art gave new resonance to such imagery, further "naturalizing" the gendered and biological roles assigned to male and female bodies. In vivid terms, influential metaphors provided the language and imagery

[117] Brown, *Private lives*, p. 185, fig. 207. [118] Castiglione, *Cortegiano*, p. 197.

by which to think about and articulate desire and sexual action. The end point of virility and patriarchal assertion was sometimes not so much penetration or impregnation as the enjoyment of abundant pleasures and potent ministration to women's bodies that depended on men for health reasons. From jokes between lovers in London to carnival songs in Florence, court gossip in Paris to love magic in Friuli, metaphors rendered familiar and concrete a gendered ideology of power disparities based on differently sexed bodies.

8 Implements in action

Action was central to the logic of sexual metaphors and hence familiar labor and tools were integrated with the humoral understanding of the body's workings. Concentrating mainly on Italian words and images but discussing cultural patterns that were widespread, this chapter adumbrates the double entendre of several implements and their uses before turning to the case of the kitchen, a metaphorical locale like the field or the garden in which were situated inventive, often humorous, sexual motifs and figures. The body was a cooking or concocting machine in which heat was essential, men's pneumatic ejaculations were compared with air and sound blown from musical instruments, copulatory movements were akin to repetitive motions like spinning or stirring and the release of seed was likened to fluid flowing from a spigot or barrel. Seemingly discordant modes of discourse such as the medical and poetic, the obscene and the learned, shared an understanding of how visual imagery and words could effectively frame and interpret bodily experience.

Morphology and action

Sexual metaphors relied on the common foundations of morphology and action, often combined, as in the case of the bagpipes. Composed of a large sack to which penile extensions are attached, bagpipes were squeezed and fingered, thereby emitting both sound and air (*pneuma*). The genital association was exploited in images of rustic, animal, grotesque or devilish musicians, including a ruffian fiddling on his instrument while sitting on the latrine, depicted on a fifteenth-century Italian copper engraving plate (fig. 55).[1] To accentuate the demeaning joke, a bauble of drooping penis and testicles hangs from the drone.

[1] Boggione and Casalegno, *Dizionario*, pp. 253–55, 405, 406, 510 (*cornamusa, piva, zampogna*). Since this chapter concentrates on Italian images and word play, references to other languages are kept to a minimum. But objects like bagpipes, bells, bottles, hoods, organs, ovens, spigots, spindles and taps, along with actions such as broaching, eating, mingling, spinning and stirring, will be found in Williams, *Dictionary*, et al.

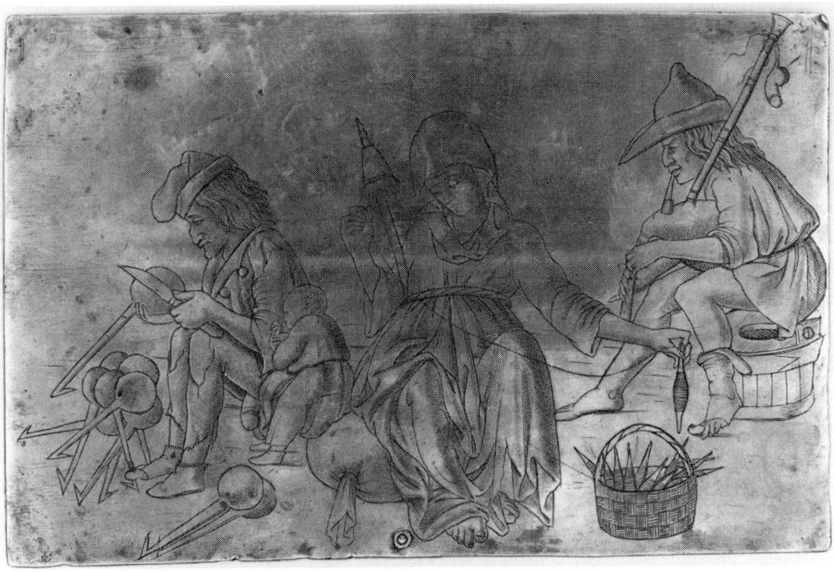

Figure 55 Anonymous northeast Italian, *Various occupations*, last quarter of the fifteenth century, recto, engraved copper plate, 150 × 224 mm, Washington DC, National Gallery of Art, Rosenwald Collection

On occasion, trumpets expelled more than air. Those blown by putti, many atop fantastical helmets, and drawn in Marco Zoppo's homoerotically inflected "Parchment book" of the mid-fifteenth century sometimes exude emphatic lines of air/sound but also drops of moisture that evoke more than humorously excessive spit.[2] Raucous trumpets are often coupled with or near pissing putti, in the margins of manuscripts for example, and the male ejection of one kind of fluid was frequently elided with ejaculation. In the case of Donatello's adjacent bronze reliefs below the statue of Judith and Holofernes, frenzied dancing and trumpeting feature on one panel, debauchery at the wine press on another, and in the latter scene a stream of urine is aimed directly into a drunkard's ear, perhaps indicating the combination of fluid and air (which carries sound) that forms semen.[3]

[2] On the heads, see Lilian Armstrong, "Marco Zoppo e il libro dei disegni del British Museum: riflessioni sulle teste 'all'antica,'" in Berenice Giovannucci Vigi (ed.), *Marco Zoppo cento 1433–1478 Venezia* (Bologna: Nuova Alfa Editoriale, 1993), pp. 79–96. A man's erection resembled the *trombone* flourished by the angel at Castel Sant'Angelo in Aretino, *Ragionamento*, p. 46.

[3] Simons, "Bodily fluids," 345, 353–54.

The male "member" was not always composed of undifferentiated parts, and metaphors like "acorn" for the *glans*, "hood" for the foreskin and "bells" for testicles led to visual and poetic jokes.[4] The uncircumcised prepuce signified controlled, decorous manliness to the ancient Greeks and Romans, and its retraction continued to be amusing to later European viewers. Cheap badges displayed a phallic-nosed face with a testicular chin peeking out from an enveloping hood, and the elite artist Michelangelo wrote a satirical poem that made a sexual joke about the hood. Around 1533–34, in response to a burlesque poem sent by Francesco Berni to the painter Sebastiano del Piombo that was filled with mock-praise of their mutual friend Michelangelo, the latter artist replied to Berni as though in Sebastiano's name.[5] Michelangelo promises to respond in kind to "la foia," to the lusty passion in Berni's poetry, and he goes on to more than hold his own in a clever set of sexual allusions and obscene double entendres. Unfortunately, his word play has escaped translators, presumably because they were unfamiliar with the period's burlesque poetry modeled after Berni's influential verse.[6] The seeming voice of the friar-painter Sebastiano addresses Berni: "To you, who are numbered among the rarest things, / I offer myself completely; do not think / that I will fail you, unless my hood falls off" (lines 52–54).

What the poetic speaker offers is allusively sexual. He will not fail – there will be no lacks or defects – unless the "cappuccio" falls. The senses are multiple here. Although he had fathered children, in November 1531 Sebastiano became a friar in order to take up the lucrative office of keeper of the papal seal ("Piombo").[7] This friar, the *capitolo* relates, will not sin (fall) unless his cowl falls, and baring a man's head was understood sexually (fig. 1).[8] Likewise, removing the hood from a hunter's falcon was a metaphor for uncapping an erect phallus so that it was ready for action.[9] Ancient Romans had already made the joke: the tops of statuettes of human figures with hooded heads could be removed, to reveal an erect phallus

[4] For hoods see Sarah Stanbury Smith, "*Game in myn hood*: the traditions of a comic proverb," *Studies in Iconography* 9 (1984), 1–12; van Beuningen, and Koldeweij (eds.), *Heilig en Profaan*, pp. 258, 304; Jones, *Secret middle ages*, pp. 70, 109, 269; Koldeweij, *Geloof & Geluk*, p. 114.

[5] Francesco Berni, *Rime*, ed. Danilo Romei (Milan: Mursia, 1985), pp. 183–85; [Michelangelo Buonarroti], *The poetry of Michelangelo*, trans. James M. Saslow (New Haven: Yale University Press, 1991), pp. 199–202.

[6] For example, Michelangelo plays on the name of the papal official Pietro Carnesecchi to imply his sodomitical activities (lines 19–21); Berni, *Rime*, p. 186.

[7] Barocchi and Ristori (eds.), *Carteggio di Michelangelo*, vol. III, p. 342; Michael Hirst, *Sebastiano del Piombo* (Oxford: Clarendon Press, 1981), pp. 122, 153.

[8] Boggione and Casalegno, *Dizionario*, pp. 234, 391 (*cappello*); François Rabelais, *Le quart livre*, ed. Robert Marichal (Geneva: Droz, 1947), p. 19 (*capussion*); Rubinstein, *Dictionary*, p. 128, citing *The merchant of Venice*, 2.6.51.

[9] Bruscagli, *Trionfi*, pp. 226, 406; Aretino, *Ragionamento*, p. 410.

underneath.[10] Late medieval lovers, male or female, indicated their amorous interest by tugging at a man's hood; in Renaissance Florence a man stealing a boy's hat or a prostitute snatching a man's hat engaged in "a sort of ritual extortion for sex."[11] The sexual innuendo of such games and gestures becomes clear if one understands the genital reference. Thus the foreskin remains unretracted and the penis limp in an anonymous Italian song written before 1508 about an aged, impotent husband: "you fall toward the ground with your head / [Still] covered with its hood."[12] To ensure that the nobleman Vincenzo Gonzaga was in no such state and could generate children, in 1583 a surgeon's examination of his genitals entailed, amongst other procedures, inspection of the testicles and manual "un-hooding" of his glans.[13]

Shape and action are also importantly combined in pendulous objects, dangling and capable of swaying backwards and forwards like a plumb line (fig. 2). Hence, the large bell in Salviati's *Triumph* (fig. 25) has a tongue or clapper with *glans*, a commonly drawn analogy that makes of the partner's body a resounding vessel.[14] Renaissance bells with sexual implications might ultimately derive from ancient tintinnabulae (fig. 7), and I suspect the profusion of bells hanging from the larger, penile elements of Roman chimes suggests a proliferation of testicles and semen, their tinkling in the wind evoking the scattering of seed. In medieval and Renaissance times, smaller, round bells containing a jingling "seed" inside were often invoked for the testicles. Indeed, in 1612 the French doctor Duval thought that semen was "full of little bells (*petites clochettes*), in which working spirits (*esprits ouvriers*) are enclosed, knowledgeable builders and makers of the human body" akin to artisans or *spiritus mechanicos*.[15] Industriously trotting along, the phalli represented on badges, some prints and a few drug jars often have a round bell around their necks (figs. 12, 14); these busy creatures surely inspired Duval's later metaphor.[16] In a case such as this, the social iconography of bells, as objects signifying more than the making of sound, percolates from popular language and imagery into medical discourse, from oral to textual registers.

To the mock-threat of castration, a character in one of Bandello's mid-sixteenth-century stories retorts that his lover should transform roosters into

10 Peter Webb, *The erotic arts*, rev. edn. (New York: Farrar Straus Giroux, 1983), figs. 39–40; Johns, *Sex or symbol?*, p. 72. Adams, *Latin sexual vocabulary*, pp. 73–74, has the foreskin being the "hood" of a "head."

11 Michael Rocke, *Forbidden friendships: homosexuality and male culture in Renaissance Florence* (Oxford University Press, 1996), p. 155; Camille, *Medieval art of love*, pp. 32, 64.

12 Prizer, "Games of Venus," 32.

13 Cipolla and Malacarne (eds.), *Più soave*, p. 436 ("lo scapellai con la mia mano").

14 Boggione and Casalegno, *Dizionario*, pp. 251–52 (*battaglio*); Jones, *Secret middle ages*, p. 269 (addressing sound but not morphology or action).

15 Duval, *Hermaphrodits*, pp. 34–35.

16 Hess, "Pleasure, shame," p. 17, fig. 1.6 (the bells are considered purely apotropaic).

capons but leave him alone, for what would he do "with the hawk without its bells?"[17] As with jokes about a genital "hood," the art of falconry informed men's erotic language in medieval and Renaissance Europe, but the image was not restricted to the aristocratic pursuit. Glass "fruits" (dildoes) delivered to the licentious nunnery in Aretino's *Ragionamento* (1534) each had "two large dangling bells that would have done honor to a tambourine."[18] Sound was singled out around 1525–26 when Vignali described in passing "great pricks [that] are always depicted with a rattle, or rather 'bell.'"[19] It is, I think, likely that the belled phallic beast represented on badges and elsewhere suited raucous moments of celebration and mockery like carnival and charivari. Bells were amongst the main noise-making objects in such "rough music" moments, which were put on to mock second marriages, especially when there was an age disparity so that the widow was thought indulgent if she was no longer able to bear children, or the remarrying widower was taking a young woman away from suitors closer to her age. The rowdy activities marked the temporary "world upside down" moment of excess at any time of the year, and in other ways re-established normative parameters.[20]

Rattles connoted not only disruption but the scattering of seed and the shaking of larger bells projected a noise caused by repetitive collision within a uterine vessel. Low-life celebrants illustrated in a fourteenth-century French manuscript of the satire *Roman de Fauvel* resort to domestic objects to create a din, shaking bells and also striking pots and pans, thereby regularly beating round forms with long, penile objects like clappers and spoons.[21] When shown in the margins of French Books of Hours, boisterously swung in groups of three by boys while those youths are being fellated, the carillon performs what a priest does in one of Firenzuola's sixteenth-century stories, "sound out a blow of glory on his bells."[22] Similarly, a friar urged marriage in Rabelais' *Pantagruel* so that

17 Bandello, *Novelle*, vol. I, p. 487.

18 Aretino, *Dialogues*, pp. 21–22; Aretino, *Ragionamento*, p. 20. For testicular bells see also Bruscagli, *Trionfi*, pp. 202–04, 225, 406; Boggione and Casalegno, *Dizionario*, pp. 372–73 (*sonagli*), 404–05. The tambourine was long considered a lascivious instrument: Seneca, *Hercules furens*, line 470; Boccaccio, *Decameron*, pp. 474, 478; Aretino, *Ragionamento*, p. 40. Annibale Carracci's timbrel in the Hercules and Omphale scene of the Galleria Farnese was "il rotondo timpano lascivo": Giovan Pietro Bellori, *Le vite de' pittori, scultori e architetti moderni*, ed. Evelina Borea (Turin: Einaudi, 1976), p. 69.

19 Vignali, *Cazzaria*, p. 125.

20 Christiane Klapisch-Zuber, *Women, family, and ritual in Renaissance Italy*, trans. Lydia Cochrane (University of Chicago Press, 1985), pp. 262, 263. For the disruption of second marriages, see also Platter, *Journal*, pp. 172–73; Natalie Zemon Davis, *Society and culture in early modern France*, rev. edn. (Cambridge: Polity Press, 1987), pp. 105–07.

21 Margaret Bent and Andrew Wathey (eds.), *Fauvel studies: allegory, chronicle, music, and image in Paris, Bibliothèque Nationale de France, MS française 146* (Oxford: Clarendon Press, 1998), Pls. VI–VII.

22 Firenzuola, *Opere*, pp. 125, 126. For the marginal figures, one in a manuscript for the young bride Jeanne d'Evreux, see Camille, "'For our devotion and pleasure'," 181, 183, figs. 5–6.

the groom could "ring out a double peal on your balls."[23] The sexual joke about bells combines morphological reference with physical action, and the metaphor also had an embodied history of lived experience because bells were familiar, rung in spires, streets and squares. To the enjoyment of sound and physical movement the pleasure of sensual touch was added on occasion, when bronze handles of small bells were cast in the form of naked, sensually curved women.[24] The limp penis and bereft state of the man carving ladles on the Italian engraving plate (fig. 55) is all the more evident because the bells on his tattered jacket have no reason to ring out.

Hoods and bells are two examples of genital metaphors which focused on shapes and actions that are not commensurate with a modern, martial and commercialized concentration on penile penetration. Removing someone's hood or ringing a bell at raucous public moments were often disruptive, eroticized acts, understood in the context of underlying historical conceptions of the body and of sexual deeds. Like tin cans tied to the back of cars marked "just married," ringing bells could mark but also release sexual tensions, although double entendre added bite to the early modern effect.

Another metaphor likened semen to ink, intercourse to writing. Cicero noted with disapproval the habit of his day that made *penicillus* (pencil) a euphemism for *penis* (a word that meant tail but had come to refer to the male organ too).[25] Censorship was allied with castration by Martial (1.35) in the first century, and his satirical picture of "the virgin sheet" of papyrus (1.66.5–8) was just one in a long line of metaphors that especially associated the codex or book with the sexually subservient and usually female but at times male body, to be opened and written upon. A riddle from Verona, dating from the eighth or early ninth century, fashions the link between writing and sexual activity by playing on the double sense of ploughing: "He yoked the oxen, ploughed white fields, and held a white plough, and sowed black seeds."[26] Having organized his fingers/testicular pair, the male body sexually "ploughs" the white parchment with a quill and his act of writing thus sows the semenotic black ink onto the feminine page. The pens and brushes of writers and artists were frequently envisaged as sexualized instruments, impressing wax tablets or directing fluids onto receptive surfaces.[27]

Despite their lesser education, women were active figures in some joking tales about writing. The empowerment of literacy was a telling synecdoche for

23 Rabelais, *Gargantua*, p. 362.
24 *Donatello e il suo tempo: il bronzetto a Padova nel Quattrocento e nel Cinquecento* (Milan: Skira, 2001), pp. 220–21; Brown, *Private lives*, p. 17 fig. 19.
25 Cicero, *Ad familiares*, 9.22.2.
26 *"The fiore" and the "Detto d'amore,"* pp. 15–16, with earlier bibliography. The identification of the plural oxen with testicles is my suggestion.
27 For example, Aretino, *Ragionamento*, p. 29, has the male brush dipped into a female "color cup."

women's sexual pleasure in one of Sermini's *novelle*, in which women learned to "guide a pen in such sweet and skillful ways (*modi*) and with such fine strokes, following all the proper rules of writing."[28] Their tutor's "inkwell (*calamajo*) was always ready, [but] the point of the pen couldn't bear so much writing." Later that century, a shorter reference to similar metaphors in Poggio's *Facetiae* represented a woman aware of jokes about the pen, and she was praised for it.[29] Asked if she wanted to send a letter to her husband, who was away on an ambassadorial mission, a noblewoman quipped: "How can I write, when my husband has taken his pen (*calamus*) away with him, and left my little writing tablets empty?" Without his semen-centric ministrations, her bivalve "book" is unwritten and she becomes illiterate in one sense, but hardly speechless, for Poggio admires her verbal wit. Women of the upper classes in such stories are represented as legitimately capable of understanding phallic and semenotic symbolism, and of using it to display their own linguistic abilities. Such women were probably in the sixteenth-century audience of a Venetian comedy, to hear the joke that a female character who wanted euphemistically to write a letter really needed the man to write with "another kind of pen than the one dipped into [literal] ink."[30]

Most often, metaphors relied on common acts and everyday technologies, focusing on repetitive, back and forth, rhythmic, abrasive motions like bowing (across a string), brushing, combing, sweeping and other acts of cleansing, filing (nails), grating, grinding, milling, pounding, digging, horse riding or scratching. Spinning and carving are two key activities endowed with a sexual sense when engraved on the fifteenth-century copper plate (fig. 55). The sexual turn given to every occupation represented there suits the verso where a copulating male–female couple is observed by a phallus bird (fig. 14). Next to the bagpiper, a woman works her distaff to spin wool onto a spindle, but this is more than a simple reference "to the opposite sex."[31]

The engraving plate's swollen spindle with its central rod projecting at either end is relatively penile in shape, and the rhythmic back-and-forth action of

28 Sermini, *Novelle*, vol. I, pp. 289–93; Valerie Martone and Robert Martone (eds. and trans.), *Renaissance comic tales of love, treachery, and revenge* (New York: Italica Press, 1994), pp. 37–41.

29 Bracciolini, *Facezie*, p. 392; trans from Bowen (ed.), *One hundred Renaissance jokes*, p. 9, though "mihi pugillare" is there given as "my inkwell."

30 Anonymous, *Venexiana*, p. 29. Toscan, *Carnaval*, p. 1134, reads *calamaio* in a sodomitical sense, and does not have an entry for *inchiostro* (ink), cf. Boggione and Casalegno, *Dizionario*, pp. 354, 381.

31 The quotation is from Konrad Oberhuber's entry on the plate, in Jay Levenson, Konrad Oberhuber and Jacquelyn Sheehan, *Early Italian engravings from the National Gallery of Art* (Washington, DC: National Gallery of Art, 1973), p. 526. The sexual potential of spinning wool is alluded to in Catherine Hess, *Italian maiolica: catalogue of the collections* (Malibu: J. Paul Getty Museum, 1988), pp. 78, 81 n. 31.

spinning alludes to coitus, the manual work to delicate fingering.[32] Inserting the man's spindle (*fuso*) into a woman's "ring," or "wheel" with a "rolling twist" had a sexual sense for Aretino.[33] Engraved into the copper is an image of a basket filled with spindles, evoking a feminine container overflowing with a penile collection, somewhat akin to a German woodcut of around the same time in which a sorceress amasses phalli in her half-open vessel.[34] Behind the spinning woman on the plate, a boy tightly holds either an actual bird or a wooden one, but this plaything has a double sense because the Italian "uccello" or bird was colloquial for the penis. This is no ordinary scene of family life on the margins.

On the left, wooden ladles are being carved, but this is about more than a generic allusion to sexual appetite, as is suggested by the shape of his drooping (jester's?) hat and the limp state of his penis. What he cannot do with a partner, he performs alone, for his menial labor with a knife alludes to sexual activity. Like Parmigianino's erotic painting of *Cupid carving his bow*, a sexually effective implement is being repetitively stroked by the knife, a tool that acts in the Aristotelian sense of masculine initiative in human reproduction, providing the form to mere matter as though its user is an artisan shaping raw materials into something greater.[35] However, the joke is exacerbated because these are people down on their luck, downcast in mien, close to the ground, despondent and disconnected, intently involved in solitary labor that is not bringing pleasure. By appreciating jokes made at the expense of the oblivious figures, the viewer is elevated to a more successful, witty status.

Each figure on the recto represents both genital morphology and sexual action. The bagpiper simultaneously expels from his genital instrument and his body, probably farting into the bucket's hole (which is itself a metaphorical *tondo*); the woman spins, fingers and inserts in a double sense; the boy clasps a "bird"; and the action of carving on the left was understood sexually, as was the phallic shape and semenotic function of the objects he fabricates. The figures are emblematic and linguistic signs more than everyday characters. The resultant

[32] For the first, but not the second point, see Alison Stewart, "Distaffs and spindles: sexual misbehavior in Sebald Beham's *Spinning bee*," in Jane Carroll and Alison Stewart (eds.), *Saints, sinners, and sisters: gender and northern art in medieval and early modern Europe* (Aldershot: Ashgate, 2003), pp. 127–54, esp. 130, 137–42. To her list of suggestive sixteenth-century portraits one can add Maerten van Heemskerck's *Portrait of a spinner* (*c.* 1529–31) from the Thyssen-Bornemisza collection: Susan Foister's entry, in Miguel Falomir (ed.), *El retrato del Renacimiento* (Madrid: Museo Nacional del Prado, 2008), pp. 264–65, 483.

[33] Aretino, *Ragionamento*, pp. 143, 228. The "crooked spindles" of wives referred to cuckoldry: Aretino, *Marescalco*, in *Commedie*, p. 56. See also Toscan, *Carnaval*, pp. 1293–95 (*filare*, *fuso* and *rocca*), 1336 (*cesta*) and passim; Boggione and Casalegno, *Dizionario*, pp. 235, 395.

[34] Zika, *Appearance of witchcraft*, fig. 2.3.

[35] On carving and knives in a sexual sense, see Bowen, "Metaphorical obscenity," 336; Simons, "Bodily fluids," 350, with further references.

print is not a rebus but it is a pictorial riddle about the multiplicity of erotic metaphor.

Cooking and eating

Examination of metaphors attached to the preparation and consumption of food continues the project of discerning patterns of social iconography, in which the interweaving of words, images and embodied practices created a logic or continuity between different metaphors and registers of discourse, far beyond the merely Latinate, learned or allegorical. Rather than regarding images of foodstuffs, market scenes and cooking as either high-flown allegory (presumptively asexual and sober) or straightforward genre scenes, recently art historians concentrate on them as astute statements about the value and commercialization of art and artistic identity.[36] Some of the pictures examined here are hybrids, combining artistic commentary with low life *and* with sexual humor that is informed by mainstream medical learning and cultural habits going back to antiquity. The act of coitus was associated with ingredients, heat, motions and implements from the technological sphere of the kitchen. It entailed more than straightforward penetration by a simple or single organ, for the spit skewering delectable, heated flesh was not the only kind of metaphor cooked up in the kitchen. Hunger or sexual appetite was assuaged by a variety of objects performing numerous actions.

In premodern medical theory, the body was a cooking machine producing a variety of fluids infused with different "spirits" (*pneumata*). Through "concoction" or "digestion" the body was nourished and excess blood transmuted into seed (discarded menses in the case of women, valuable semen in the instance of men). Jean Fernel's cookery analogy was particularly vivid, having the semen "clotted and whitened by heat" and becoming foamy with "vital spirit" though "bubbles can barely be seen in it, anymore than in butter."[37] The basic Hippocratic model presented sperm as having "the power of humidifying and heating" female bodies and characterized the gravid uterus as an oven.[38] Furthermore, diet was one of the most important non-naturals in complexional medicine, a factor that people could manage in their everyday lives as well as with the guidance of health manuals and professional consultations.

36 See, in particular, Honig, *Painting and the market*, and Silver, *Peasant scenes and landscapes*. For a recent overview of "erotic appetites" in paintings of food see John Varriano, *Tastes and temptations: food and art in Renaissance Italy* (Berkeley: University of California Press, 2009), pp. 118–40.

37 Fernel, *Physiologia*, p. 547. On diet in humoral medicine, see Ken Albala, *Eating right in the Renaissance* (Berkeley: University of California Press, 2002), esp. pp. 143–54.

38 "On generation" (4.3), in *Hippocratic treatises*, p. 3; Lemay, *Women's secrets*, p. 147.

To "eat" or "devour" sometimes alluded to oral sex but the verbs also worked as metaphors for the greedy consumption of sexual pleasures more broadly. In ancient Greece, bread and cakes were baked in genital shapes; many foods and the act of eating provided sexual metaphors. Female pudenda were edibles like figs, roast meat or pastries, their fluids compared to soups, sauces or juices.[39] "To eat" in a sexual sense was vulgar slang in ancient Latin due to the presumptive taboo against oral sex, which continued for millennia.[40] Christian discourse paired the sins of Gluttony and Lust since both were material indulgences that required the pleasuring of the physical body for their enactment. Lust and concupiscence were fueled by the sustenance of the body, just as the Fall resulted from the eating of forbidden fruit. In some Italian poems and songs, the very space of the *cucina*, the kitchen, was metaphorically the locale for sodomy ("a dish for the great masters" according to Aretino), while reproductive sex was confined to the *camera*, or bedroom.[41]

Regardless of Church disapproval, the pagan gods partied on in elite circles, pictorially brought to life in paintings like Giovanni Bellini's *Feast of the gods* for the Duke of Ferrara (1514), Raphael's banquet for the wedding of Cupid and Psyche on the ceiling of the garden loggia of the Chigi villa in Rome (*c.* 1519), or Giulio Romano's fresco of the same subject in the Marquis of Mantua's palace on the outskirts of town, the Palazzo del Te (*c.* 1525–35). Sensual pleasures were accentuated by sexual metaphors, like Bellini's satyr carrying on his head a vase with a genital neck, or the vegetal joke about genitals in Raphael's border (fig. 53). In palaces and taverns, the pleasures of meals consumed by courtiers, scholars and artisans could include sexual companionship, obscene jokes and after-dinner speeches. The word play, high jinks, music either refined or rudimentary and theatrical buffoonery on stage or between courses engendered a pleasant mood of indulgence and amusement, which might or might not lead on to sexual activities or abuse. The appetite for food was considered interchangeable with the desire for sex, and a pleasurable feast was the answer for each. In the words of a Roman gentleman in Aretino's comedy *Cortigiana* first staged in 1525, "I feed myself with the memory of my lady. I crave nothing else to satisfy my hunger."[42] And the courtier-poet Ariosto warned that an unmarried man's foraging for sex would escalate from "pecking

[39] Henderson, *Maculate muse*, pp. 47, 61, 65, 117–20, 134–36, 144–45, 180.

[40] Adams, *Latin sexual vocabulary*, pp. 138–41; Toscan, *Carnaval*, pp. 1152–53 (*appetito*), 1212–13 (*mangiare*), 1219–20 (*gusto*), 1299–1300 (*montone*), 1436–51 (various fruits), 1663 (*arrosto*), 1676 (*carne*), 1692 (*fame*) and passim; Boggione and Casalegno, *Dizionario*, pp. 11–24, 328, and passim; Ch. 6 above for female sexual appetite.

[41] Aretino, *Ragionamento*, p. 49; Toscan, *Carnaval*, pp. 1351–53.

[42] Aretino, *Cortigiana*, ed. Innamorati, p. 115; *Cortigiana*, trans. Douglas Campbell and Leonard Sbrocchi (Ottawa: Dovehouse, 2003), p. 125.

at someone else's meat" to ever-increasing gluttony, lusting after richer and larger game birds day by day.[43]

Accompanied by witty or bawdy entertainments and conversation, much of the eating primarily enabled male bonding, which had both homosocial and homoerotic possibilities. These elements are evident in a Latin poem from early sixteenth-century Rome, filled with double entendres and even some Greek loan words used for genital allusions.[44] Yet this verse of Fabio Vigile, later bishop of Spoleto, has been read as merely a "sort of mock satire" or "mock invective" on the genre of banquet speeches, without any sexual connotations. Taken at face value, the poem celebrates a gathering of humanists who have forced Blosio Palladio (also later a bishop) to mount a lavish *symposium* in reparation for having been caught by Paolo Giovio "dining alone upon a huge pheasant."

But the bird was more than a bird. The text's five references to the always-capitalized Pheasant gratuitously add that it is a bird. One can imagine special, even drawn-out vocal emphasis at these points in the recitation, emphasizing what was not obvious to its twentieth-century readers. Not only was the generic Italian "bird" slang for cock, but the male pheasant was a vernacular staple too for the male genitals.[45] Emphatically, Blosio has been seen – that witnessing is emphasized by *vidi ego . . . vidi* – "alone" in an act of pleasure. This most likely means masturbation, though that deed could hardly have been remarkable, so it might indicate that Blosio had not shared his latest conquest and was caught performing oral sex with a well-endowed youth. The imprecision is part of the poem's witty suggestiveness. Around the same time, both Aretino and Ariosto attacked the hypocrisy of elite men in Rome, such as clerics, who greedily dined sumptuously and alone in order to avoid sharing, so Blosio's selfishness was of political and ethical import too.[46]

For this ambiguous *crimen* (also repeated), *stigma* or stain (*macula*) Blosio has to endure the mock humiliation of a convivial banquet with friends. There was to be no more supping alone for Blosio. Never again should he commit "so foul a deed / As to devour a bird of Phasis, by yourself alone, / In secret voraciousness, forgetful of your old friend Jovius / Nor mindful of any of

[43] *Ludovico Ariosto, The satires of Ludovico Ariosto*, trans. Peter DeSa Wiggins (Athens: Ohio University Press, 1976), pp. 124–25.

[44] See T. C. Price Zimmermann and Saul Levin, "Fabio Vigile's *Poem of the pheasant*: humanist conviviality in Renaissance Rome," in P. A. Ramsey (ed.), *Rome in the Renaissance: the city and the myth* (Binghamton: Medieval and Renaissance Texts and Studies, 1982), pp. 265–78, including 273–77 for the poem; T. C. Price Zimmermann, *Paolo Giovio: the historian and the crisis of sixteenth-century Italy* (Princeton University Press, 1995), pp. 64–65. It can be dated between 1512, when Giovio arrived in Rome, and the Sack of Rome in 1527.

[45] Bruscagli, *Trionfi*, pp. 438–40; Toscan, *Carnaval*, pp. 231, 798, 1544–45. Palladio's pheasant is an *avis* or winged (*volucrem*) at lines 38, 43, 67, 161, 180. At these points, the *privata* and *solus* nature of the offense is also stressed (and at lines 2, 53). The verbs for "dining" are all about voracious consumption and wastage (*voro*, *comedo*, *exedo* and *abstuleris*, lines 2, 38, 44, 69, 181).

[46] Ariosto, *Satires*, pp. 32–33 (*c.* 1517); Aretino, *Cortigiana*, ed. Innamorati, p. 65.

your companions!" (lines 42–46). To avoid public humiliation and eternal blight (creeping vines will reject his "stakes," "fish" will not swim, and so on), he will have to pay dearly. Hence, the banquet will lay before them delicacies such as sausages and pigs' balls. Like the represented feast, the poem is a rhetorical exercise in ironic periphrasis, piling on more words than necessary in order to conceal, as Quintilian understood, "something which would be indecent (*deformia*), if expressed in so many words."[47] In general, the plethora of words and depicted edibles, evident also in market stalls and kitchen scenes, provide delectable "feasts" which have more than one meaning.

Sex in the kitchen

Due to its necessary heat and supply of liquids as well as the types of motions and metamorphoses performed there, the kitchen was a locus for sexual metaphors. Hence, for instance, a secular badge depicts the male genitals turning on a spit over a vulval fire that also serves as a grease trap for the released "juices" (fig. 13). Spoons and ladles were sexual signs, carved by the deflated fellow in the northeast Italian engraving plate (fig. 55). The ladle resembles a phallus because it has a long stem and a larger, curved bulb at one end. The hooks of the pictured ladles result from easy, cheap manufacture, though in the *Decameron* and elsewhere they refer to genital cleaving by male barbs.[48] What has not been understood is that morphological resemblance is complemented by function: the ladle dipped in and out, in and out, transferring fluids to a vessel. The action is metaphorically appropriate for the fundamental semen-centric pattern, upheld in Hippocratic, Aristotelian and Galenic systems, that the female vessel was irrigated, watered, refreshed, by liquid that was delivered by male genitals. In the comedic version of a rural Dionysia in Aristophanes' *Acharnians*, performed on the Athenian stage in 425 BCE, at the beginning of a scene in which a phallus will be raucously processed, a nubile woman requests: "Mother, hand me up the broth ladle, so I can pour broth over this cake" (245–46). The lines continue the phallus joke, ensuring that the processed object is regarded in a sexual and earthy sense rather than with ritual piety. The ladle will transfer "sauce" or "soup" and pour the fluid over her "cake" or genitals.[49] The theatrical

[47] Quintilian, *Institutio Oratoria*, 8.6.60.

[48] Florio, *Queen Anna's new world of words*, p. 46 (*attaccare l'uncino*); Boggione and Casalegno, *Dizionario*, p. 227 (*uncino*) (and for foods and food preparation, see pp. 11–24, 289–303, 313–19 and passim). I thank Maureen Cox for her point about the economics of the handiwork.

[49] For the various words in ancient Greek see Henderson, *Maculate muse*, p. 145. There is also the call for a wine ladle immediately after a phallic alabastron has been handled: Aristophanes, *Acharnians*, 1069–70. For the Latin ladle, see Adams, *Latin sexual vocabulary*, p. 23, and for "soup" in Italian and Dutch, Boggione and Casalegno, *Dizionario*, p. 352; Dekker, *Humour in Dutch culture*, p. 102.

joke worked with equipment and innuendo that were present in contemporary Dionysian imagery. Several fifth-century BCE Greek vase paintings show women attending to the mixing and distribution of liquids, one or more with a ladle in hand. Some stand either side of a large Dionysian herm but all dip into stamnoi that rest on a table, which occasionally has round cakes heaped high in front of the herm. The stamnos was a pot for liquids, chiefly used for storage and mixing, and it was the very form of the red-figure pot on which these ladles are depicted.[50] On the one hand showing women engaged in a serious ritual, on the other hand the image of ladling women could amuse wine drinkers using the actual stamnos, entertaining them with double entendres during their own feast.

The evocative ladle survived beyond ancient Greece, along with the basic medical model of sexual concourse. In Florio's Italian–English dictionary of 1598, "a skope [scoop] or a ladle" was *cazza*, providing the potential for plays with *cazzo*, the word for "a mans privie member."[51] *Cazzuto* meant "a man that hath a pricke" (presumably the men without one were being addressed more decorously); *cazzuola* and *cazzetta* meant "a little ladle. Also a bricklayers trowell." The combination of phonetic concurrence and morphological similarity with the male genitals was cleverly tied in at the lexical level with the instrumental function of transferring fluid or wet substances like semen, soup, plaster or mortar.

Sexual play with words and images characterized the Florentine Compagnia della Cazzuola, a convivial sodality formed in 1512 to stage fancy-dress banquets and theatrical entertainments such as Pluto's wedding to Persephone in hell or racy comedies like Bibbiena's *Calandra*, Ariosto's *Suppositi* and Machiavelli's *Mandragola*. Musicians and artists who provided the stage backdrops and other devices were "minore" members or associates (*aderenti*).[52] Class distinctions were marked by costumes that members donned for the Cazzuola's parties, and their club's emblem, as recorded by the artist Giorgio Vasari, represented a trowel or small ladle (*cazzuola*) surrounded by little tadpoles (*cazzuole* in Tuscan) so it visually suggested a hierarchy between a

[50] There are at least eleven surviving stamnoi showing the Dionysian ladles listed in the Beazley Archive (www.beazley.ox.ac.uk/) as numbers 207187–90, 207192–93, 207195, 207286–87, 214430, 215254.

[51] Florio, *Worlde of wordes (1598)*, p. 65. For the ladle as a metaphor of the penis/genitals, see Williams, *Dictionary*, pp. 775–76; Toscan, *Carnaval*, pp. 92, 591–92; Boggione and Casalegno, *Dizionario*, pp. 215–16, 236–37.

[52] Giorgio Vasari, *Le vite de' più eccellenti pittori, scultori ed architettori*, ed. Gaetano Milanesi, 8 vols., 1878–85, rpt. (Florence: Sansoni, 1906, and Florence: Sansoni, 1973), vol. VI, pp. 437, 609–19. For the Compagnia della Cazzuola, and that of the Paiuolo, see Tommaso Mozzati, *Giovanfrancesco Rustici: le Compagnie del Paiuolo e della Cazzuola: arte, letteratura, festa nell'età della maniera* (Florence: Olschki, 2008), pp. 191–331; Sanne Wellen, "*La Guerra de' topi e de' ranocchi* attributed to Andrea del Sarto: considerations on the poem's authorship, the Compagnia del Paiuolo, and Vasari," *I Tatti Studies* 12 (2009), 181–232.

large center and smaller acolytes. Vasari noted that tadpoles "have a large head and a tail" (*capo* and *coda*), which alludes to penile morphology and terminology (*coda* meant both tail and penis), as well as echoing the basic shape of a ladle, so erotic byplay was implied by a larger *cazza* amidst busily attentive *cazzuole*.[53]

The more usual name for tadpoles, *botticine*, could also mean small barrels or "the hole of a privy or jakes" and just such a hole is visible under the bagpipe player in the engraving plate (fig. 55), which indicates yet another one of the image's verbal jokes to be deciphered by the discerning viewer.[54] Bodily types of the round form or *tondo* (buttocks and anus) intimately meet another kind. Visual and word play with the company's emblem created various combinations and suggestions, one of them being the homoerotic allusion that big "ladles" were dipped into the holes or barrels of those with smaller "ladles."

The ladle/trowel was adopted as their name when a group at a garden party in 1512 enjoyed the sight of a trowel shoveling lime instead of ricotta into a man's mouth. Their instant delight, as they shouted "cazzuola, cazzuola," indicated that a witticism came to mind. The founding members of the banqueting society of artisans were doing more than punning on a combination of food and craft. The trowel (*cazzuola*) featured as one of the chief sexual allusions in the carnival song of *muratori* or masons, as a phallic instrument "cleaning up" old "houses," filling in "holes" and applying a fresh coat of "plaster."[55] The song is usually attributed to the surgeon and herald Jacopo da Bientina, who was associated with the group.[56] I suggest that a similar double or even triple entendre was at work in 1512. A literal builder's trowel should indeed handle lime, whereas the ladle would be an appropriate utensil for ricotta, which had been a metaphor for semen since at least the 1430s.[57] The butt of the joke should have remembered the double meaning of the word *cazzuola* and therefore been wary of the white substance headed for his mouth, all the time alert to the phonetic hint that a *cazzo* can deposit yet a third kind of white matter.

This word play likely informs a painting attributed to Vincenzo Campi (1580s), which shows three peasants taking large scoops from a mound of

[53] Vasari, *Vite*, vol. VI, p. 612. As their name implies, the Compagnia del Paiuolo (cauldron) excelled in fancy culinary preparation, at which double entendre was sometimes in play: Vasari, *Vite*, vol. VI, pp. 609–13 passim; Toscan, *Carnaval*, pp. 1414–15 (*paiuolo*), 1578 (*chiavare* and *chiave*), and passim. The goldsmith and engraver Cristofano Robetta turned a calf's head into an anvil, and that object was understood as the recipient of genitally masculine blows (see below). Artists could have merrily hammered on the anvil with their spoons or ladles before carving the meat.

[54] Florio, *Worlde of wordes (1598)*, p. 47.

[55] Bruscagli, *Trionfi*, p. 228. See Ch. 7 for "cleaning" metaphors.

[56] Vasari, *Vite*, vol. VI, p. 613; Mozzati, *Rustici*, pp. 299–303, 369–70.

[57] Boggione and Casalegno, *Dizionario*, p. 357.

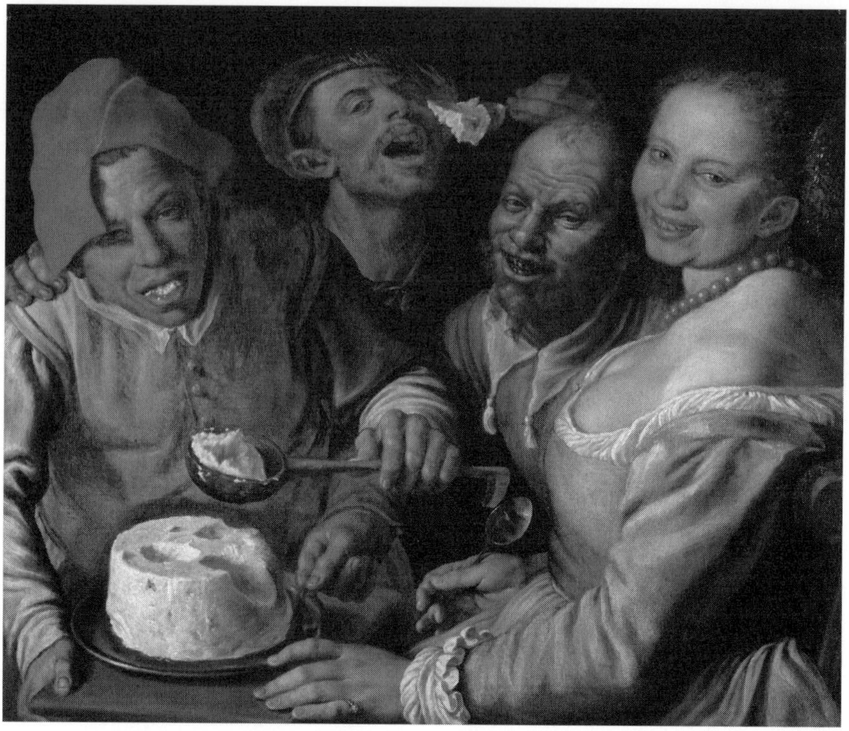

Figure 56 Vincenzo Campi, *The ricotta eaters*, 1580s, oil on canvas, 770 × 890 mm, Lyon, Musée des Beaux-Arts

ricotta, about to be joined by a voluptuous woman whose dress, rouge and familiarity with the viewer suggests she may be a prostitute (fig. 56).[58] Three of the characters hold spoons, but the dullard on the far left has been so greedy that he has used a ladle and hence his mouth overflows with the white cheese. Popular enough to exist in at least six copies, the seemingly inconsequential genre scene is probably the one identified as a "buffonaria" in the will of the painter's widow in 1611. The fly pictured on the ricotta dares viewers to attempt to brush it away, and the manner in which the figures look out at

[58] Barry Wind, "Pitture ridicole: some late Cinquecento comic genre paintings," *Storia dell'arte* 20 (1974), 27–28, 30; Franco Paliaga and Bram de Klerck, *Vincenzo Campi* (Soncino: Edizioni del Soncino, 1997), pp. 140, 145, 176–77, 184–85, 195, 270 ("una buffonaria"), figs. 46, 59, Pls. XXIV, XXXV; Franco Paliaga (ed.), *Vincenzo Campi: scene del quotidiano* (Milan: Skira, 2000), pp. 21, 26, 160–61, 220; Stefania Biancani's entry, in Martina Corgnati (ed.), *Le immagini affamate: donne e cibo e nell'arte: dalla natura morta ai disordini alimentari* (Aosta: Museo Archeologico Regionale, 2005), p. 178 (the restored version in a private collection).

viewers while grinning further involves the audience in what is presented as an especially witty joke focused on low-life habits. The buffoonery may consist of straightforward class ridicule, but a sexual subtext probably came to the mind of most viewers as well. Many associated ricotta with semen, an idea surely derived from the widely known medical analogy between the production of semen and cheese, along with similarities in the properties of color and consistency.[59]

The ladle served another joint sexual and culinary function, that of mixing. In both Greek and Latin a verb for sexual intercourse also meant the mixing of liquids.[60] The Italian word *mescola* begins to make this evident, defined by Florio as "a masons or carpenters squire ruler or plummet, a bricklayers trowell. Also a plummers melting ladle, anie kind of ladle or great spoon . . . Also a medlie, a mixture, a blending, a mesh, a hochpoch. Also taken for a foolish idle huswife."[61] In the semenotic system, sexual intercourse was likened to the mixing of liquids, and the "ladle" facilitated this blending, of two seeds in the uterine vessel. Such was the model in the Hippocratic treatise on the seed and in Galenic theory, continuing into anatomical texts from medieval Salerno and Avicenna's *Canon* and on to sixteenth- and seventeenth-century texts like Marinello's gynecological text and Sharp's midwifery.[62] Explaining the sex determination of the embryo according to ratios of the mixture of male and female seed, the *Anatomia Magistri Nicolai Physici* made the analogy with everyday experience especially clear, observing that "the same thing can be seen in water and wine." Spoons were also understood as sexual, though their action was more a matter of stirring than mixing two different fluids. Stirring a stew or polenta involved the insertion of a long object into a pot, but it also alluded to repetitive motion and swaying hips, the addition of heat and the slow concoction of an appetizing reward.[63]

59 For example, Boggione and Casalegno, *Dizionario*, p. 357. As an example of the metaphor, see *Problemes of Aristotle*, E 2v: "The seede of the father and the mother doth goe into the substance of the childe in the wombe: because that as creame doth goe into the substance of cheese, so the seede of man into the fruite in the wombe like unto the creame, and the flowers [menses] of the woman doth enter in like unto the milke." See below for more on cheese.

60 "On generation," in *Hippocratic treatises*, p. 3; Adams, *Latin sexual vocabulary*, pp. 180–81.

61 Florio, *Worlde of wordes (1598)*, p. 224; Florio, *Queen Anna's new world of words*, p. 310; Aretino, *Ragionamento*, p. 47; Toscan, *Carnaval*, pp. 373 (*mischia*), 1299 (*mescola*), 1413–14 (*mestola*); Boggione and Casalegno, *Dizionario*, pp. 55–58, 220–21.

62 See Ch. 6 above; also Adams, *Latin sexual vocabulary*, pp. 180–81; Avicenna, *Liber canonis*, 351v (Bk. III, fen. 20, tr. 1, ch. 1, "commixiione"); *Anatomia Magistri Nicolai Physici*, in Corner, *Anatomical texts*, p. 86; *Anatomia vivorum*, in Corner, *Anatomical texts*, p. 105; Lemay, *Women's secrets*, p. 65; Marinello, *Medicine*, fol. 56r ("si mescola"); Sharp, *Midwives book*, p. 75; Jacquart and Thomasset, *Sexuality and medicine*, pp. 62–63.

63 For the penile spoon see, for example, Williams, *Dictionary*, p. 1291; Christa Grössinger, *Humour and folly in secular and profane prints of northern Europe, 1430–1540* (London: Harvey Miller, 2002), p. 91. For the stew see Vasvari, "Battle," 7, for the polenta, anonymous, *Venexiana*, p. 61.

An especially inventive invective by an English medical practitioner demonstrates the ubiquity and memorable nature of the ladle metaphor. In 1597, the barber and surgeon Richard Lichfield used the ladle for one of his satirical metaphors to suggest how much he was going to "trim" his opponent Thomas Nashe, virtually castrating him with razor, lance and pen. "I will stirre thee up and make thee seething hot, and when thou art in thy heate, I will then quell thee by mooving of thee more and more, as when a pot seetheth if we lade it and moove the liquor up and down, even while it seetheth, wee shall make it quiet."[64] First the phallic ladle will stir his opponent into passion, and then it will bring the rage off the boil. The image of erotic "mooving" may have particularly struck him as apposite because he had medical training and would have known the Hippocratic image of pouring spermatic fluid on a heated woman's womb to cool her passion (*On generation*, 4). Lichfield will "quell thee" by inserting his phallic instrument into a youngster's heated fluid and move it around so much that the lad will quieten. Rather than the anticipated orgasm, Lichfield suggests that Nashe will feel a lesser pleasure, more akin to that of the penetrated, poured-upon woman.

Imagery played an active part in disseminating the unequal two-seed theory. For instance, the placement of a thin-necked, wide-bodied flask near a ladle at a refreshing well in the engraving of the *Large Garden of Love* by Master E. S. (*c.* 1465) probably refers to the feminine vessel that will be filled by the masculine ladle.[65] Stirring the waters is a central feature in Titian's reinvention of the Garden of Love theme, his so-called *Sacred and profane love* (fig. 52). The winged god of love directly performs the vital mixing of male and female fluids. The ladle, like the distaff, was also deployed as a sign of female domesticity and simultaneously as a "phallic" symbol of appropriated power, put to use in a topsy turvy world. Thus, a woman can be shown acting perversely when she beats her husband with a ladle. On a ballad sheet collected by Pepys, a female scold raises her hefty ladle when fighting with her husband over possession of the symbolic breeches, outweighing his far less effectual stick.[66]

Amusing stories and visual jokes were also told about the tapping of barrels or the turning of a tap's stop-cock (valve). In Albrecht Dürer's woodcut of the *Men's bath-house* (fig. 57) a man's genitals are wittily placed immediately behind a tap that is decorated in the form of a cock (in German, *Hahn* meant cockerel, tap and

64 Richard Lichfield, *The trimming of Thomas Nash 1597*, facsimile (Menston, Yorkshire: Scolar Press, 1973), E1r.

65 Grössinger, *Humour and folly*, fig. 44. The cook's spoon ("Kochlöffel") was sexual: Mezger, *Narrenidee und Fastnachtsbrauch*, pp. 207, 540 n. 61.

66 *The jolly widower* (Pepys, *Diary*, vol. IV, p. 102); also *The cuckold's complaint*, in which the refrain runs "the world is turn'd upside down" (*ibid.*, p. 132); for other examples, including a misericord, see Jones, *Secret middle ages*, pp. 97, 102, 230, 236.

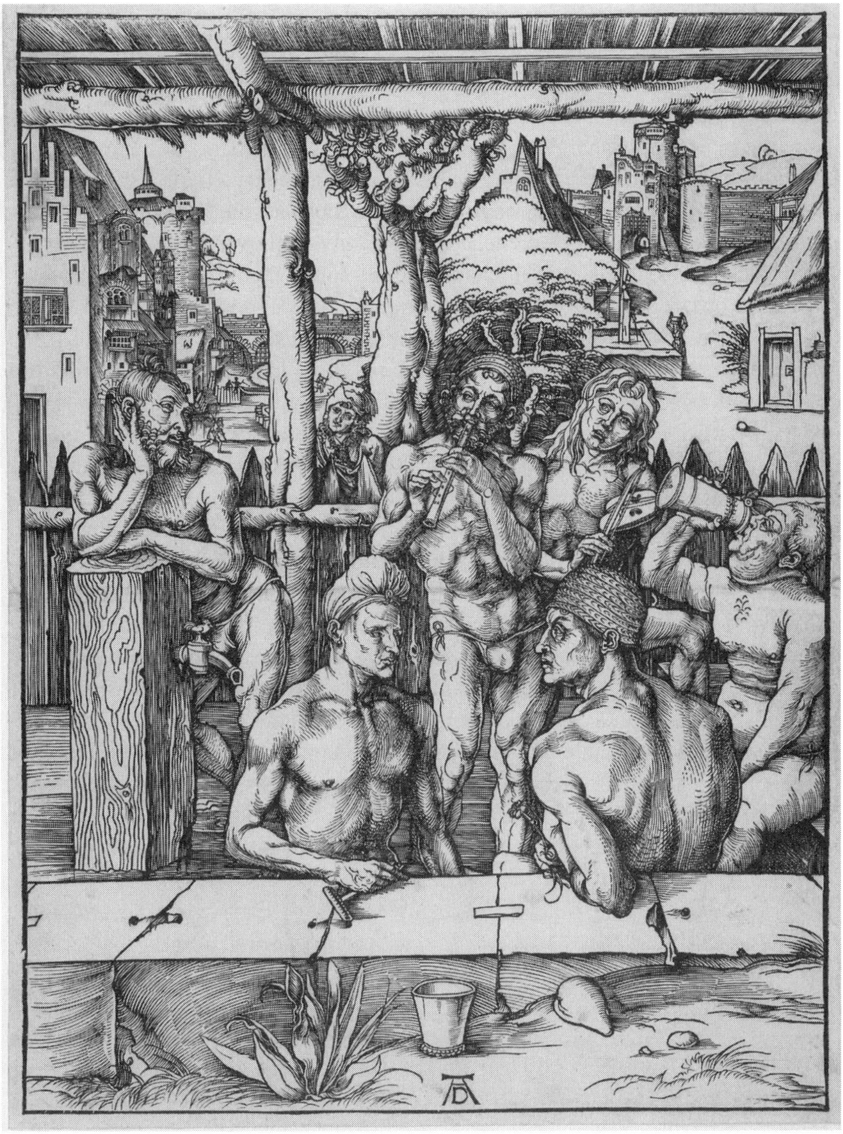

Figure 57 Albrecht Dürer, *Men's bath-house*, *c*. 1496, woodcut, 388 × 282 mm, London, British Museum

penis).[67] Actual faucets in the shape of cockerels survive; using these mechanisms would have set up a feedback loop between linguistic, medical and practical connotations. Ostensible masking or coyness performed by the depicted cockerel-topped outlet is overcome in Dürer's woodcut by the punning layers of the pictorial metaphor that resonate with linguistic multivalence. The print almost flirts wittily with viewers, teasing them with allusions (including the tree with "arms" raised behind the enclosure as well as the punning *Hahn* and the silent music) just as erotic gazes are exchanged between men within the image.

Rabelais' fictive character Gargantua referred to his "petite dille" in adolescence (1.11), a word defined by Cotgrave's French–English dictionary of 1611 as "the Quill, or Fawcet of a Hogshead," that is, a feather pen with ink or the spigot of a large cask.[68] The underlying logic of such jokes assumed that erotic activity could be conceived in terms of the expulsion and transfer of liquids. Semen was represented metaphorically in a variety of other bodily substances, especially blood, marrow, milk, spit or urine, and it was likened to such fluids as oil, sap, sauce, water and wine.[69] Sometime in the mid-1630s to late 1640s, the Le Strange family of Norfolk was entertained with a joke about an adulterous husband's beer "barrel" drained dry by his servant who claimed that she merely enjoyed "a draught of the Best."[70]

One of the double entendres that amused the ladies at the end of the fifth day in Boccaccio's *Decameron* relied on the image of a pipe inserted into a large vessel. All that the entertainer Dioneo did was deliver a line from a popular song, "Monna Simona, *imbotta imbotta*" (embarrel, that is, fill the barrel, put wine in your cask) and yet the Queen told him to change his tune.[71] Readers of Boccaccio's infamous tale gained a clear notion that coitus was about inserting funnels or pipes into casks or bottles for the purpose of transferring fluids, and that to take virginity was akin to unsealing or tapping a keg. Thus, for instance, Vignali's scabrous *Cazzaria* used the metaphor of placing a tap in a barrel.[72]

[67] Baskett, *Parts of the body*, p. 109; Edgar Wind, "Dürer's *Männerbad*," *Journal of the Warburg Institute* 2 (1939), 269; Jones, *Secret middle ages*, p. 50 (for a surviving tap).

[68] Cotgrave, *Dictionarie*, s.v. Erhard Schön wittily makes the joke literal by depicting a pissing fountain figure who lifts his garments to reveal that the fluid is pouring from the beak of a long-necked bird/cock: Walter Strauss, *The illustrated Bartsch 13 (Commentary): German masters of the sixteenth century: Erhard Schoen, Niklas Stoer* (New York: Abaris Books, 1984), pp. 358–59.

[69] Toscan, *Carnaval*, pp. 1243–44, 1595–96, 1658, 1723–24, 1753, 1755, and passim; Boggione and Casalegno, *Dizionario*, pp. 351–62. For urine, water and wine see Simons, "Bodily fluids"; for foamy beer, see Ch. 1 above.

[70] Le Strange, *Merry passages and jeasts*, pp. 77–78.

[71] Boccaccio, *Decameron*, p. 381. For Italian, see Toscan, *Carnaval*, pp. 1666 (*barile*), 1607 (*botte*), 1695 (*fiasco*), 1705 (*imbottare*); Boggione and Casalegno, *Dizionario*, pp. 127, 213, 218–19, 390.

[72] Vignali, *Cazzaria*, p. 65. For two views of women being tapped by devils, see James Mills, "Sexuality in the Danish medieval wall-paintings," in Helen Rodnite Lemay (ed.), *Homo carnalis: the carnal aspect of medieval human life* (Binghamton: Center for Medieval and Early Renaissance Studies, State University of New York at Binghamton, 1987), pp. 133 (*c.* 1450), 138 and fig. 5.

And, adapting the Hippocratic metaphor about a woman's flaming fluids cooled by the application of male liquid, the French courtier Brantôme imagined that an aroused woman was dosed by her lover's "little pipette" (*petite burette*) with "that good water that is sweet enough without sugar."[73] Numerous putti represented as cheerfully filling their drinking bowls with wine pouring forth from a cask are thus, in one sense, about to savour the fruits of a "virginal" harvest, though the all-male merriment and the multivalence of flowing fluids also allow a same-sex interpretation of the indulgence.[74] The long-necked glass flask filled with red wine that rests on a peasant's lap in a composition of *Bean eaters* attributed to Vincenzo Campi's design is placed so that the vessel's neck rears up like a large erection.[75] His smiling female companion points across at the man, whose wide-open mouth is ready to receive another spoonful of beans, the food renowned for its capacity to produce the kind of "wind" or *pneuma* that is a key component of semen (along with the flask's fluid) and produces an erection. More commonly, a vessel or vase was a medical metaphor for the uterus, informing visual representations from Praxiteles' Knidian *Aphrodite* standing beside a large jug holding water for her bath, to Parmigianino's *Madonna of the long neck* replete with a bulbous vase echoing her form. If to be female was to have an interior vessel for receiving fluids, to be male was to produce, eject and deliver those liquids.

Vessels of various kinds complement hanging sausages in the background of a kitchen scene engraved in Rome by Ambrogio Brambilla in 1583 (fig. 58).[76] Characters reminiscent of the theatrical repertoire of the *commedia dell'arte* are busy preparing what an inscription calls the "feast of Zan Trippu when he marries"; both the explicit occasion and the performative tradition readily lend themselves to sexual innuendo, further signaled by a fumbling attempt at seduction by the character labeled Zan Zaccagni on the right. Oversized noses on the three male characters are shaded darkly, as though they are fake, red

[73] Brantôme, *Dames galantes*, p. 30.

[74] See, for example, Marco Zoppo's "Parchment book" in the British Museum and Michelangelo's red chalk drawing of *The children's bacchanal* in Windsor; for the theme of wine, water and semen see Simons, "Bodily fluids."

[75] Paliaga and de Klerck, *Vincenzo Campi*, pp. 121–22, 201, 203–04, 231–32, 266; *Rabisch. Il grottesco nell'arte del Cinquecento: L'Accademia della Val di Blenio Lomazzo e l'ambiente milanese* (Milan: Skira, 1998), pp. 196, 203–04 (for various copies, including an early seventeenth-century one by an anonymous Netherlandish artist); Paliaga (ed.), *Vincenzo Campi: scene del quotidiano*, pp. 156–59 (for the figure and his flask in a signed painting of *Fish sellers* in a private collection).

[76] For the print, but not its sexual humor, see Wind, "Pitture ridicole," 30–31; M. A. Katrizky, "Italian comedians in Renaissance prints," *Print Quarterly* 4 (1987), 246–48; Franco Paliaga's entry on the print in *Rabisch*, pp. 176, 183; Stefania Biancani's entry, in *Le immagini affamate*, pp. 178–79; M. A. Katritzky, *The art of 'Commedia': a study in the 'Commedia dell'Arte' 1560–1620 with special reference to the visual records* (Amsterdam: Rodopi, 2006), pp. 114–17, 189, 190, 207, 248, 257.

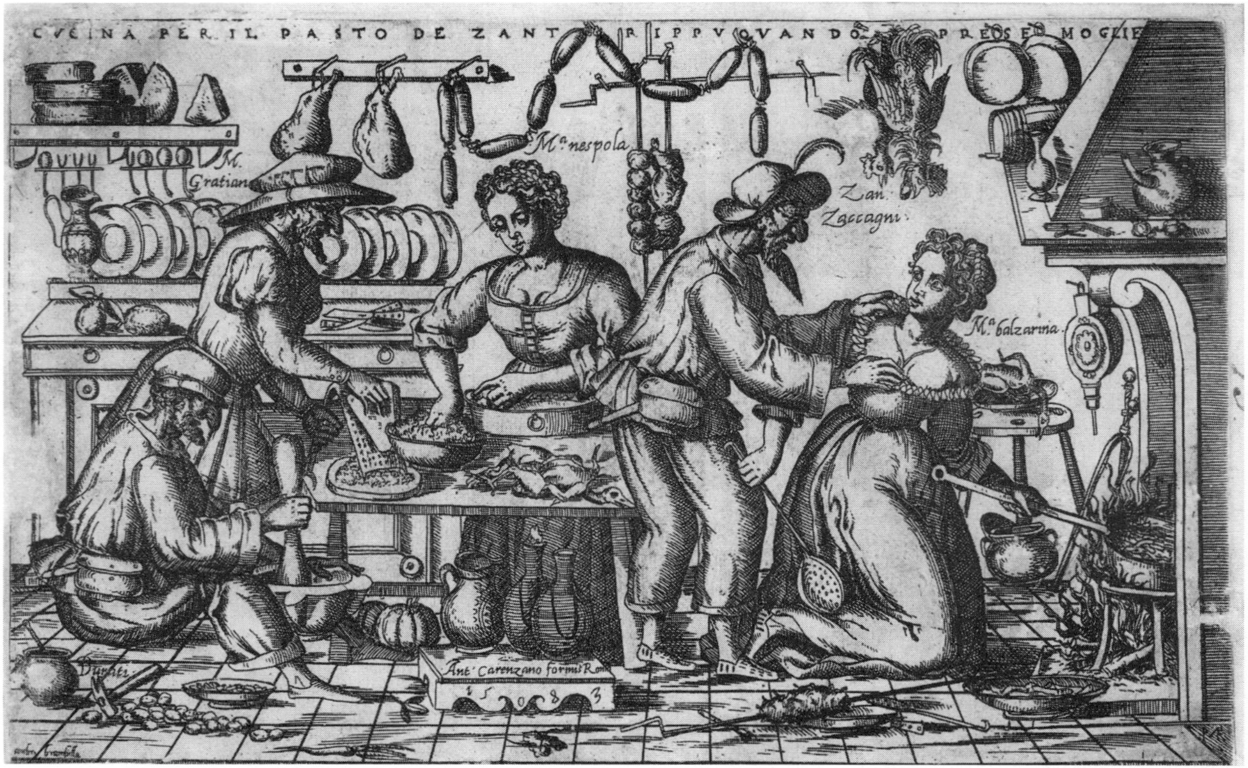

Figure 58 Ambrogio Brambilla, *Kitchen for the feast of Zan Trippu when he marries*, signed and dated 1583, Rome, Biblioteca Teatrale del Burcardo

protuberances, befitting the common association of the penis with the nose. Most of the objects and actions displayed call sexual double entendres to mind, including the barrel with a spigot on the mantelpiece, the dried and skewered meats, the panoply of birds in general and their various drooping necks in particular, several spits, the hanging cockerels (or capons?) and a pot with a spoon inserted on the floor to the far left. Sausages were notoriously penile, represented detached and limply hanging over a cooking spit by Hans Baldung Grien at the witches' Sabbath meal (fig. 59) to indicate the women's dangerously voracious hunger.

At the far right, the draining or skimming spoon that Madonna Balzarina might soon use to defend herself is a linguistic cousin of the ladle.[77] Frying pans hanging side by side on the right cheekily emphasize the doubleness of the buttocks to which they refer.[78] Seated on the floor at the far left, a man pounds away with a large pestle, and this equipment was another standard in the sexual lexicon. Boccaccio's epilogue to the *Decameron* had drawn attention to the metaphor when he defended his language against the supposed objections of prudish ladies, pointing out that words like "mortar, and pestle, and sausage, and mortadella" were used every day.[79] Brambilla's print employs a similar strategy, ostensibly presenting an ordinary scene while loading it with as many sexual allusions and metaphors as he can, for reasons of amusement rather than arousal.

The pestle was penile in morphology but action is key to its sexual meaning; it not only entered the mortar in a steady rhythm but its function was to grind. The friction and exertion of grinding, especially of milling flour or grating cheese, was sexually charged and relates to the medical as well as practical understanding of coitus. Holding to the two-seed theory and commenting on the conversion of blood into male and female seed, the English barber-surgeon Thomas Vicary noted that "by the labour and chafing of the testikles or stones this blood is turned into another kinde, and is made sparme."[80] Hence, coitus was likened to grinding corn or grain between millstones to produce the white substance of flour, familiar in such languages as classical Latin (*molo*), Renaissance Italian (*macinare*), French (*moudre*) and Shakespearean English.[81]

77 Florio, *Worlde of wordes (1598)*, pp. 65 ("*Cazzaforata*, skimmer"), 224 ("*Mestola, Mestela*, a skimmer. Also a ladle or a trowel, as *Mescola*. Also a foolish simple idle huswife, that can do nothing but skum a pot").

78 Bruscagli, *Trionfi*, p. 329; Agnolo Bronzino, *Rime in burla*, ed. Franca Petrucci Nardelli (Rome: Istituto della Enciclopedia Italiana, 1988), pp. 89–102; Toscan, *Carnaval*, pp. 1415–16, 1482–83; Deborah Parker, "Towards a reading of Bronzino's burlesque poetry," *Renaissance Quarterly* 50 (1997), 1027–28.

79 Boccaccio, *Decameron*, pp. 673, also 175, 478.

80 Vicary, *Anatomie*, M iii verso.

81 B. Rowland, "The mill in popular metaphor from Chaucer to the present day," *Southern Folklore Quarterly* 33 (1969), 69–79; Boggione and Casalegno, *Dizionario*, pp. 128–32, 353, 354; Simons, "Bodily fluids," 348–50; Simons, "Agostino Carracci's wit," 212 (for filing nails).

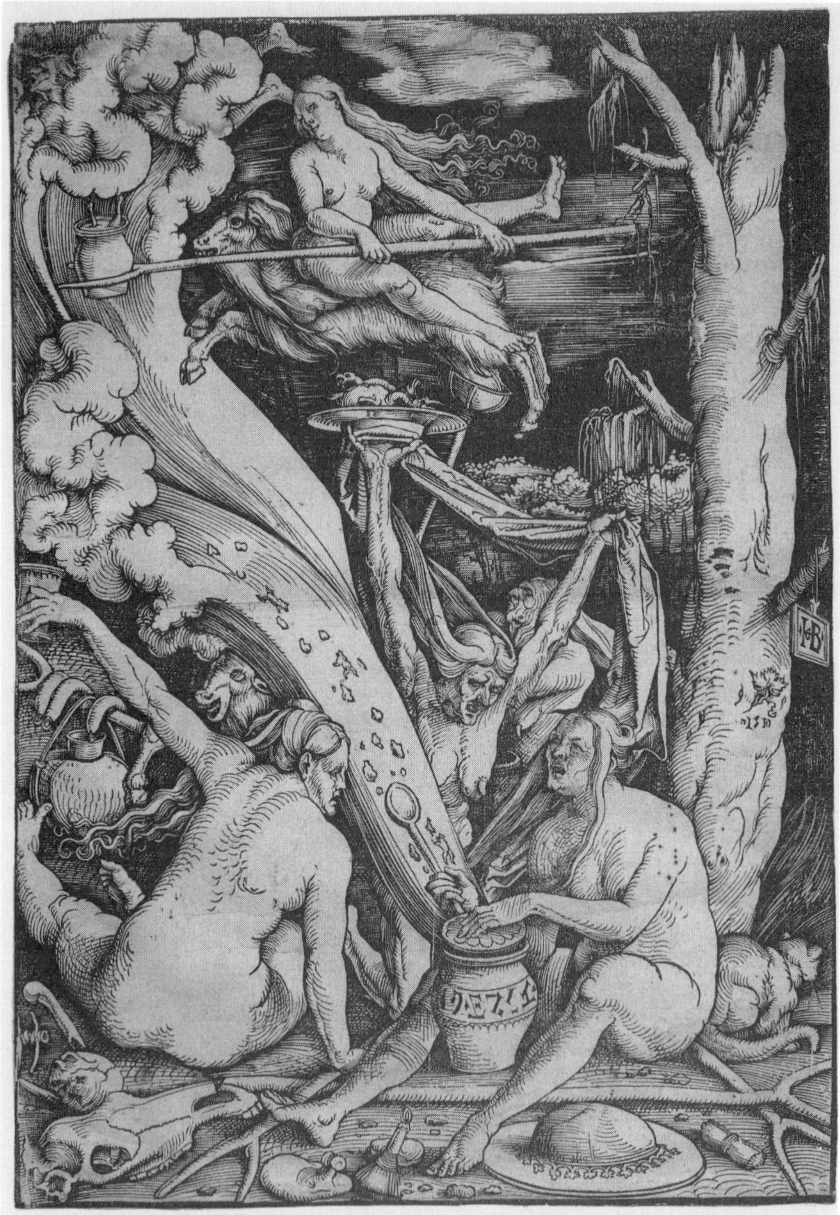

Figure 59 Hans Baldung Grien, *Witches' Sabbath*, 1510, woodcut, 375 × 259 mm, London, British Museum

Urine or ejaculate masquerading as water supplied the power necessary to drive mill wheels and mix with the "flour" to make a paste. The typically impotent husband in Italian stories was, in the case of one of Firenzuola's tales (written by 1543) so aged that his "donkey" could scarcely carry "grain to the mill one time per month," yet he fantasized about an attractive servant, "discharging a load into her hopper."[82] Grain was an appropriate metaphor for seed-laden semen, represented as a more literal substitute for masculine presence in Sercambi's tale "De libidine" of *c.* 1400 where millet appears as the stuffing of a dildo manufactured by an abbess.[83]

Brambilla's engraving highlights the labor of grating cheese, performed by a character labeled "Messer Gratian," whose role is explained in Florio's dictionary as "a gull, a foole or clownish fellowe in a play or comedie."[84] The pedantic physician Dottor Graziano was a familiar guise in the *commedia dell'arte*, but his name may be amusingly deployed in the print because the Latin *gratarium* meant grater and the Italian verb *gratare* was "to grate." His depicted action follows the now familiar pattern: repetitive, rhythmic, back and forth motion that entails friction. Florio defined the grater thus: "*Gratuggia*, any kind of grate or grater. Also a shaving iron that Tanners use. Also an itching or manginesse. Also used for a womans quaint."[85] A man satisfied his sexual itch in a vaginal grater.

The abbess in Aretino's orgiastic nunnery lusted after a young man's genitals and wanted "to grate this cheese with my grater."[86] Hard cheeses, stacked in plentiful amounts on a shelf in Brambilla's kitchen, allude to male genitals, in one Neapolitan type even taking phallic form according to an allusion in the obscene Macaronic verse written in 1498 by the physician Gian Giacomo Bartolotti, associate of Giorgione and Titian.[87] More often, medical analogies between male semen and the coagulating agents that produced cheese or an embryo were about softer cheeses like ricotta. Aristotle drew a parallel between male semen and rennet or fig-juice, a fluid containing "vital heat," that "set" or

[82] Firenzuola, *Opere*, p. 109. [83] Sercambi, *Novelle*, vol. I, no. 30.

[84] Florio, *Worlde of wordes (1598)*, p. 155.

[85] Florio, *Queen Anna's new world of words*, p. 219. For its ironic use regarding sex between women see Matteo Maria Boiardo, *Orlando innamorato*, trans. Charles Stanley Ross (Berkeley: University of California Press, 1989), pp. 846–47; Luca Contile's comedy *Cesarea Gonzaga* of 1550, in Laura Giannetti, *Lelia's kiss: imagining gender, sex, and marriage in Italian Renaissance comedy* (University of Toronto Press, 2009), p. 104.

[86] Aretino, *Ragionamento*, p. 40; Aretino, *Dialogues*, p. 36.

[87] The name of the poem's character Caseus Cabalus, "is a Latin rendering of *caciocavallo*, a phallic-shaped Neapolitan cheese": Schupbach, "Doctor Parma's medicinal macaronic," 152. His organ, "similis figura Priapo," resembled that of Priapus, for it was a "long, large and hard *priapo*" (128, 131). Cheese indicates the male genitals in Berni, *Rime*, p. 56, but for Williams, *Dictionary*, p. 232, it is "allusive of women." For an obscene joke, told by a seventeenth-century Englishwoman, which associates cheese with semen, see Le Strange, *Merry passages and jeasts*, pp. 43–44.

curdled female milk so that an embryo was formed.[88] Pliny likened rennet to male semen too, Galen quoted Aristotle and also compared the early stages of fetal formation with the molding of cheese, and Avicenna repeated the comparison with cheese making. The analogy influenced metaphors about creation and sex, not all necessarily drawn from the Greek tradition. Job asked God, "didst thou not pour me out like milk and curdle me like cheese?" (10.10); the twelfth-century theologian and abbess Hildegard von Bingen conceptualized creation by way of an analogy between milk as seed and the resulting humans as cheese.[89] According to the Friulian miller Menocchio, whose ideas were first reported to the Inquisition in 1583, the creation of the cosmos began when "the water of the sea was whipped into a foam and coagulated like a cheese," from which worms and angels were born.[90] The making of cheese remained a relatively familiar technology and also a comforting, homespun process. The analogy still appeared in English midwiferies of the 1660s (as well as Jane Sharp's book of 1671), and the autobiography published in 1695 by the widow of a Dutch clergyman.[91] The metaphorical relationship between coitus and cheese making was well established, doubtless bolstered by the repetitive, rhythmic motion of churning.

Buxom Madonna Nespola, working at the same table as Gratian, is named after medlar (*nespola*), a fruit that has to be rotting and split open before it can be eaten, and thus the word has sexual connotations of accessibility and over-use, even prostitution.[92] Its alternative English name, known to Chaucer, Shakespeare and Florio, was "open-arse."[93] She is intent on making an open pie in a tall-sided, round pan, the form of which may allude to the sexual connotations of her name. With one hand, she takes ingredients from a bowl and with the other she places them around the edge of a high *tortiere*, a "pan to

88 Aristotle, *GA*, 739b23, also 729a10, 737a14–16, 771b23, 772a22–25. See also Pliny, *NH*, 7.66; Galen, *Semen*, pp. 69, 187; Jacquart and Thomasset, *Sexuality and medicine*, p. 59; Cadden, *Sex difference*, pp. 128–29.

89 Barbara Newman, *Sister of wisdom: St. Hildegard's theology of the feminine* (Berkeley: University of California Press, 1987), pp. 137–40.

90 Andrea Del Col (ed.), *Domenico Scandella detto Menocchio: i processi dell'Inquisizione (1583–1599)* (Pordenone: Edizioni Biblioteca dell'Immagine, 1990), p. 19; Del Col, *Menocchio: his trials*, p. 9. Menocchio's reading, ideas and oral culture are analyzed in Carlo Ginzburg, *The cheese and the worms: the cosmos of a sixteenth-century miller*, trans. John and Anne Tedeschi (Harmondsworth: Penguin, 1982), esp. pp. 28–58, 152–56; Del Col, *Domenico Scandella*, pp. l–lxxxiii (which stresses Cathar roots). Only the latter mentions Aristotle, and in passing. Ginzburg thinks the "foam" too recondite to be invented, but can only find a precedent in a legend from the Kalmucks in Mongolia (pp. 53, 58). For the foamy sea, see Ch. 5 above.

91 Sharp, *Midwives book*, pp. 106–07; Fissell, *Vernacular bodies*, pp. 203–04; Roodenburg, "Autobiography of Isabella De Moerloose," 530–31.

92 Bruscagli, *Trionfi*, p. 53; Boggione and Casalegno, *Dizionario*, p. 291.

93 Norman Davis, et al., *A Chaucer glossary* (Oxford: Clarendon Press, 1979), p. 104 (Reeve's Tale, 3871); Partridge, *Shakespeare's bawdy*, p. 147; Williams, *Glossary*, pp. 204–05; Williams, *Dictionary*, pp. 871–72; Florio, *Worlde of wordes (1598)*, p. 239.

bake a tart or pudding pye in," as Florio put it.[94] A very similar pan is shown in Bartolomeo Scappi's cookery book of 1570 (possibly illustrated by Brambilla), amongst the *padelle da torta alte*, pans for a high torta. A *padella*, round pan or frying pan, often referred to the anus in erotic verse, as it did in Bronzino's burlesque poem on the common kitchen item. Nespola appears to be filling or stuffing her "open-arse." The pie is likely to be savory, using the grated cheese, nearby fowl and other ingredients for a *pasticcio*, a medley chiefly of meat and pasta. A mainstay of banqueting kitchens, *pasticci* of various kinds occasionally occur in burlesque literature as objects of desire.[95] Alternatively, she may be preparing a stuffing for the bird, which has sexual connotations but also brings in witty word play because "farsa" meant both stuffing and theatrical merriment, of just the sort depicted in the print.[96] It may be that the stuffed bird will then be placed in the pie dish and baked, just as Scappi described. Nespola and Gratian are making a "medley" or "farce" together, an eroticized mixture, he with his phallic cheese, she with her round and open form.

Balzarina's leaky ladle, on the other hand, cannot mix or transfer fluids and is instead a skimmer refusing the man's advances, clearing off the "scum." Yet a round pan bakes on the intense fire, the pot handle pointing at her genitals, to suggest that her lust is stoked and she might find interest in another man, the sort of byplay that could lead to much improvised humor on the *commedia* stage. A bellows hangs at the ready near the already blazing fire, and these too could be sexual props. In terms of morphology and materials, bellows were doubled containers made from leather and hence they were similar to scrota (as were moneybags).[97] In relation to function, they added air (chiefly to a fire or a musical organ), akin to the *pneuma* that mixed with heated bodily fluid to produce semen.

Bellows were also associated with the forerunner of modern "hot air," for Florio gave the following definition: "*Folle*, a pair of bellowes. Also vain, fond, or foolish. Also a foole, an idiot, a sotte, a gull, a coxcombe."[98] The windy

[94] Florio, *Worlde of wordes (1598)*, p. 425; illustrated in *The 'Opera' of Bartolomeo Scappi (1570): l'arte et prudenza d'un maestro Cuoco*, trans. Terence Scully (University of Toronto Press, 2008), Pl. 9, and similarly in the later edition, Bartolomeo Scappi, *Opere ... dell'arte del cucinare* (Venice: Alessandro Vecchi, 1610), Book 3, n.p.

[95] Berni, *Rime*, p. 152; Toscan, *Carnaval*, pp. 478, 1364.

[96] Florio, *Queen Anna's new world of words*, p. 182: "*Farsa*, a merry tale, a pleasant discourse. Also an enterlude or stage-play. *Farsare*, to farce or to stuffe meat. *Farsata*, a farcing or stuffing of meat." I am grateful to Chip van Dyck for this suggestion. Grated cheese was often an ingredient for the stuffing of fowl and other meats: *'Opera' of Bartolomeo Scappi (1570)*, pp. 147, 193–94, 452.

[97] Adams, *Latin sexual vocabulary*, p. 75 (*follis*); R. E. Latham, *Revised medieval Latin word-list from British and Irish sources* (London: British Academy, 1965), pp. 195–96 (*folles*). The pairing of bellows and distaff is suggestive in a secular badge: van Beuningen, and Koldeweij (eds.), *Heilig en Profaan*, p. 241.

[98] Florio, *Worlde of wordes (1598)*, p. 134.

instrument thus lent itself to satirical humor, delivering in several images an enema that acted as a humorous reversal of farting, and mocking what was a regular medical procedure.[99] A purgative for many ills, an enema was sometimes specifically prescribed to improve an erection as though the inserted *pneuma* had a Viagra-like effect.[100] It was also familiar to anatomists, used to inflate the womb for inspection according to Massa in 1536.[101] One can well imagine that obscene double entendre came to the fore in an after-dinner speech delivered by the physician Giuseppe Cincio during carnival season sometime in the 1530s to a Roman "academy" or feasting sodality "On the nature of winds (*venti*)."[102] Musical jokes were also possible. The bellows were evocative instruments used to power a musical organ, as when two bellows are at work in a print by Israhel van Meckenem, near a woman who listens to a man fingering his organ, the bedroom in the background soon to be their destination.[103] Titian's paintings from the 1550s that show men serenading a reclining nude woman on an organ similarly joke with the double sense of "organo," a word play employed by his good friend Aretino as well as other Italian writers, and made especially evident in two of the canvases through the men's gaze at the female figure's genital region.[104]

Sexual meaning was not oblique in Ariosto's poetic, mainstream representation of two men enjoying one woman "like two bellows each blowing alternately upon the furnace."[105] Michelangelo's poetry similarly put to inventive use the erotic convention of locating desire in the heated environs of a forge, where hammer blows rained down on an anvil that was the receptive element and thus envisaged as feminine or homoerotically "passive" in the language of the time. One of his unfinished sonnets, of around 1524–25, addressed an

99 For illustrations, see Laurinda Dixon, "Some penetrating insights: the imagery of enemas in art," *Art Journal* 52 (1993), 28–35; Hugo Chapman and Marzia Faietti, *Fra Angelico to Leonardo: Italian Renaissance Drawings* (London: British Museum Press, 2010), 146–49 no. 25; Jones, *Secret middle ages*, pp. 292–93.

100 Jacquart and Thomasset, *Sexuality and medicine*, p. 136. 101 Lind, *Studies*, p. 204.

102 Luigi Sbaragli, *Claudio Tolomei, umanista senese del cinquecento* (Siena: Accademia per le arti e per le lettere, 1939), pp. 50–51, takes the topic seriously, but for the sexual humor enjoyed by the "Accademia della virtù" see Patricia Simons and Monique Kornell, "Annibal Caro's after-dinner speech (1536) and the question of Titian as Vesalius' illustrator," *Renaissance Quarterly* 61 (2008), 1069–97.

103 Koreny, *Israhel van Meckenem*, vol. XXIV, p. 195, vol. XXIV A, Pl. 507; Achim Riether, *Israhel van Meckenem (um 1440/45–1503). Kupferstiche – Der Münchner Bestand* (Munich: Staatliche Graphische Sammlung, 2006), pp. 164, 262.

104 For the paintings see Miguel Falomir (ed.), *Tiziano* (Madrid: Museo Nacional del Prado, 2003), pp. 248–51; Humfrey, *Titian*, pp. 258–59, 306, 235 (for two later variants with a lutenist, see pp. 308–09). On "organs," see for example Aretino, *Ragionamento*, p. 143; Toscan, *Carnaval*, pp. 644–46; Boggione and Casalegno, *Dizionario*, pp. 254, 535; Jones, *Secret middle ages*, p. 265.

105 Ariosto, *Orlando furioso*, vol. II, p. 858; trans. Guido Waldman (Oxford University Press, 1974), p. 345. Furnace imagery is also present in 20.38.5–8.

unnamed beloved: "my heart I made an anvil, my breast a bellows, / for forging sighs with the flame you kindle in me."[106] Smitten with darts entering his eyes from the object of his desire, Michelangelo wrote of himself as a receptive agent, simultaneously stoking with his own bellows the fire of passion. By doing so, he spurned the conventional role of the hammering male figure, and the verse's lack of gender specificity further rebuffed the usual homophobic point of the literary metaphors established by Alan of Lille and the *Roman de la rose*. While the pilgrim in the latter poem was obedient, and continued searching for his rose, neither Michelangelo's sonnet nor Brambilla's print is focused on reproductive or marital labor.

In Brambilla's print a carpenter's hammer lies on the floor at the left, its ordinariness almost a parody of the blacksmith's tools. An item such as this could be exploited during buffoonery on stage with the bellows, but in the print it is purportedly used to crack open walnuts. The character's name Burati is inscribed just above the hammer, which is related to the stage name Buratino, defined by Florio as "a silie gull in a Comedie," and *burattino* was, among other things "a millers or bakers man."[107] The solitary laborer, having hammered at his nuts, now clasps a rod and pounds away at an open, round object between his legs. Brambilla's scene is replete with sexual innuendo, so much were friction, heat, liquids and air part of the general erotic lexicon and performative repertoire.

Some of the same amusing, salacious references are made in Vincenzo Campi's oil painting of a kitchen scene from the 1580s (fig. 60).[108] While the viewers' eyes might first be captivated by the acknowledging gaze of the woman looking out from the center, or the butcher at the left also aware of the spectator, the canvas offers a panoply of activities and generates pleasurable anticipation for the banquet. The indulgence is sexual as well as gustatory, the fire producing the heat of concoction but also desire. A feast of assorted colors and detailed vignettes is arrayed over an inconsistent space of discordant orthogonals, illogical proximities and shifting scale. This does not pretend to be the realistic view of an ordinary kitchen. It is abruptly situated next to an arbor where aristocratic diners will sup out of doors once the sun sets, enjoying

[106] [Buonarroti], Saslow, *Poetry of Michelangelo*, p. 199. Veronica Franco warned a critic that he had better watch his back, "in case someone wants to do with a hammer / what's usually done to the anvil instead": Franco, *Poems and selected letters*, p. 239. For more on the forge and bellows, see Ch. 4 above.

[107] Florio, *Worlde of wordes (1598)*, p. 71.

[108] Paliaga and de Klerck, *Vincenzo Campi*, pp. 54, 135–36, 143–44, 180, 270, 271, 273, fig. 52 (a contemporary copy), Pl. XXVII; Paliaga (ed.), *Vincenzo Campi: scene del quotidiano*, pp. 40–43, 152–55; McTighe, "Foods and the body," 311–12; Vera Fortunati, "Tracce per un tema iconografico poco indagato: la donna e il cibo nella pittura dell'età moderna in Europa," in Corgnati (ed.), *Le immagini affamate*, p. 59; Marta Ajmar-Wollheim and Flora Dennis (ed.), *At home in Renaissance Italy* (London: V & A Publications, 2006), p. 333.

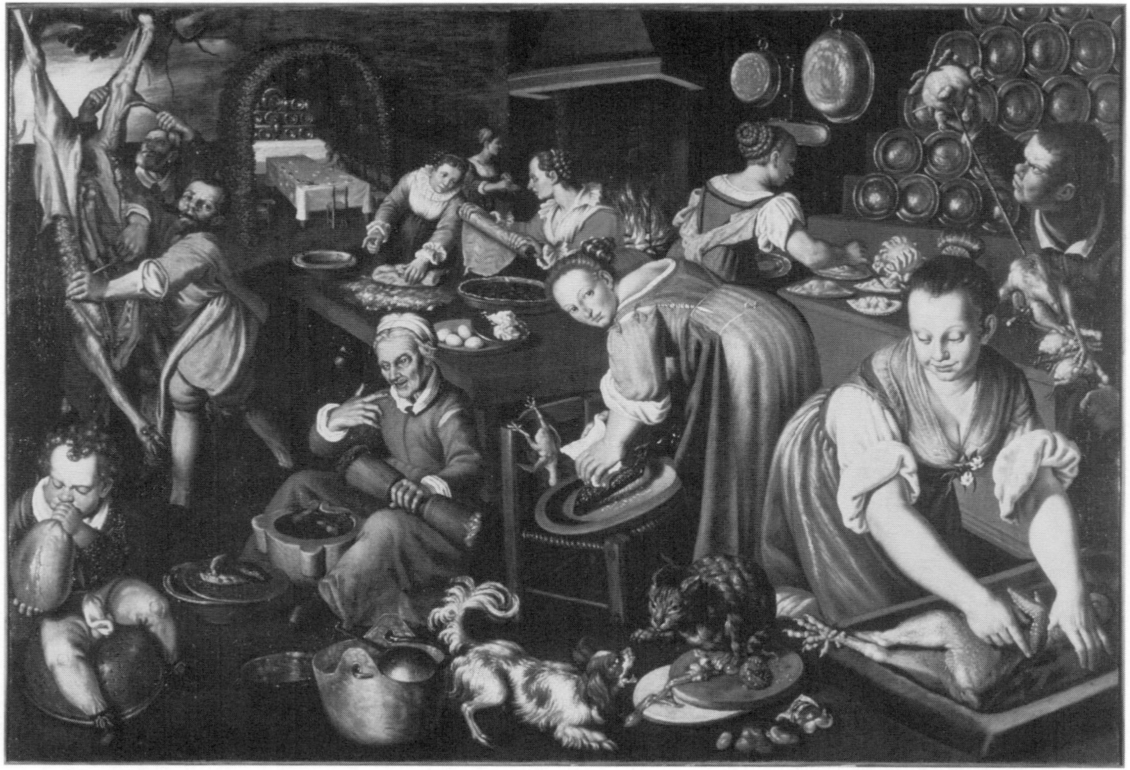

Figure 60 Vincenzo Campi, *Kitchen scene*, 1580s, oil on canvas, 145 × 220 cm, Milan, Pinacoteca di Brera

the song of caged birds and probable ripostes about the well-known sexual connotations of "birds" (male genitals) within (female) "cages." The nearby butchers flaying a calf that is suspended from a tree are too close to the interior kitchen, asserting the immediacy of blood, viscera and masculine labor. That the spread legs of the foreground butcher echo those of the animal demonstrates the closeness between all humans and beasts, though the creatures snarling in the foreground enable the painting's primary audience of members of the elite to be amused at the antics of their inferiors. Fighting over food (including aphrodisiac oysters), the cat and dog encapsulate the necessity of survival and the ferocity of lust, but the kitchen is preparing an indulgent meal so the battle catalyzes an amusing contrast between animal world and high table, mediated through the bodies of laboring servants.

The actions of those human actors highlight pleasures of taste and sensuality. On the far right, for instance, a doltish kitchen assistant draws attention to his action of skewering birds on a spit, and at the table a woman clasps a penile rolling pin that is wrapped in dough as though in a vaginal sheath while her companion pounds repetitively at the yielding, folding substance of feminized dough. On the lower left a brass ladle lies across a copper bowl, each highly polished due to frequent rubbing. Next to it, a boy inflates the slaughtered cow's bladder while his own innards, that is, his genitals, protrude from his pants. Spheres, bubbles and blown-up bladders were part of the carnivalesque equipment of fools, so the boy's action alerts the viewer to the painting's double sense.[109] Furthermore, the inflation alludes to the role of *pneuma* in semen, which enlarged the penis and caused an erection, likened by the English anatomist Crooke to "a gutte filled with winde, presently swelling and growing hard."[110] In the foreground, a woman prepares a large bird that is seen from the back as she leans over to display her décolletage. An old woman avidly tastes the pesto produced by her labor with the mortar and pestle, anticipating much of

[109] For spheres, bubbles and balloons see Mezger, *Narrenidee und Fastnachtsbrauch*, pp. 281–95. A young boy blows up the bladder of a butchered animal in several northern paintings, including Maerten van Cleve's *Slaughtered ox* of 1566 (Vienna, Kunsthistorisches Museum), but his clothing is not disarranged and the scene is about domestic industriousness rather than sensual indulgence. There may also be a reference to the vanitas theme *Homo bulla* (man is a bubble). Campi probably knew one of the versions of the *Return of the prodigal son* by Jacopo and Francesco Bassano, for it has the boy blowing up a bladder, the butcher, a cat and a dog eager for food (albeit at opposite ends of the canvas), and the spatial incongruity between exterior and interior. See Francesca Rossi, "Una cucina di Jacopo Bassano e il suo modello nordico," *Verona illustrata* 7 (1994), 57–64; Bernard Aikema and Beverly Louise Brown (eds.), *Renaissance Venice and the north: crosscurrents in the time of Bellini, Dürer, and Titian* (New York: Rizzoli, 1999), pp. 578–81. No matter how Campi collected such motifs, he took them to a satirical level and added sexual innuendo, which has not been recognized.

[110] Crooke, *Mikrokosmographia*, p. 212. An English ballad of *c.* 1690 has a bridegroom using "a Sheep's gut / blow'd up very stiff, as a Bladder" as a dildo on his wedding night: Toulalan, *Imagining sex*, pp. 144, 226.

the imagery in a song printed in 1612, in which a kitchen maid aroused by music ejaculates sauce from her vessel's interior: "I take the pestle in my hand / And in the mortar / I pound with such fury / That I throw the garlic paste and the relish / out of the pot."[111]

At the painting's center, a plucked bird with a penile neck hangs over a chair, its implausible placement drawing attention to the visual pun. At that chair, in the painting's center, a woman is suggestively seen from behind and she attracts the eye by gazing out over her shoulder while grating a large lump of cheese. Viewers are invited to feel superior to the simple, earthy butchers and servants, amused more than aroused, entertained by elements that were often informed by Flemish paintings, such as Aertsen's view of fondling in the kitchen (fig. 23), which were being described in Italy at the time as pleasingly "ridiculosi" and "bizaria."[112] Campi's popular painting of the ricotta eaters was of the same kind (fig. 56), and at least some of these scenes were hung in the convivial space of an elite household's dining room.

To see "bawdy humour" in Campi's paintings, Robert Miller has claimed recently, is to discern "a pornographic joke."[113] However, he means this in a dismissive sense, assuming that any sexual material must be merely pornographic and, furthermore, that humor and erotic reference are mutually exclusive. The drastically broad definition of pornography and adoption of value-laden terminology does not accord with early modern attitudes towards erotic wit, which was rarely aimed primarily at physical arousal. In 1584, the Lombard painter Gian Paolo Lomazzo opened his chapter on pleasing and amusing pictures by advising that they needed to move the viewer to laughter by showing the cause for such mirth, and his first example was the depiction of lovers engaged in their customary flirtatious, wanton dalliance.[114] The now-lost market and kitchen scenes ordered in 1588 by the Spanish governor of Cremona in a contract with the painter Giulio Calvi were filled with details like an attractive woman exposing her breasts ("una donna bella et gratiosa con il petto scoperto") while plucking a goose and laughing at a boy who is, with exaggerated effort (his puffed up cheeks emphasizing the role

[111] Flora Dennis, "Unlocking the gates of chastity: music and the erotic in the domestic sphere in fifteenth and sixteenth-century Italy," in Matthews-Grieco (ed.), *Erotic cultures*, p. 236. For seminal basil see Boggione and Casalegno, *Dizionario*, p. 352.

[112] Claudia Goldstein, "Vincenzo Campi's kitchen and market scenes: the cultural pull of Antwerp in early-modern Lombardy," in *Italian art, society, and politics: a Festschrift in honor of Rab Hatfield presented by his students on the occasion of his seventieth birthday* (Florence: Syracuse University in Florence, 2007), pp. 194–208. For the language in a contract of 1588 see Robert Miller, "'Diversi personagii molto ridiculosi': a contract for Cremonese market scenes," in Andrea Bayer (ed.), *Painters of reality: the legacy of Leonardo and Caravaggio in Lombardy* (New York: Metropolitan Museum of Art, 2004), p. 159, referred to below. See also Wind, "Pitture ridicole," 25–35; Francesco Porzio, *Pitture ridicole: scene di genere e tradizione popolare* (Geneva: Skira, 2008).

[113] Miller, "'Diversi personagii,'" p. 157; also McTighe, "Foods and the body," 321.

[114] Gian Paolo Lomazzo, *Scritti sulle arti*, ed. Roberto Paolo Ciardi (Florence: Centro Di, 1974), vol. II, pp. 314–16.

of *pneuma*), wringing a duck's penile neck between his legs, the bird's gasping beak placed in front of his genitals.[115] The contract's description of a kitchen scene included two of the main actions represented by Brambilla five years earlier, the woman making a *torta* and another attending a frying pan at the fire. Perhaps not every viewer understood the word plays and double entendres of these sorts of paintings, for they have escaped some scholars, and certain viewing circumstances such as the visit of a moralizing matron or priest might have muted the delight. But the humor was widespread, and even naïve viewers would have found the social satire appealing and the colorful abundance provided sensual delight.

Although saying little about this particular painting and concentrating on contemporaneous Italian images of butchers and food vendors, Sheila McTighe has persuasively argued that they all assert a biological as well as social hierarchy between those who produce, sell and prepare refined food and members of the leisured elite who consume it.[116] While agreeing that Campi's *Kitchen* is neither allegory nor everyday snapshot, and that medical and verbal cultures are central to its meaning, I think more can be said. The *Kitchen scene* works as more than a lesson in "moral edification" and "moral warning" about excess and the "dangerous intimacy with foods that would transgress the boundaries of a working person's diet." The *Ricotta eaters* (fig. 56) is about more than the unhealthy eating habits of poverty-stricken, greedy louts.[117] So too Campi's characters in his popular *Bean eaters*, which reappear at either end of one of his canvases of *Fish vendors*, might be about dietary influence on "the sexual generation of noble or low children" in which doltish infants naturally result from their parents' gross nutrition.[118] But the figures (crying babe, grinning mother, gluttonous man) also invite the viewer to enjoy amusing contrasts in open orifices and the expulsion of pneumatic breath, wind or ejaculate, in which fertility is less central than other sorts of corporeal processes and jokes made by way of comedic figures who consciously address their viewers. The central female fruit vendor peeling a *nespola* while looking directly out of the signed canvas once owned by the Fugger family is not only accompanied by a man making obscene gestures in several variants but sits near emphatically opened rotund fruits, and the bell-like weight suspended from the penile end of a scale dangles between her legs.[119] Such pictorial abundance presents the availability of food and flesh, natural wonders and wit.

[115] Campi painted just such a scene several times, showing a woman with a plunging neckline and displaying a female turkey's breast and genitals; it was often copied: Paliaga and de Klerck, *Vincenzo Campi*, pp. 176, 179, figs. 18 (the Fugger castle at Kirchheim), 45 (a copy), Pl. XXIII (Milan); Paliaga (ed.), *Vincenzo Campi: scene del quotidiano*, pp. 27–28, 152–55.

[116] McTighe, "Foods and the body," 301–23, hereafter quoted from 304, 312.

[117] Cf. ibid., 308, 320. [118] Ibid., 318, fig. 3. On the *Bean eaters* see above.

[119] Ibid., 317–19 passim; Paliaga and de Klerck, *Vincenzo Campi*, pp. 178, 181–82, 207–08, Pls. xxix–xxx, fig. 15.

Considered a virtual document of culinary practice, an entertaining anecdotal scene, a warning against gluttony or lower-class contamination, or an allegory of the element of fire or of the season of winter, Campi's painting (fig. 60) also belongs to kitchen scenes (fig. 23) in which sexual references wittily appease more than one kind of bodily appetite.[120] Terence's maxim "Sine Cerere et Baccho friget Venus" (Without Ceres [goddess of grain] and Bacchus [god of wine], Venus [goddess of sexual pleasure] grows cold), oft cited and illustrated during the Renaissance, linked food, wine and desire, an idea to be alternately celebrated in the voice of pleasure or denigrated in moralizing mode.[121] Yet images had the capacity to operate between these two extremes. Much art historical discussion of kitchen and market scenes used to insist on the importance of their depiction of genre and still life, and on their moralizing aspects, sometimes finding the two to be in opposition, as though reportage of presumed "low life" is incompatible with broader meaning. To elevate them to a purely "serious" plane does not do justice to the pictorial lavishness, sensuality and wit either. They are images of consumption and market forces, of social hierarchy and dietary restrictions, and more. It is possible to understand the paintings as pleasurable while also working in didactic mode, enabling viewers to grasp and enjoy yet distance themselves from sexual innuendo. They can laugh at the depicted figures but also take pleasure in "getting the joke" and assuming their own moral superiority, while nevertheless feeling beguiled by the pictorial lushness.[122] For the lesson to have purchase, temptation must be truly enticing. Depending on the audience and context, the virtuosity and sensuality of the paint and the direct address to the viewer or libidinous gestures made by certain figures as well as the offered comestibles (some of which were thought to have aphrodisiac properties) all tend to counterbalance the moralizing with the voluptuary.[123] Artists, artisans and servants in dining halls might feel put in their place, but it is more likely that they too enjoyed the visual jokes because

120 Sexual readings of other kitchen or market scenes include Ardis Grosjean, "Toward an interpretation of Pieter Aertsen's profane iconography," *Konsthistorisk Tidskrift* 43 (1974), 120–43; Barry Wind, "Vincenzo Campi and Hans Fugger: a peep at late cinquecento bawdy humor," *Arte lombarda* 47–48 (1977), 108–14; Ethan Matt Kavaler, "Erotische Elementen in de Markttaferelen van Beuckelaer, Aertsen en hun Tijdgenoten," in *Joachim Beuckelaer: Het Markt- en Keukenstuk in de Nederlanden, 1550–1650* (Ghent: Gemeentekrediet, 1986), pp. 18–26; Honig, *Painting and the market*, pp. 42–44, 46, 48–52, 58–60, 95–96.

121 Terence, *The Eunuch*, 4.732; cited, for example, by Aretino, *Marescalco*, 5.10.

122 Honig, *Painting and the market*, p. 95 and passim, argues for peasant satire serving to assure rich burghers of their superiority. The issue of satire is elucidated in Margaret Sullivan, "Aertsen's kitchen and market scenes: audience and innovation in northern art," *Art Bulletin* 81 (1999), 236–66, esp. 244–50, 258–59.

123 On aphrodisiac foods and sexual gestures see Reindert Falkenburg, "Matters of taste: Pieter Aertsen's market scenes, eating habits, and pictorial rhetoric in the sixteenth century," in Anne Lowenthal (ed.), *The object as subject: studies in the interpretation of still life* (Princeton University Press, 1996), pp. 19–20.

they shared the language and the dynamic of satire, welcoming the chance to join with making the depicted characters inferior yet engaging. Patrons like the Spanish governor of Cremona or the wealthy German merchant Hans Fugger (in the case of a series of market paintings by Campi of around 1580–81), or the multiple purchasers of Brambilla's print, could enjoy jokes at someone else's expense, having their cake and eating it too.

The heat of passion, suggested by kitchen fires, was associated with overly desirous women, as is the case with Ariosto's image of men stoking a woman's furnace, or the readily available woman with "a really hot oven" according to the Italian version of the *Roman de la rose*.[124] But kitchen metaphors about heat also relate to medical discourse. Concoction was the body's technology in the humoral system of medicine; heat characterized basic masculine nature, yet the uterus was like an oven. When attending Aristophanes' comedy *Peace* in the year 421 BCE, the audience would have been amused to hear the boast about "toasting the pease, and roasting some acorn" (1136–37), that is, warming up the testicles and baking the *glans* in a warm oven. In the words of the second-century dream analyst Artemidorus, "both a hearth and a baking-oven are similar to a woman in that they receive things that are productive of life. Seeing fire in them means that a man's wife will become pregnant."[125] The bun was already in the oven in Hippocratic theory, for there the womb was a heated container slowly cooking the seed. In particular, the embryo was coated in a membrane, "in just the same way as a thin membrane is formed on the surface of bread when it is being baked: the bread rises as it grows warm and inflates."[126]

Aristotle also used the word "oven," but Galen, who gave greater weight to complexional temperatures, adapted the metaphor more often. For him, too, the analogy for the amniotic sac was baked goods, the flat cake or pastry that "bakers make by gently pouring moist dough on a hot flat pan," which then smoothly separates from the uterus, "like the cake from the bronze pan."[127] The membrane was like the "crust [that] forms on dough when a hot iron is brought near it" in one of the Salernitan anatomical texts, and the very action of male sperm upon female seed caused "bubbling like yeast in dough" according to the *Anatomia vivorum* of *c.* 1225.[128] Adapting the metaphor to yet another process, Crooke's anatomical volume of 1615 and Jane Sharp's midwifery of 1671

124 *"The fiore" and the "detto d'amore,"* pp. 98–99 (sonnet 32); see also sonnets 221–22.

125 Artemidorus, *Dreams*, p. 92; Adams, *Latin sexual vocabulary*, p. 86.

126 "On generation" (4.2, 12.2–6, 30.1–9), in *Hippocratic treatises*, pp. 2–3, 6–7, 18–20, here quoted from p. 7. See also Aristotle, *GA*, 764a15–20; Henderson, *Maculate muse*, pp. 142–43.

127 Galen, *Semen*, p. 79.

128 *Second Salernitan demonstration*, in Corner, *Anatomical texts*, p. 65, and *Anatomia vivorum*, p. 105. In a German surgical text of 1518 "the fruit is guarded from destruction as the bread crust protects the crumbs" in the sac: Laqueur, *Making sex*, p. 120.

referred to the placenta as "cake."[129] Commonly said to be a vessel like the tabernacle housing the Body of Christ or Eucharist, the Virgin Mary's body was at other times likened to an oven, concocting the body and thence Eucharistic wafer.[130]

Baking was adapted by erotic literature: a white paste was usually involved in a man's sexual activity, and something soft rose up and became hard in the warm oven.[131] The carnival song of the wafer makers, attributed to Lorenzo de' Medici and dated to the 1470s or 1480s, described their art in erotic terms. Women were essential for the recipe to work well, and then "you place water in the vessel (*vaso*), and place as much flour in it as will fit (*entra*), then beat it until it is ready: when you have beaten it, it becomes an unguent, a liquid almost like meat paste (*maccheroni*)."[132] The mixing of male and female seed was the goal and pregnancy implied, but semenotic ingredients and motion are the song's focus. *Menare*, the verb translated here as "to beat" or vigorously mix, also meant "to lead," and was used for the groom's act of taking his bride to their new home, but it was especially fitting for carnival time because the stirring movement also referred to the rhythmic motion of coitus (and hence implied marital consummation).[133] Lorenzo's song of the bakers used *menare* for the motion of a pestle in the mortar, and the feminine "oven" (*forno*), kept clean with an oven-brush (*spazzatoio*), baked various goods including bread, but through a smaller opening (the anus) the baker sodomitically cooked roast meat.[134] One of the clients of Aretino's prostitute Nanna thrust "his bread-shovel into my oven," another man's *spazzatoio* "swept out all their ovens."[135] Cooking, roasting and heating over a fire or forge were activities singled out on badges: a man and a woman roast a phallus on a spit and she bastes it with a ladle, for instance, and in another badge male genitals bake on a spit in the heat radiating from a vulva

[129] Crooke, *Mikrokosmographia*, p. 227; Sharp, *Midwives book*, p. 106.

[130] Isa Ragusa and Rosalie Green (eds.), *Meditations on the life of Christ: an illustrated manuscript of the fourteenth century*, trans. Isa Ragusa (Princeton University Press, 1961), p. 21; Miri Rubin, *Corpus Christi: the Eucharist in late medieval culture* (Cambridge University Press, 1991), pp. 144–45 (citing an English Franciscan carol of *c.* 1492).

[131] See, for example, Boccaccio, *Corbaccio*, p. 272; Giovanni della Casa's *Sopra il Forno*, in Francesco Berni, *Il primo libro dell'opere burlesche* (Rome: Jacopo Broedelet, 1726), pp. 119–24.

[132] Bruscagli, *Trionfi*, p. 8; Florio, *Worlde of wordes (1598)*, pp. 209–10: "*Maccaroni*, a kinde of paste meate boiled in broth, and drest with butter, cheese, and spice."

[133] Florio, *Worlde of wordes (1598)*, p. 221: "*Menare*, to leade, to bring, to conduct, to direct, to guide, to frig, to wriggle, to iumble, to wag or stirre to and fro." For frig meaning to masturbate or copulate, see Williams, *Dictionary*, pp. 554–56.

[134] Bruscagli, *Trionfi*, pp. 24–26.

[135] Aretino, *Ragionamento*, pp. 119, 143, 370; Aretino, *Dialogues*, pp. 93, 110, 281; see also Toscan, *Carnaval*, p. 1697 (*forno*); Boggione and Casalegno, *Dizionario*, pp. 449, 544; Jones, *Secret middle ages*, pp. 238–39.

(fig. 13), while in a third example a female blacksmith hammers away at a phallus on her anvil.[136]

Flour was milled, cheese was grated, pots were stirred, the pestle ground in the mortar, the dough rose in the oven, the roast was carved, the barrel was tapped, liquid was transferred and mixed by ladles and spoons, fires were stoked; in medical literature, semen was concocted, friction created sexual pleasure, the male and female seeds were blended and the embryo was cooked in a crust. Other implements and actions in the sexual lexicon, like the shaking of bells, the pumping and expulsion from bellows or writing with ink, also accorded with medical emphases regarding corporeal experience. From Hippocratic theory in ancient Greece to carnivalesque images of the fifteenth century, from prints, paintings and poems of the sixteenth century to contemporary colloquialisms, the heat of desire and the processes of everyday technologies and familiar practices have been embedded in medical and lay culture alike, inflecting notions and metaphors of sexual activity.

[136] For the first and second see Koldeweij, *Geloof & Geluk*, p. 116, figs. 7.52 and 7.53, for the third, Koldeweij, "'Shameless and naked images,'" p. 500, fig. 240.

Conclusion: metaphors and embodiment

Despite its materiality, the human body is largely conceptualized by way of metaphor or, rather, the daunting complexity and vulnerability of fleshly substance generates metaphor. Sexual activities and fantasies especially lead to logorrhea, as though the very excess of the words themselves stays decay and answers desire. As Labé and Lacan independently recognized more than four centuries apart, "speaking of love is in itself a *jouissance*," a heightened pleasure.[1] Wit, misdirection and connotation ostensibly mask, yet add to the thrill. Writing about the management of marriageable women in 1526, Erasmus believed that erotic songs and tales were made even more shocking by the addition of "words of such obscenity, through euphemisms and innuendo, that pure filth could not be filthier."[2] Belying their professed purpose, Castiglione's "veil" that cloaks obscene humor from women, or Cicero's wordy coverage of "deformity" by periphrasis, simultaneously draw attention to the underlying impropriety and to the wit of its ostensible concealment (for example, figs. 2–3, 6, 22–24, 27, 33–37, 49, 51–54, 56–58, 60). In a related vein, Montaigne remarked that books "become all the more marketable and public by being suppressed," a precursor to Foucault's central point that a taboo can act as an "incitement to discourse" rather than giving rise to censorial unspeakability.[3] Whether euphemism, "dirty talk" or sophisticated metaphor, whether music, words, images or objects, cultural language is central to erotic desire and pleasure, as well as to the oppositional reaction it can spark.

Yet the Lacanian attempt to prioritize the role of language above that of the body continues the modern habit of privileging mind over matter (a binary schemata often reiterated in the Aristotelian contrast between the male and female roles in reproduction, and also a practice deeply embedded since Plato but especially since the Neoplatonists of the third century). A neat division

[1] See Ch. 2 above.

[2] Translation adapted from *Institution of Christian matrimony*, trans. Heath, p. 426. See Jeanice Brooks, "Singing the courtly body: the *Chanson lascive* and the performance of obscenity," in Hugh Roberts, Guillaume Peureux and Lise Wajeman (eds.), *Obscénités renaissantes* (Geneva: Droz, 2011), pp. 193–206.

[3] Montaigne, *Complete works*, p. 644; Foucault, *History of sexuality*, vol. I, pp. 17–35.

between the two is overdrawn, as indicated by the case of Elena/o, discussed in Chapter 1, whose psyche was affected by corporeal changes. In 1526, Erasmus went on to rail against suggestively mimed actions and the character of the performed music itself. As his disquiet about performance suggests, there was always the risk that the proverbial divide between words and deeds could be blurred, that representation and action would feed into each other and that authoritative control would fail in its project of containment. Humoral medicine inextricably linked *complexio* with physical conditions of health, for example, and the element of soul or spirit was as vital as mind and body.[4] Citing the Aristotelian tradition when writing in the mid-sixteenth century, physician Jean Fernel observed that body and mind were chained in concert by *spiritus*, which intervened "to reconcile and hold opposed natures together." Furthermore, "Aristotle was right to hold that spirit [*pneuma* in Greek] was enclosed in seed (*semine*) and a foamy body, and that a nature was enclosed in spirit that by analogy corresponds to the element of the stars." The Lacanian phallus needs to remain disconnected from actual bodies to remain potent as a sign of psycho-linguistic and political order, but the theory, despite valiant attempts, relies on a corporeal, gendered scheme of sexual desire and symbolism. Representational language, evocative imagery and experiential corporality intersect in inextricable, countless ways.

Before the era of sperm and ova, in European thought and practice the male genitals and their output of semen were determining signs of power and pleasure in a manner that is rarely recognizable today, whether in psychoanalytic theory or cultural history. The penis was a means to an end, that purpose being the release and delivery of semen to another body, aided in its forceful ejection by innately masculine heat and the pressure of built up *pneuma* or essential spirit. As producers or repositories of semen, the testicles were more vital to a man's virility than any other genital part. These fundamental ideas about the properly male body were disseminated in poems and songs, tavern talk and graffiti, medical tomes and public spectacles, artifacts like glass vessels or wax votives, oral habits like puns and turns of phrase, expensive paintings and cheaper prints.

Images, texts and objects (mostly but not entirely male-authored), in a variety of genres and contexts, accentuated humor, inequality and physical satisfaction, while relying on basic medical knowledge that did not accord with what modern presumptions have since naturalized. The best model for early modern masculine anatomy and patriarchal action is projection, from corporeal signs like

[4] See, for instance, Jean Fernel, *Medicina* (Paris: Wechel, 1554), pp. 84–85, 87–89, 104–05 (first published 1542); hereafter quoted from Fernel, *Physiologia*, p. 263. More broadly, see Caroline Bynum, "Why all the fuss about the body? A medievalist's perspective," in Victoria Bonnell and Lynn Hunt (eds.), *Beyond the cultural turn* (Berkeley: University of California Press, 1999), pp. 241–80.

ejaculation, urination, facial hair and external genitals to forceful and pervasive action in such public arenas as commerce, agriculture, governance and chivalric spectacle. Throwing coins in Baden or flinging beer in Somerset, firing cannon or proclaiming laws, men were performing what was understood to be their complexional, semenotic nature. Less solely penetrative, this model demonstrates that masculinity and patriarchy are not immutable and that biology can be rethought in historical terms. In conjunction with the attendant unequal two-seed theory, the projective model envisaged male bodies as necessary for and superior to female bodies, which nevertheless had more agency (of a receptive and dependent kind) than is construed by the archetypal pattern of penetrative men and passive women.

By means of sexual metaphors, one could effectively conceive and communicate assertive ideas about such diverse matters as international relations, military strategy or business dealings. It is striking how much double entendre exists in Nofri Tornabuoni's reports from Rome back to the head branch of the Medici bank in Florence. From 1487 to 1491, the client Pope Innocent VIII was stirred, fingered, hammered, plucked like fruit, labored over as though a field, caressed and ridden, all terms replete with masculine boasting about the sexual conquest and thence feminization of a powerful man.[5] In the financial as in the physiological and anatomical worlds, the masculine epitome of perfection was projective, aggressive action.

Metaphors are vivid in effect, but not naïve: one's sexualized organ does not become or literally resemble a ladle or a vase, for instance, and nor do the male genitals match a phallus in permanence, authority or effect. The process of constructing and deploying metaphors is predicated upon a double vision, a human, poetic ability to place the material and the symbolic in tandem or in a dialectical relationship. Hence, it works especially well for erotic double entendre, and the wit is in the invention, the reassemblage, the layering. And the sense. In terms of internal logic, but also in relation to corporeal experience and cultural expectations, metaphors about bodies have to make a degree of sense. They have to resonate with contemporary technologies and experiences as well as medical epistemology, and they have to fit within somatic and social parameters. To then exaggerate – suggest a relationship between roasting and sex, say, or log dragging and sexual expenditure (figs. 13, 48, 58, 60) – is amusing and inventive but relies on familiar objects and practices, and builds on what is historically situated common knowledge about bodies.

Hence, metaphors are essential when trying to find the texture of corporeal experience in the past. Materiality and textuality connect. The premodern notion that male sexual action and semen carried curative properties to a female

[5] For the terminology, but not the sexual implications, see Bullard, "'Hammering away at the Pope,'" pp. 383–98.

sex partner is both the stuff of jokes and the ideology of Hippocratic medicine. To believe or joke about the metaphor is to affirm fundamental patriarchal ideas about the superiority of the male body and the dependence of the female one. Hearing or seeing the metaphor creates a feedback loop that continues to institute and engrave the idea in cultural memory, bodily experience and medical knowledge. An early modern woman might, for instance, comprehend what today is considered the adrenalin rush of sexual pleasure as an infusion of semen-delivered moisture and refreshment. A man could understand postcoital lassitude to be a consequence of depleting his valuable resource of semen. Observing common effects of castration confirmed what was considered a given, that virility was inherent to the testicles; no wonder that the military family of the Colleoni assertively adopted eponymous testicles (*coglioni*) for their coat of arms (fig. 19). Coin pouches on the sides of bags (fig. 35) reminded men and women that their anatomical "purses" contained "seed" of value. For most people, the pneumatic paradigm sufficiently explained the processes of erection and ejaculation, as well as the foamy appearance of male semen (fig. 33). Everyday deeds like coagulating or grating cheese, ploughing a field, watering a garden, tapping a beer keg or wine barrel, blowing on a fire or into a balloon, turning a tap, stirring or ladling a pot, or urinating while standing up, could bring to mind an old joke or spur the formation of a new quip, a novel image, all the while reinforcing standard biological knowledge.

Seeking to understand the constitutive effect of visual and metaphorical representation, and to trace its embeddedness in material reality, I have found it useful to think of "social iconography," an explanatory matrix that existed in words and images but also practices. It gets to the long life of such metaphors and ways of understanding the premodern body, before modern anatomy, physiology, embryology and psychoanalysis began to redirect the focus to a one-seed, more solely penetrative, penile model. Rather than posit that the phallus is pure symbol, as is attempted by Lacan, or address chiefly the medico-legal aspects of the history of the body, as Foucault did to such illuminating effect, I find that metaphors about bodies have material presence and everyday effect. They are lived, in a variety of forms including practice, spectacle, object and sign. The embodied history of women was equally engaged, practicing and commissioning love magic that put symbolic objects to powerful, erotic effect, for instance, or struggling with a husband about the placement of his semen in the case of Isabella De Moerloose who insisted on making sense of her life by publishing an autobiography.

More evidence survives about the dominant class of literate men. Yet, Duval's "bells" within semen, or common metaphors in medical discourse like purses and roses had efficacy well beyond the learned elite. Professional men such as anatomists, surgeons, artists and writers assumed and put to use a range of metaphors that were often in operation at illiterate levels too, many of them conveying an understanding of eroticized bodies that differs from a modern framework. Hence, even well-known works of art for the elite, viewed with an eye to these metaphors and their logic, can yield new meanings or resonances. The foamy sea repetitively painted by Botticelli (fig. 33), the expulsion of air from a musical organ or a shower of heated gold in paintings by Titian (fig. 34), the spilt wine and flowing gold of Carracci's rebus (fig. 41) or the full import of sexualized ladles (fig. 55) are semen-centered references rarely recognized today. So too in jokes and word plays, whether about ink, breaking lances or medicinal cures, the implications for rethinking phallic power have been overlooked.

Judged according to a scale of variables focused on semen, testicles and humoral heat, the ideal adult male body was reassuringly and aggressively on top. Women experienced justifiable desire, craving the curative refreshment of male semen. Their amorous agency was misogynistically cast as rapacious, or legitimized as dependent (though not always reproductive), in either case operating to reinforce the biological parameters that supported patriarchal power. Male anxiety was ameliorated and norms affirmed by medical knowledge, cultural metaphors and strategies of humor. As with the contradictions inherent in any dominant ideology, seeds of subversion, transgression and adjustment were present, enabling women to satisfy their sexual desire, for example, or carnivalesque groups to mock moral boundaries.

Even Christ's body, incarnated as ideal male flesh yet chaste, was understood in terms of semen, testicles and heat. As an infant his genitals proved his human manhood, as an adult a beard often did the same. His now-clothed loins frequently sprouted exuberant protuberances that Steinberg likened to "wings of excess."[6] The "flaring forth" of drapery from the genital center trumpets a "fanfare of cosmic triumph" in images like Lucas Cranach's *Crucifixion* of 1503 (fig. 61). Steinberg concentrates on the animation that signifies Christ's conquest of mundane death in such imagery, to which I would add that the victory is manifest in an expansive projection of dynamic cloth akin to ejaculation on a grand and godly scale. Cranach's light reddish ground underlain across the panel, and the loincloth's sharp white highlights, significantly bring the efflorescent fabric closer in color to Christ's flesh, already turning waxen. The gnarled, elongated material acts like the independent genital animal mistrusted by Plato and Augustine.

Yet it is more, contrasted with those whose mortality is truly human. Mary's hands clasped in grief in front of John the Evangelist's groin form a knotted and downward-pointing form, suggesting the erotic loss suffered by Christ's beloved disciple and contrasting human fallibility with divine victory. The

[6] On the enhanced loincloth, see Steinberg, *Sexuality of Christ*, pp. 91–94, 199–201.

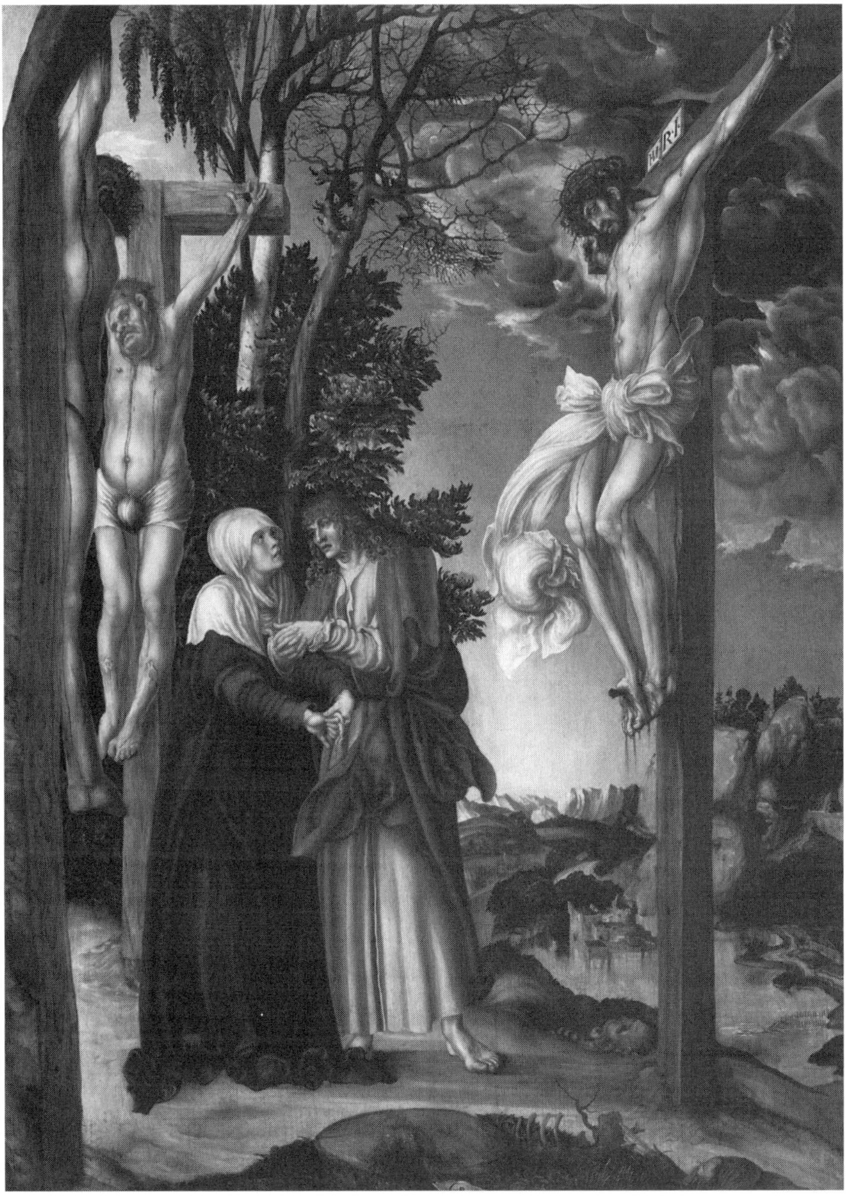

Figure 61 Lucas Cranach the Elder, *Crucifixion*, 1503, oil on pine wood, 138 × 99 cm, Munich, Alte Pinakothek

bad thief crucified at the left margin in profile, his face covered by hair, is even more eclipsed by the black strip that turns his genitals invisible. The good thief, closer to Christ and seen frontally, wears white pants that have the usual undifferentiated bulge of a cup or codpiece. Christ's outpouring, on the other hand, is not only fleshly but fluid and almost aerial in its roiling eddies and florid streams, a portent of the oncoming storm of darkness approaching Golgotha at the upper right but also an analogy for the extrusion of his vital *pneuma* in ejaculatory if not orgasmic death. By metaphorical, ecstatically visual means, Cranach paints the Christian paradox about a male body that encapsulates yet transcends its semen-centric nature. Mortal flesh expires while the eternal *spiritus* will rise in life everlasting.

Select bibliography

PRIMARY SOURCES

Accademici Intronati di Siena. *Gl'ingannati* (Bologna: Arnaldo Forni, 1984).

Albertus Magnus. *De animalibus*, ed. Hermann Stadler, vol. XV (Münster: Aschendorffsche Verlagsbuchhandlung, 1916); Vol. XVI (1921).

Anonymous. *The mirror of coitus: a translation and edition of the fifteenth-century "Speculum al foderi,"* trans. and ed. Michael Solomon (Madison: Hispanic Seminary of Medieval Studies, 1990).

Anonymous. *La venexiana*, ed. Ludovico Zorzi (Turin: Einaudi, 1982).

Aretino, Pietro. *Aretino's "Dialogues,"* trans. Raymond Rosenthal (New York: Stein and Day, 1971).

Cortigiana, ed. Angelo Romano (Milan: Biblioteca Universale Rizzoli, 1989).

La cortigiana, ed. Giuliano Innamorati (Turin: Giulio Einaudi, 1970).

Lettere, ed. Paolo Procaccioli. 6 vols. (Rome: Salerno, 1997–2002).

Ragionamento: dialogo, ed. Paolo Procaccioli (Milan: Garzanti, 1984).

Tutte le commedie, ed. G. B. De Sanctis (Milan: Mursia, 1968).

Ariosto, Ludovico. *Orlando furioso*, ed. Lanfranco Caretti, 2 vols. (Turin: Einaudi, 1966).

Artemidorus. *The interpretation of dreams: Oneirocritica*, trans. Robert J. White (Park Ridge, NJ: Noyes Press, 1975).

Augustine. *Concerning the city of God against the pagans*, trans. Henry Bettenson (Harmondsworth: Penguin, 1984).

Avicenna. *Liber canonis* (Venice, 1507), rpt. (Hildesheim: Georg Olms, 1964).

Bandello, Matteo. *Le novelle*, ed. Demo Maestri, 4 vols. (Alessandria: Edizioni dell'Orso, 1992).

Banister, John. *The historie of man, sucked from the sappe of the most approved anathomistes* (London: John Day, 1578).

Barocchi, Paola and Renzo Ristori (eds.). *Il carteggio di Michelangelo*, 5 vols. (Florence: SPES, 1965–83).

Bartholin, Caspar. *Anatomicae institutiones corporis humani* (Oxford: William Turner, 1633).

Bartholin, Thomas. *Anatome*, 4th edn. (Lyon: Joan. Ant. Huguetan, & Soc., 1677).

[Bartholin, Thomas]. *Bartholinus anatomy; made from the precepts of his father, and from the observations of all modern anatomists, together with his own* (London: John Streater, 1668).

Bauhin, Gaspard. *Theatrum anatomicum* (Frankfurt: Matthäus Becker, 1605).

Benedetti, Alessandro. *Historia corporis humani sive Anatomice*, ed. Giovanna Ferrari (Florence: Giunti, 1998).
Benivieni, Antonio. *De abditis nonnullis ac mirandis morborum et sanationum causis*, trans. Charles Singer (Springfield: Charles C. Thomas, 1954).
Berengario da Carpi, Jacopo. *Isagogae breves*, 2nd edn. (Bologna: Benedict Hector, 1523).
Berni, Francesco. *Rime*, ed. Danilo Romei (Milan: Mursia, 1985).
Biagi, Maria Luisa Altieri, Clemente Mazzota, Angela Chiantera and Paola Altieri (eds.). *Medicina per le donne nel cinquecento: testi di Giovanni Marinello e di Girolamo Mercurio* (Turin: UTET, 1992).
Bibbiena. *La calandria*, ed. Paolo Fossati (Turin: Einaudi, 1967).
Boccaccio, Giovanni. *The corbaccio*, trans. and ed. Anthony K. Cassell (Urbana: University of Illinois Press, 1975).
Decameron, ed. Cesare Segre (Milan: Mursia, 1966).
Elegia di Madonna Fiammetta: Corbaccio, ed. Francesco Erbani (Milan: Garzanti, 1988).
Borris, Kenneth (ed.), *Same-sex desire in the English Renaissance: a sourcebook of texts, 1470–1650* (Routledge: New York, 2004).
Bowen, Barbara C. (ed.). *One hundred Renaissance jokes: an anthology* (Birmingham, AL: Summa Publications, 1988).
Bracciolini, Poggio. *Facezie*, ed. Marcello Ciccuto (Milan: Biblioteca Universale Rizzoli, 1983).
[Brantôme] Pierre de Bourdeille, Seigneur de Brantôme, *Les dames galantes*, ed. Maurice Rat (Paris: Éditions Garnier Frères, 1965).
Bronzino, Agnolo. *Rime in burla*, ed. Franca Petrucci Nardelli (Rome: Istituto della Enciclopedia Italiana, 1988).
Bruno, Giordano. *Candlebearer*, trans. Gino Moliterno (Ottawa: Dovehouse, 2000).
Opere italiane, ed Giovanni Aquilecchia (Turin: UTET, 2002).
Bruscagli, Riccardo (ed.). *Trionfi e canti carnascialeschi del Rinascimento* (Rome: Salerno, 1986).
[Bunworth, Richard]. *The doctresse* (London: JF, 1656).
[Buonarroti, Michelangelo]. *The poetry of Michelangelo*, trans. James M. Saslow (New Haven: Yale University Press, 1991).
Castiglione, Baldassare. *The book of the courtier: the Singleton translation*, ed. Daniel Javitch (New York: W. W. Norton, 2002).
Il libro del cortegiano, ed. Giulio Carnazzi (Milan: Biblioteca Universale Rizzoli, 1987).
Cellini, Benvenuto. *Autobiography*, trans. George Bull (Harmondsworth: Penguin, 1956).
Vita, ed. Ettore Camesasca (Milan: Biblioteca Universale Rizzoli, 1985).
Del Col, Andrea. *Domenico Scandella known as Menocchio: his trials before the Inquisition (1583–1599)*, trans. John and Anne Tedeschi (Binghamton: Medieval and Renaissance Texts and Studies, 1996).
Colombo, Realdo. *De re anatomica* (Venice: Nicolai Bevilacquae, 1559 [sic: 1560]).
[Constantinus Africanus]. Enrique Montero Cartelle. *Constantini "Liber de coitu": el tratado de andrología de Constantino el Africano* (Santiago de Compostela: Secretariado de Publicaciones de la Universidad de Santiago, 1983).
Corner, George W. *Anatomical texts of the earlier middle ages* (Washington: Carnegie Institution of Washington, 1927).
Cotgrave, Randle. *A dictionarie of the French and English tongues* (1611), facsimile (Menston: Scolar Press, 1968).

Crooke, Helkiah. *Mikrokosmographia: a description of the body of man. Together with the controversies thereto belonging. Collected and translated out of all the best authors of anatomy, especially out of Gasper Bauhinus and Andreas Laurentius* (London: William Jaggard, 1615).

Culpeper, Nicholas. *A directory for midwives* (London: Peter Cole, 1651).

Delany, Paul. "Constantinus Africanus' *De coitu*: a translation," *Chaucer Review* 4 (1969), 55–65.

Dryandrum, Ioannem (ed.), *Anatomia Mundini* (Marburg: Christiani Egenolphi, 1541).

du Laurens, André. *Historica anatomica humani corporis* (Paris: A. Mettayer et Ourry, 1600).

Opera anatomica (Lyon: Ioannis Baptistae Buysson, 1593).

Duval, Jacques. *Des hermaphrodits* . . . (Rouen: David Geuffroy, 1612).

Erasmus, Desiderius. *Institution of Christian matrimony*, trans. Michael J. Heath, in John W. O'Malley and Louis A. Perraud (eds.), *Collected works of Erasmus*, vol. LXIX: *Spiritualia* and *pastoralia* (University of Toronto Press, 1999), pp. 214–438.

Fernel, Jean. *Medicina* (Paris: Wechel, 1554).

The Physiologia of Jean Fernel (1567), trans. John M. Forrester (Philadelphia: American Philosophical Society, 2003).

Ferrand, Jacques. *Erotomania, or, a treatise discoursing of the essence, causes, symptomes, prognosticks, and cure of love, or erotique melancholy* (Oxford: L. Lichfield, 1640).

De la maladie d'amour ou mélancholie érotique (Paris: Denis Moreau, 1623).

Ficino, Marsilio. *Opera omnia* (Basel: Henrici Petrina, 1576), 2 vols., facsimile (Turin: Bottega d'Erasmo, 1959).

"The fiore" and the "Detto d'amore": a late thirteenth-century Italian translation of the "Roman de la rose" attributable to Dante, trans. Santa Casciani and Christopher Kleinhenz (University of Notre Dame Press, 2000).

Firenzuola, Agnolo. *Opere*, ed. Adriano Seroni (Florence: Sansoni, 1958).

Florio, John. *Queen Anna's new world of words* (1611), facsimile (Menston: Scolar Press, 1968).

A worlde of wordes (1598), facsimile (Hildesheim: Georg Olms Verlag, 1972).

Franco, Veronica. *Poems and selected letters*, ed. and trans. Ann Rosalind Jones and Margaret F. Rosenthal (University of Chicago Press, 1998).

Galen. *On the affected parts*, trans. Rudolph E. Siegel (Basel: Karger, 1976).

On semen, ed. and trans. Phillip De Lacy (Berlin: Akademie Verlag, 1992).

On the usefulness of the parts of the body, 2 vols., trans. Margaret Tallmadge May (Ithaca: Cornell University Press, 1968).

Giannetti, Laura and Guido Ruggiero (eds. and trans.). *Five comedies from the Italian Renaissance* (Baltimore: Johns Hopkins University Press, 2003).

Giovio, Paolo. *Lettere*, ed. Giuseppe Guido Ferrero, 2 vols. (Rome: Istituto Poligrafico dello Stato, 1956–58).

Goodich, Michael (ed.). *Other middle ages: witnesses at the margins of medieval society* (Philadelphia: University of Pennsylvania Press, 1998).

Gorosch, Max. *La notomia de Anric de Mondavilla* (Avignon: Centre d'Études Occitanes, 1975).

Guy de Chauliac. *The Cyrurgie of Guy de Chauliac*, ed. Margaret S.. Ogden (Oxford University Press, 1971).

[Guy de Chauliac] Guigonis de Caulhiaco. *Inventarium sive Chirurgia Magna*, ed. Michael R. McVaugh, vol. I: *Text* (Leiden: Brill, 1997).

Hanson, Ann Ellis (trans.). "Hippocrates: *Diseases of women* 1," *Signs* 1 (1975), 567–84.

Henri de Mondeville. *Die Chirurgie des Heinrich von Mondeville: nach Berliner, Erfurter und Pariser Codices*, ed. Julius Leopold Pagel (Berlin: A. Hirschwald, 1892).

The Hippocratic treatises "On generation," "On the nature of the child," "Diseases IV," trans. and commentary Iain M. Lonie (Berlin: Walter de Gruyter, 1981).

Hooke, Robert. *The diary of Robert Hooke M.A., M.D., F.R.S. 1672–1680*, ed. Henry W. Robinson and Walter Adams (London: Taylor & Francis, 1935).

Isidore of Seville: the medical writings, trans. William Sharpe, *Transactions of the American Philosophical Society* n.s. 54 no. 2 (1964).

Joubert, Laurent. *Des erreurs populaires*, ed. Madeleine Tiollais, 2 vols. (Paris: Éditions L'Harmattan, 1997).

Popular errors, trans. Gregory David de Rocher (Tuscaloosa: University of Alabama Press, 1989).

Kagan, Richard and Abigail Dyer (ed. and trans.). *Inquisitorial inquiries: brief lives of secret Jews and other heretics* (Baltimore: Johns Hopkins University Press, 2004).

Kramer, Heinrich and James Sprenger. *The hammer of witches: a complete translation of the "Malleus maleficarum,"* trans. Christopher Mackay (Cambridge University Press, 2009).

Lanfranco of Milan. *Lanfrank's "Science of Cirurgie,"* ed. Robert von Fleischhacker (New York: Scribner, 1894).

Lemay, Helen. *Women's secrets: a translation of Pseudo-Albertus Magnus's "De secretis mulierum" with commentaries* (Albany: SUNY Press, 1992).

Lemnius, Levinus. *Occulta naturae miracula* (Antwerp: G. Simonem, 1559).

The secret miracles of nature (London: Jo. Streater, 1658).

Le Strange, Nicholas. *Merry passages and jeasts: a manuscript jestbook of Sir Nicholas Le Strange (1603–1655)*, ed. H. F. Lippincott (Salzburg: Institut für Englische Sprache und Literatur, Universität Salzburg, 1974).

Liébault, Jean. *Trois livres des maladies et infirmitez des femmes* . . . (Rouen: Jean Berthelin, 1649).

Lind, L. R. *Studies in pre-Vesalian anatomy* (Philadelphia: American Philosophical Society, 1975).

de Lorris, Guillaume, and Jean de Meun. *Le roman de la rose*, ed. Félix Lecoy. 3 vols. (Paris: Honoré Champion, 1965).

The romance of the rose, trans. Charles Dahlberg (Hanover: University Press of New England, 1986).

Marinelli, Giovanni. *Thresor des remedes secrets pour les maladies des femmes* [trans. Jean Liébault] (Paris: Jacques Du Puys, 1585).

Marinello, Giovanni. *Le medicine partenenti alle infermità delle donne* (Venice: Giovanni Valgrifio, 1574).

Massaria, Alessandro. *De morbis foemineis: the woman's counsellour*, trans. R. Turner (London: John Streater, 1657).

Medici, Lorenzo de'. *Tutte le opere*, ed. Paolo Orvieto, 2 vols. (Rome: Salerno, 1992).

Mercurio, Scipione. *La commare* (Venice: Giovanni Battista Ciotti, 1601).

Merrick, Jeffrey and Bryant T. Ragan Jr. (eds.). *Homosexuality in early modern France: a documentary collection* (Oxford University Press, 2001).

Montaigne, Michel de. *The complete works of Montaigne: essays, travel journal, letters*, trans. Donald M. Frame (Stanford University Press, 1958).

Les essais, 3 vols, 2nd edn., Pierre Villey (Paris: Quadrige/PUF, 1992).
Paré, Ambroise. *The collected works of Ambroise Paré translated out of the Latin by Thomas Johnson from the first English edition, London, 1634* (Pound Ridge, NY: Milford House, 1968).
On monsters and marvels, trans. Janis L. Pallister (University of Chicago Press, 1982).
Des monstres et prodiges, ed. Jean Céard (Geneva: Droz, 1971).
Œuvres complètes, ed. J.-F. Malgaigne, 3 vols, 1840–41, rpt. (Geneva: Slatkine Reprints, 1970).
Pepys, Samuel. *The diary of Samuel, Pepys*, ed. Robert Latham and William Matthews, 11 vols. (London: G. Bell and Sons Ltd., 1970–83).
Samuel Pepys' penny merriments: being a collection of chapbooks, full of histories, jests, magic, amorous tales of courtship, marriage and infidelity, accounts of rogues and fools, together with comments on the times, ed. Roger Thompson (London: Constable, 1976).
Platter, Thomas. *Journal of a younger brother: the life of Thomas Platter as a medical student in Montpellier at the close of the sixteenth century*, trans. Seán Jennett (London: Frederick Muller, 1963).
Poliziano, Angelo. *Detti piacevoli*, ed. Tiziano Zanato (Rome: Istituto della Enciclopedia Italiana, 1983).
The Priapus poems: erotic epigrams from ancient Rome, trans. Richard W. Hooper (Urbana: University of Illinois Press, 1999).
The problemes of Aristotle (Edinburgh: Robert Waldgrave, 1595).
Rabelais, François. *The histories of Gargantua and Pantagruel*, trans. J. M. Cohen (Harmondsworth: Penguin, 1955).
Œuvres complètes, ed. Mireille Huchon and François Moreau (Paris: Gallimard, 1994).
Raynald [also Raynold], Thomas. *The byrth of mankynde* (London: Thomas Raynold, 1545).
Rocco, Antonio. *L'Alcibiade fanciullo a scola* (Rome: Salerno, 1988).
Rösslin, Eucharius. *De partu hominis* (Frankfurt: Ch. Egen, 1556).
Ruzante. *Teatro*, ed. Ludovico Zorzi (Turin: Einaudi, 1967).
Sanudo, Marin. *Venice: città excelentissima. Selections from the Renaissance diaries of Marin Sanudo*, ed. Patricia H. Labalme and Laura Sanguineti White, trans. Linda L. Carroll (Baltimore: Johns Hopkins University Press, 2008).
Sanuto, Marino. *I diarii*, ed. Rinaldo Fulin et al., 59 vols. (Venice: F. Visentini, 1879–1903).
Sercambi, Giovanni. *Novelle*, ed. Giovanni Sinicropi, 2 vols. (Bari: Laterza, 1972).
Sermini, Gentile. *Novelle*, ed. Giuseppe Vettori (Rome: Avanzini e Torraca Editori, 1968).
Shakespeare, William. *The poems*, ed. John Roe (Cambridge University Press, 1992).
Sharp, Jane. *The midwives book or the whole art of midwifry discovered (1671)*, ed. Elaine Hobby (Oxford University Press, 1999).
The "Trotula": a medieval compendium of women's medicine, ed. and trans. Monica H. Green (Philadelphia: University of Pennsylvania Press, 2001).
[Vasari-Milanesi] Vasari, Giorgio. *Le vite de' più eccellenti pittori scultori ed architettori*, ed. Gaetano Milanesi, 8 vols., 1878–85, Rpt. (Florence: Sansoni, 1906, and Florence: Sansoni, 1973).
Vesalius, Andreas. *The epitome of Andreas Vesalius*, trans. L. R. Lind (New York: Macmillan, 1949).

On the fabric of the human body: a translation of "De humani corporis fabrica libri septem," Book V: the organs of nutrition and generation, trans. William Frank Richardson and John Burd Carman (Novato, CA: Norman Publishing, 2007).
De humani corporis de fabrica libri septem (Basel: Johannes Oporinus, 1543).
Humani corporis fabrica librorum Epitome (Basel: Johannes Oporinus, 1543).
Vesling, Johann. *The anatomy of the body of man: wherein is exactly described every part thereof, in the same manner as it is commonly shewed in publick anatomies*, trans. Nicholas Culpeper (London: Peter Cole, 1653).
Syntagma anatomicum, 2nd edn. (Padua: Pauli Frambotti, 1651).
Vicary, Thomas. *A profitable treatise of the anatomie of mans body* (London: Henry Bamforde, 1577).
Vignali, Antonio. *La cazzaria*, ed. Pasquale Stoppelli (Rome: Edizioni dell'Elefante, 1984).
Villon, François. *The poems of François Villon*, new edn., trans. Galway Kinnell (Hanover: University Press of New England, 1977).
Wieri, Ioannis. *Opera omnia* (Amsterdam: Peter van den Berge, 1660).

SECONDARY SOURCES

Adams, J. N. *The Latin sexual vocabulary* (Baltimore: Johns Hopkins University Press, 1982).
Adelman, Janet. "Making defect perfection: Shakespeare and the one-sex model," in Viviana Comensoli and Anne Russell (eds.), *Enacting gender on the English Renaissance stage* (Urbana: University of Illinois Press, 1999), pp. 23–52.
Bach, Rebecca Ann. "Tennis balls: *Henry V* and testicular masculinity, or, according to the OED, Shakespeare doesn't have any balls," *Renaissance Drama* 30 (2001), 3–23.
Bajada, Joseph. *Sexual impotence: the contribution of Paolo Zacchia (1584–1659)* (Rome: Editrice Pontificia Università Gregoriana, 1988).
Baldwin, John W. *The language of sex: five voices from northern France around 1200* (University of Chicago Press, 1994).
Barbazza, Marie-Catherine. "Un caso de subversión social: el proceso de Elena de Céspedes (1587–1589)," *Criticón* 26 (1984), 17–40.
Bartrum, Giulia. *German Renaissance prints 1490–1550* (London: British Museum Press, 1995).
Baskett, William Denny. *Parts of the body in the later Germanic dialects* (University of Chicago Press, 1920).
Bayer, Andrea (ed.). *Art and love in Renaissance Italy* (New York: Metropolitan Museum of Art, 2008).
Behrend-Martínez, Edward. *Unfit for marriage: impotent spouses on trial in the Basque region of Spain, 1650–1750* (Reno: University of Nevada Press, 2007).
Bertelli, Sergio. *The king's body: sacred rituals of power in medieval and early modern Europe* (1999), trans. R. Burr Litchfield (University Park: Pennsylvania State University Press, 2001).
van Beuningen, H. J. E. and A. M. Koldeweij (eds.). *Heilig en Profaan: 1000 Laat-middeleeuwse insigne suit de collectie H. J. E. van Beuningen* (Cothen, Netherlands: Stichting Middeleeuwse Religieuze en Profane Insignes, 1993).
Bildhauer, Bettina. "The *Secrets of women* (c. 1300): a medieval perspective on menstruation," in Andrew Shail and Gillian Howie (eds.), *Menstruation: a cultural history* (New York: Palgrave Macmillan, 2005), pp. 65–75.
Boardman, John. "A curious eye cup," *Archäologischer Anzeiger* 3 (1976), 281–90.

Boggione, Valter and Giovanni Casalegno, *Dizionario storico del lessico erotico italiano* (Milan: Longanesi, 1996).

Bowen, Barbara C. "Metaphorical obscenity in French farce, 1460–1560," *Comparative Drama* 11 (1977), 331–44.

Boyarin, Daniel. "Who wrote the dominant fiction? On the history of the early phallus," in Mieke Bal, et al. (eds.), *Brief: intellectual traditions in movement* (Amsterdam: Amsterdam School for Cultural Analysis, Theory and Interpretation, 1998), 41–83.

Boylan, Michael. "The Galenic and Hippocratic challenges to Aristotle's conception theory," *Journal of the History of Biology* 17 (1984), 83–112.

Breitenberg, Mark. *Anxious masculinity in early modern England* (Cambridge University Press, 1996).

Brinkmann, Bodo (ed.). *Cranach* (London: Royal Academy of Arts, 2007).

Brown, Pamela Allen. *Better a shrew than a sheep: women, drama, and the culture of jest in early modern England* (Ithaca: Cornell University Press, 2003).

"Jesting rights: women players in the manuscript jestbook of Sir Nicholas Le Strange," in Pamela Allen Brown and Peter Parolin (eds.), *Women players in England, 1500–1600: beyond the all-male stage* (Aldershot: Ashgate, 2005), pp. 305–14.

Brown, Patricia. *Private lives in Renaissance Venice: art, architecture, and the family* (New Haven: Yale University Press, 2004).

Brown, Peter. *The body and society: men, women and sexual renunciation in early Christianity* (London: Faber and Faber, 1989).

Brumble, David. *Classical myths and legends in the middle ages and Renaissance: a dictionary of allegorical meanings* (Westport, CT: Greenwood Press, 1998).

Brundage, James. *Law, sex, and Christian society in medieval Europe* (University of Chicago Press, 1987).

Bullard, Melissa Meriam. "'Hammering away at the Pope': Nofri Tornabuoni, Lorenzo de' Medici's agent and collaborator in Rome," in David Peterson and Daniel Bornstein (eds.), *Florence and beyond: culture, society and politics in Renaissance Italy* (Toronto: Center for Reformation and Renaissance Studies, 2008), pp. 383–98.

Burshatin, Israel. "Elena alias Eleno: genders, sexualities, and 'race' in the mirror of natural history in sixteenth-century Spain," in Sabrina Petra Ramet (ed.). *Gender reversals and gender cultures* (London: Routledge, 1996), pp. 105–22.

"Interrogating hermaphroditism in sixteenth-century Spain," in Sylvia Molloy and Robert McKee Irwin (eds.), *Hispanisms and homosexualities* (Durham: Duke University Press, 1998), pp. 3–18.

"Written on the body: slave or hermaphrodite in sixteenth-century Spain," in Josiah Blackmore and Gregory Hutcheson (eds.). *Queer Iberia* (Durham: Duke University Press, 1999), pp. 420–56.

Butler, Judith. *Bodies that matter: on the discursive limits of "sex"* (New York: Routledge, 1993).

Cadden, Joan. *Meanings of sex difference in the middle ages: medicine, science, and culture* (Cambridge University Press, 1993).

Camille, Michael. "'For our devotion and pleasure': the sexual objects of Jean, Duc de Berry," *Art History* 24 (2001), 169–94.

The medieval art of love (New York: Harry N. Abrams, 1998).

Canning, Kathleen. *Gender history in practice: historical perspectives on bodies, class, and citizenship* (Ithaca: Cornell University Press, 2006).

Cipolla, Costantino and Giancarlo Malacarne (eds.). *El più soave et dolce et dilectevole et gratioso bochone: amore e sesso al tempo dei Gonzaga* (Milan: FrancoAngeli, 2006).

Clarke, John R. *Looking at laughter: humor, power, and transgression in Roman visual culture, 100 B.C.–A.D. 250* (Berkeley: University of California Press, 2007).

Cortelazzo, Manlio and Paolo Zolli. *Dizionario etimologico della lingua italiana*, 5 vols. (Bologna: Zanichelli, 1980).

Crawford, Patricia. "Sexual knowledge in England, 1500–1750," in Roy Porter and Mikulás Teich (eds.), *Sexual knowledge, sexual science: the history of attitudes to sexuality* (Cambridge University Press, 1994), pp. 82–106.

Darmon, Pierre. *Le tribunal de l'impuissance* (Paris: Éditions du Seuil, 1979).

Daston, Lorraine and Katharine Park. "The hermaphrodite and the orders of Nature: sexual ambiguity in early modern France," in Louise Fradenburg and Carla Freccero (eds.), *Premodern sexualities* (New York: Routledge, 1996), pp. 117–36.

Dekker, Rudolf M. *Humour in Dutch culture of the Golden Age* (New York: Palgrave, 2001).

Dempsey, Charles. *Inventing the Renaissance putto* (Chapel Hill: University of North Carolina Press, 2001).

Derbes, Anne and Mark Sandona. *The usurer's heart: Giotto, Enrico Scrovegni, and the Arena Chapel in Padua* (University Park, Pennsylvania: Pennsylvania State University Press, 2008).

Dixon, Laurinda S. *Perilous chastity: women and illness in pre-Enlightenment art and medicine* (Ithaca: Cornell University Press, 1995).

duBois, Page. *Sowing the body: psychoanalysis and ancient representations of women* (University of Chicago Press, 1988).

Durling, Richard J. "A chronological census of Renaissance editions and translations of Galen," *Journal of the Warburg and Courtauld Institutes* 24 (1961), 230–92.

Ferraro, Joanne. *Marriage wars in late Renaissance Venice* (Oxford University Press, 2001).

Ferroul, Yves. "Abelard's blissful castration," in Jeffrey Jerome Cohen and Bonnie Wheeler (eds.), *Becoming male in the middle ages* (New York: Garland, 1997), pp. 129–49.

Finucci, Valeria. *The manly masquerade: masculinity, paternity, and castration in the Italian Renaissance* (Durham: Duke University Press, 2003).

Finucci, Valeria and Brownlee, Kevin (eds.). *Generation and degeneration* (Durham: Duke University Press, 2001).

Fisher, Will. *Materializing gender in early modern English literature and culture* (Cambridge University Press, 2006).

Fissell, Mary. "Gender and generation: representing reproduction in early modern England," *Gender and History* 7 (1995), 433–56.

Vernacular bodies: the politics of reproduction in early modern England (Oxford University Press, 2004).

Foucault, Michel. *The history of sexuality*, 3 vols., trans. Robert Hurley (New York: Pantheon Books, 1981–86).

Foyster, Elizabeth. *Manhood in early modern England: honour, sex and marriage* (London: Longman, 1999).

Fraccari, Claudio. "Per amore di metafora: linguaggio erotico e travestimenti dell'osceno nella corrispondenza gonzaghesca," in Costantino Cipolla and Giancarlo Malacarne (eds.), *El più soave et dolce et dilectevole et gratioso bochone: amore e sesso al temo dei Gonzaga* (Milan: FrancoAngeli, 2006), pp. 265–89.

Freud, Sigmund. *Jokes and their relation to the unconscious* (1905), in *Standard edition*, vol. VIII (London: Hogarth Press, 1960).

The standard edition of the complete psychological works of Sigmund Freud, ed. James Strachey, in collaboration with Anna Freud, assisted by Alix Strachey and Alan Tyson, 24 vols. (London: Hogarth Press, 1953–74).

Friedländer, Max and Jakob Rosenberg. *The paintings of Lucas Cranach* (Secaucus, NJ: Wellfleet Press, 1978).

Friedman, David M. *A mind of its own: a cultural history of the penis* (New York: The Free Press, 2001).

Giannetti, Laura. *Lelia's kiss: imagining gender, sex, and marriage in Italian Renaissance comedy* (University of Toronto Press, 2009).

Goubitz, Olaf. *Purses in pieces: archaeological finds of late medieval and 16th-century leather purses, pouches, bags and cases in the Netherlands* (Zwolle: Stichting Promotie Archeologie, 2007).

Gowing, Laura. *Common bodies: women, touch and power in seventeenth-century England* (New Haven: Yale University Press, 2003).

Domestic dangers: women, words, and sex in early modern London (Oxford: Clarendon Press, 1996).

Green, Monica H. "Bodies, gender, health, disease: recent work on medieval women's medicine," *Studies in Medieval and Renaissance History* 3rd ser., 2 (2005), 1–49.

"Flowers, poisons and men: menstruation in medieval western Europe," in Andrew Shail and Gillian Howie (eds.), *Menstruation: a cultural history* (New York: Palgrave Macmillan, 2005), pp. 51–64.

Making women's medicine masculine: the rise of male authority in pre-modern gynaecology (Oxford University Press, 2008).

Women's healthcare in the medieval west: texts and contexts (Aldershot: Ashgate Variorum, 2000).

Hacke, Daniela. *Women, sex and marriage in early modern Venice* (Aldershot: Ashgate, 2004).

Hanson, Ann Ellis. "The medical writers' woman," in David M. Halperin, John J. Winkler and Froma I. Zeitlin (eds.), *Before sexuality: the construction of erotic experience in the ancient Greek world* (Princeton University Press, 1990), pp. 309–38.

Henderson, Jeffrey. *The maculate muse: obscene language in Attic comedy*, 2nd edn. (Oxford University Press, 1991).

Hess, Catherine. "Pleasure, shame and healing: erotic imagery on maiolica drug jars," in Allison Levy (ed.), *Sex acts: practice, performance, perversion and punishment in early modern Europe* (Aldershot: Ashgate, 2010), pp. 13–25.

Hewson, M. Anthony. *Giles of Rome and the medieval theory of conception* (London: Athlone Press, 1975).

Hodges, Frederick Mansfield. "The ideal prepuce in ancient Greece and Rome: male genital aesthetics and their relation to *lipodermos*, circumcision, foreskin restoration, and the *kynodesme*," *Bulletin of the History of Medicine* 75 (2001), 375–405.

Honig, Elizabeth Alice. *Painting and the market in early modern Antwerp* (New Haven: Yale University Press, 1998).

Humfrey, Peter. *Titian: the complete paintings* (Ghent: Ludion, 2007).

Jacquart, Danielle. "Medical explanations of sexual behavior in the middle ages," in Helen Rodnite Lemay (ed.). *Homo carnalis: the carnal aspect of medieval human life* (Binghamton: Center for Medieval and Early Renaissance Studies, State University of New York at Binghamton, 1987), pp. 1–21.

Jacquart, Danielle and Claude Thomasset. *Sexuality and medicine in the middle ages*, trans. Matthew Adamson (Cambridge: Polity Press, 1988).

Johns, Catherine. *Sex or symbol? Erotic images of Greece and Rome* (London: British Museum Publications, 1982).

Jones, Malcolm. *The secret middle ages* (Phoenix Mill: Sutton Publishing, 2002).

"Sex and sexuality in late medieval and early modern art," in Daniela Erlach, Markus Reisenleitner and Karl Vocelka (eds.). *Privatisierung der Triebe? Sexualität in der Frühen Neuzeit* (Frankfurt am Main: Peter Lang, 1994), pp. 187–304.

Jordan, Mark D. *The invention of sodomy in Christian theology* (University of Chicago Press, 1997).

Keele, Kenneth D. *Leonardo da Vinci's elements of the science of man* (New York: Academic Press, 1983).

King, Helen. *Hippocrates' women: reading the female body in ancient Greece* (London: Routledge, 1998).

"The mathematics of sex: one to two, or two to one?," *Studies in Medieval and Renaissance History* 3rd ser., 2 (2005), 47–58.

Midwifery, obstetrics and the rise of gynaecology: the uses of a sixteenth-century compendium (Aldershot: Ashgate, 2007).

Kleinhenz, Christopher. "Texts, naked and thinly veiled: erotic elements in medieval Italian literature," in Joyce Salisbury (ed.), *Sex in the middle ages* (New York: Garland, 1991), pp. 83–109.

Klibansky, Raymond, Erwin Panofsky and Fritz Saxl. *Saturn and melancholy: studies in the history of natural philosophy, religion and art* (London: Nelson, 1964).

Koldeweij, Jos. *Geloof & Geluk: Sieraad en devotie in middeleeuws Vlaanderen* (Brughes: Bruggemuseum, 2006).

"'Shameless and naked images': obscene badges as parodies of popular devotion," in Sarah Blick and Rita Tekippe (eds.), *Art and architecture of late medieval pilgrimage in northern Europe and the British Isles: texts* (Leiden: Brill, 2005), pp. 493–510.

Koreny, Fritz (comp.). *Hollstein's German engravings, etchings and woodcuts 1400–1700*, vol. XXIV: *Israhel van Meckenem, Text*, ed. Tilman Falk (Blaricum: A. L. van Gendt, 1986), and vol. XXIV A: *Plates.*

Lacan, Jacques. *Écrits: a selection*, trans. Alan Sheridan (London: Tavistock, 1977).

Feminine sexuality: Jacques Lacan and the "école freudienne," ed. Juliet Mitchell and Jacqueline Rose (London: Macmillan, 1982).

Ladurie, Emmanuel Le Roy. "The aiguillette: castration by magic" (1974), in Siân Reynolds and Ben Reynolds (trans.). *The mind and method of the historian* (University of Chicago Press, 1981), pp. 84–96.

Laqueur, Thomas. *Making sex: body and gender from the Greeks to Freud* (Cambridge, MA: Harvard University Press, 1990).

"Sex in the flesh," *Isis* 94 (2003), 300–06.
Solitary sex: a cultural history of masturbation (New York: Zone Books, 2003).
Lehman, Peter. *Running scared: masculinity and the representation of the male body*, new edn. (Detroit: Wayne State University Press, 2007).
Lemay, Helen Rodnite. "Anthonius Guainerius and medieval gynecology," in Julius Kirshner and Suzanne Wemple (eds.). *Women of the medieval world: essays in honor of John H. Mundy* (Oxford: Basil Blackwell, 1985), pp. 317–36.
Lochrie, Karma, Peggy McCracken and James Schultz (eds.). *Constructing medieval sexuality* (Minneapolis: University of Minnesota Press, 1997).
Long, Kathleen (ed.). *High anxiety: masculinity in crisis in early modern France* (Kirksville, MS: Truman State University Press, 2002).
Maclean, Ian. *The Renaissance notion of woman: a study in the fortunes of scholasticism and medical science in European intellectual life* (Cambridge University Press, 1980).
McClive, Cathy. "Masculinity on trial: penises, hermaphrodites and the uncertain male body in early modern France," *History Workshop Journal* 68 (2009), 45–68.
McGrath, Aidan. *A controversy concerning male impotence* (Rome: Editrice Pontificia Università Gregoriana, 1988).
McTighe, Sheila. "Foods and the body in Italian genre paintings, about 1580: Campi, Passarotti, Carracci," *Art Bulletin* 86 (2004), 301–23.
Matthews-Grieco, Sara (ed.). *Erotic cultures of Renaissance Italy* (Aldershot: Ashgate, 2010).
Mezger, Werner. *Narrenidee und Fastnachtsbrauch: Studien zum Fortleben des Mittelalters in der europäischen Festkultur* (Constance: Universitätsverlag, 1991).
Morel, Philippe. "Priape à la Renaissance: les guirlandes de Giovanni da Udine à la Farnésine," *Revue de l'art* 69 (1985), 13–28.
Moulton, Ian Frederick. *Before pornography: erotic writing in early modern England* (Oxford University Press, 2000).
Muir, Edward. *Ritual in early modern Europe* (Cambridge University Press, 1997).
Park, Katharine. "Itineraries of the 'one-sex body': a history of an idea," unpublished paper.
"The rediscovery of the clitoris: French medicine and the tribade, 1570–1620," in David Hillman and Carla Mazzio (eds.), *The body in parts: fantasies of corporeality in early modern Europe* (New York: Routledge, 1997), pp. 170–93.
Secrets of women: gender, generation, and the origins of human dissection (New York: Zone Books, 2006).
Park, Katharine and Robert A. Nye. "Destiny is anatomy," *The New Republic* 204 (18 February 1991), 53–57.
Partridge, Eric. *Shakespeare's bawdy*, 3rd edn. (London: Routledge, 1990).
Paster, Gail Kern. *Humoring the body: emotions on the Shakespearean stage* (University of Chicago Press, 2004).
"The unbearable coldness of female being: women's imperfection and the humoral economy," *English Literary Renaissance* 28 (1998), 416–40.
Pomata, Gianna. "Vollkommen oder verdorben? Der männliche Samen im frühneuzeitlichen Europa," *L'Homme* 6 (1995), 59–85.
Preus, Anthony. "Galen's criticism of Aristotle's conception theory," *Journal of the History of Biology* 10 (1977), 65–85.
Prizer, William F. "*Facciamo pure noi carnevale*: non-Florentine carnival songs of the late fifteenth and early sixteenth centuries," in Irene Alm, Alyson McLamore and

Colleen Reardon (eds.), *Musica Franca: essays in honor of Frank A. D'Accone* (Stuyvesant, NY: Pendragon, 1996), pp. 173–211.

"Games of Venus: secular vocal music in the late quattrocento and early cinquecento," *Journal of Musicology* 9 (1991), 3–56.

Purdie, Susan. *Comedy: the mastery of discourse* (University of Toronto Press, 1993).

Quaife, G. R. *Wanton wenches and wayward wives: peasants and illicit sex in early seventeenth century England* (London: Croom Helm, 1979).

Roach, Mary. *Bonk: the curious coupling of science and sex* (New York: W. W. Norton & Co., 2008).

Roodenburg, Herman W. "The autobiography of Isabella De Moerloose: sex, child-rearing and popular belief in seventeenth century Holland," *Journal of Social History* 18 (1985), 517–40.

Roper, Lyndal. *Oedipus and the devil: witchcraft, sexuality and religion in early modern Europe* (London: Routledge, 1994).

Witch craze: terror and fantasy in Baroque Germany (New Haven: Yale University Press, 2006).

Rubinstein, Frankie. *A dictionary of Shakespeare's sexual puns and their significance*, 2nd edn. (London: Macmillan, 1989).

Ruggiero, Guido. *Binding passions: tales of magic, marriage, and power at the end of the Renaissance* (Oxford University Press, 1993).

Machiavelli in love: sex, self, and society in the Italian Renaissance (Baltimore: Johns Hopkins University Press, 2007).

Scarborough, John. *Medical terminologies: classical origins* (Norman: University of Oklahoma Press, 1992).

Schiebinger, Londa. "Skelettestreit," *Isis* 94 (2003), 307–13.

Schleiner, Winfried. "Early modern controversies about the one-sex model," *Renaissance Quarterly* 53 (2000), 180–91.

Medical ethics in the Renaissance (Washington, DC: Georgetown University Press, 1995).

Schupbach, William. "Doctor Parma's medicinal macaronic: poem by Bartolotti, pictures by Giorgione and Titian," *Journal of the Warburg and Courtauld Institutes* 41 (1978), 147–91, 350.

Shepard, Alexandra. *Meanings of manhood in early modern England* (Oxford University Press, 2003).

Silver, Larry. *Peasant scenes and landscapes: the rise of pictorial genres in the Antwerp art market* (Philadelphia: University of Pennsylvania Press, 2006).

Simons, Patricia. "Agostino Carracci's wit in two lascivious prints," *Studies in Iconography* 30 (2009), 198–221.

"The cultural history of *Seigneur Dildoe* in Renaissance Italy," in Allison Levy (ed.). *Sex acts: practice, performance, perversion and punishment in early modern Italy* (Aldershot: Ashgate, 2010), pp. 77–91.

"Manliness and the visual semiotics of bodily fluids in early modern culture," *Journal of Medieval and Early Modern Studies* 39 (2009), 331–73.

Simons, Patricia and Monique Kornell. "Annibal Caro's after-dinner speech (1536) and the question of Titian as Vesalius' illustrator," *Renaissance Quarterly* 61 (2008), 1069–97.

Siraisi, Nancy G. *Medieval and early Renaissance medicine: an introduction to knowledge and practice* (University of Chicago Press, 1990).

Steinberg, Leo. *The sexuality of Christ in Renaissance art and in modern oblivion*, 2nd edn. (University of Chicago Press, 1996).
Stephanson, Raymond. *The yard of wit: male creativity and sexuality, 1650–1750* (Philadelphia: University of Pennsylvania Press, 2004).
Stephens, Walter, *Demon lovers: witchcraft, sex and the crisis of belief* (University of Chicago Press, 2001).
Stolberg, Michael. "A woman down to her bones: the anatomy of sexual difference in the sixteenth and early seventeenth centuries," *Isis* 94 (2003), 274–99.
Talvacchia, Bette. *Taking positions: on the erotic in Renaissance culture* (Princeton University Press, 1999).
Taylor, Gary. *Castration: an abbreviated history of western manhood* (New York: Routledge, 2000).
Tentler, Thomas N. *Sin and confession on the eve of the Reformation* (Princeton University Press, 1977).
Toscan, Jean. *Le carnaval du langage: le lexique érotique des poètes de l'équivoque de Burchiello à Marino* (Lille: Presses Universitaires de Lille, 1981).
Toulalan, Sarah. *Imagining sex: pornography and bodies in seventeenth-century England* (Oxford University Press, 2007).
Turner, James Grantham. *Schooling sex: libertine literature and erotic education in Italy, France, and England 1534–1685* (Oxford University Press, 2003).
Varone, Antonio. *Erotica Pompeiana: love inscriptions on the walls of Pompeii*, trans. Ria P. Berg, David Harwood and Roger Ling (Rome: "L'Erma" di Bretschneider, 2002).
Vasvari, Louise O. "The battle of flesh and Lent in the *Libro del arcipreste*: gastro-genital rites of reversal," *La Corónia* 20 (1991), 1–15.
Vollendorf, Lisa. *The lives of women: a new history of Inquisitional Spain* (Nashville: Vanderbilt University Press, 2005).
Wack, Mary Francis. *Lovesickness in the middle ages: the "Viaticum" and its commentaries* (Philadelphia: University of Pennsylvania Press, 1990).
Wethey, Harold E. *The paintings of Titian: complete edition*, vol. III: *The mythological and historical paintings* (London: Phaidon, 1975).
Williams, Gordon. *A dictionary of sexual language and imagery in Shakespearean and Stuart literature* (London: Athlone Press, 1994).
A glossary of Shakespeare's sexual language (London: Athlone, 1997).
Zika, Charles. *The appearance of witchcraft: print and visual culture in sixteenth-century Europe* (London: Routledge, 2007).
Zorach, Rebecca. *Blood, milk, ink, gold: abundance and excess in the French Renaissance* (University of Chicago Press, 2005).
Zucker, Mark. *The illustrated Bartsch 24 Commentary part 3: early Italian masters* (New York: Abaris Books, 2000).

Index